Milne's Dermatopathology

Milne's Dermatopathology

Revised and edited by

Rona M. MacKie MD, FRCP, FRCPath

Professor of Dermatology, University of Glasgow

With contributions by

Mary E. Catto MD, FRCPath
   Reader in Pathology, University of Glasgow
Frances M. McGregor MB, MCh, BOA, FRCPath
   Lecturer in Pathology, University of Glasgow
Alexander MacQueen MB, ChB, FRCPath
   Senior Lecturer in Pathology, University of Glasgow
Christine J. Skerrow B.Sc., M.Phil., Ph.D.
   Research Fellow in Dermatology
   University of Glasgow
   (Ultrastructural Consultant)

Edward Arnold

© Mrs J. A. Milne and Rona M. MacKie 1984

First published 1972
as *An Introduction to the Diagnostic Histopathology of the Skin*
by Edward Arnold (Publishers) Ltd
41 Bedford Square, London WC1B 3DQ

This edition first published 1984

British Library Cataloguing in Publication Data
Milne, John Alexander
   Milne's dermatopathology.
   1. Skin—Diseases—Diagnosis
   I. Title   II. MacKie, Rona M.
   III. Milne, John Alexander. Introduction to
   the diagnostic histopathology of the skin
   616.5′075   RL105

   ISBN 0-7131-4434-3

Whilst the advice and information in this book is believed to be true and accurate at the
date of going to press, neither the authors nor the publisher can accept any legal
responsibility or liability for any errors or omissions that may have been made.

Filmset in 10/12 Plantin
and printed in Great Britain by
Butler & Tanner Ltd,
Frome and London

Preface to Second Edition

Before his untimely death in 1977 John Milne had indicated his plans for a second edition of 'Milne'. Sadly these were not to come to fruition, but after some discussion a decision was made to produce a second edition, edited and revised by Glasgow colleagues. One of the strengths of the first edition was the personal and individual approach, and it is hoped that, by involving only those who had been trained by John Milne or who know well his approach to dermatopathological problems, the flavour of the first edition has been partly carried over into the second.

In the decade since publication of the first edition major changes have been made in the approach to the diagnosis of cutaneous lymphoma and in the terminology used in the reporting of melanocytic lesions. This has necessitated major restructuring of Chapters 13 and 16. Developments in cutaneous ultrastructure have advanced our understanding of the areas of involvement in epidermolysis bullosa, and new entities such as cutaneous graft versus host disease have been recognized. All of these advances have been included as well as more general revision. At the request of the publishers the word 'introduction' has been dropped from the title. This seems appropriate as the book, although not fully comprehensive, covers all major areas of dermatopathology. Selected references have been added at the end of each chapter to guide the reader to relevant literature.

Miss Una Syme has once again performed the time-consuming task of transforming handwritten notes into immaculate typescript and I am most grateful to her.

Rona M. MacKie
Glasgow

v

Contents

1
Introduction

The pathologists who wishes to interpret histopathological sections of skin disease must familiarise himself with the clinical features of at least the commoner skin disorders. The gross appearance of lesions and their distribution is as important a diagnostic aid to him as the naked eye appearance of other organs is to a general histopathologist; in other words, clinical dermatology is his morbid anatomy. The clinical dermatologist must be aware also of the potentials and limitations of the skin biopsy and above all appreciate the fact that the skin, like most other body tissues, has a limited number of reaction patterns with which it can respond to pathological stimuli. If he will appreciate this fact he will understand why clinically different lesions may show essentially similar histological patterns. The pathologist must be given the name, age, sex and occupation of the patient, the fullest possible clinical history, the precise site of the biopsy and the duration of the lesion as well as the type and, if possible, the duration, of local and systemic therapy. It is also necessary to include the possible clinical differential diagnosis. The view held by some that the tissue should be submitted 'blind' to the pathologist cannot be condemned too strongly. If significant help is to be obtained from a skin biopsy it is necessary to submit a detailed history with the specimen.

Some of these points require further emphasis. The selection of a lesion for biopsy is of prime importance. In blistering skin disease it is of little use to submit a lesion of more than 12 hours' duration, because secondary changes in the blister may obscure the diagnostic primary changes (see Chapter 12). Bullous disease apart, fully developed lesions should be chosen where possible in order to give time for the development of pathognomonic changes. In lupus erythematosus for example, a biopsy of too early a lesion may show only a non-specific dermatitis reaction (see Chapter 11). Involuting or extensively excoriated lesions rarely yield diagnostic information.

If tumour is suspected and the lesion is small enough, excision biopsy is to be preferred. In larger tumours the biopsy should be through the advancing margin only, avoiding the central portion which may be necrotic. In nodular lesions of the limbs the biopsy must go deep enough to include a generous sample of subcutaneous fat, as it is at this level that most of the changes are seen.

If a granulomatous lesion is suspected a portion of tissue should be retained unfixed for bacteriological and mycological examination (Chapter 9).

The widespread use today of potent topical steroids as anti-inflammatory agents has added considerably to the difficulties of histological diagnosis, because either they partially suppress the inflammatory response or they encourage secondary invasion by bacteria or fungi. In addition, prolonged use can cause atrophy of the skin and telangiectasia. Where possible corticosteroids should be avoided before biopsy, and where this is not advisable the pathologist should be notified of the extent and duration of such treatment.

It should be appreciated that a histology section represents a static, 5 μm 'still' of what is a continuous disease process interrupted at the very moment when the biopsy scalpel severed the blood supply. It is this that explains the many differences between the standard textbook descriptions and what is encountered in practice.

In some cases it may be necessary to repeat the biopsies at intervals of time before a definitive diagnosis can be reached. This is particularly well seen in cases of cutaneous lymphoma of mycosis fungoides type which, although clinically suspected, may not show the diagnostic histopathology for a considerable time. If clinical doubt persists in the face of a negative histological report the biopsy should be repeated at three- or six-monthly intervals until either the histological findings are diagnostic or the clinical picture has declared itself. The importance of submitting the clinical differential diagnosis with the biopsy specimen cannot be overemphasised. While in many instances an exact histological diagnosis is not possible, some at least of the conditions suspected can be excluded.

It should be remembered that the difficult clinical case almost invariably turns out to be equally difficult from the laboratory point of view. To obtain the maximum amount of useful information close co-operation between the clinician and histopathologist and understanding of each other's problems is necessary.

Confronted with a problem case the clinical dermatologist is well advised to consult his laboratory colleagues before performing a biopsy. The increased use of histochemical techniques and, in particular, of immunopathology as diagnostic aids requires the submission of either fresh or rapidly frozen tissue: sometimes special fixatives are necessary.

For those unfamiliar with interpreting skin sections it is useful to train oneself consciously to identify each of the epidermal layers in turn, then to assess the dermis, appendages, vasculature and subcutaneous fat. This is much easier to do in a formal elliptical biopsy through the edge of a lesion which includes a portion of the normal adjacent skin (Chapter 2). The entire section should first be scanned with a two-and-a-half times objective and six, eight or ten times eyepieces, depending on personal preference. This will give a general idea of whether the lesion is predominantly epidermal, dermal or affecting the subcutaneous fat, and will reveal also any gross distortion of the microanatomy of the skin. This range of magnification is probably the most useful on the microscope, as with experience the initial scan often leads to the diagnosis or triggers a train of thought which eventually will make a diagnosis possible. Higher magnifications are used to confirm the impressions gained from the low-power scan and to assess cellular detail where this is necessary. Using a ten times objective a more detailed examination of the various structures is made, and it is then that the process of elimination begins.

Starting with the stratum corneum, is it normal for the area (Chapter 3) or is it increased (hyperkeratosis, Chapter 4)? Do the cells composing it retain their nuclei (parakeratosis, Chapter 4)? Turning to the stratum granulosum, is it normal or increased in thickness (lichen planus, Chapter 7), or is it absent as it may be if associated with parakeratotic keratin? (In one type of ichtyosis (Chapter 5) there is hyperkeratosis associated with diminution or absence of the granular layer and this is very easy to miss unless the eye is trained to assess each layer of the epidermis.) Are the cells of the stratum spinosum of normal or variable size? Do any of them exhibit individual cell keratinisation (dyskeratosis, Chapter 4)? Is there intra- or intercellular oedema (balloon degeneration or spongiosis, Chapter 4)? Is there a blister in the epidermis, and, if so, is it subcorneal (pemphigus foliaceus, Chapter 12; subcorneal pustular dermatosis, Chapter 10; one of the psoriasiform tissue reactions, Chapter 6); intraepidermal (pemphigus vulgaris, Chapter 12; benign familial pemphigus, Chapter

5; some viral diseases, Chapter 8), or subepidermal (dermatitis herpetiformis, bullous pemphigoid or porphyria, Chapter 12; epidermolysis bullosa, Chapter 5)? Is the basal cell layer regular and does it retain its normal orientation to the dermis (Chapter 3)? Are the cell nuclei seen to occupy the same place in every cell or does their position within the cells vary (loss of polarity)? Are the melanocytes (clear cells) present in normal proportions (Chapter 3) or is their number increased or decreased, and are they abnormally large or shrunken (pigmented tumours, Chapter 16)? Is there any increase in mitotic activity in the epidermis and, if so, are the mitoses normal (epidermal tumours, Chapter 4)? Are there inflammatory or other cells in the epidermis (certain inflammatory dermatoses, Chapter 6; malignant lymphomata, Chapter 13; Paget's disease, Chapter 14)? Is the basal lamina intact or are epidermal cells invading the dermis? (Confusion may arise if the section is cut obliquely, especially if the epidermis is thickened (epidermal tumours, Chapter 14).)

Passing to the dermis, is the general arrangement of collagen fibres in the papillary and reticular dermis normal (Chapter 3)? Are the collagen fibres thickened and hyalinised (morphoea, Chapter 11) or are the fibres separated by oedema fluid or other abnormal substance such as mucin? Is the staining of collagen within normal limits or is there the basophilia of solar damage (Chapter 3) Where appropriate the elastic tissue network should be examined although, as pointed out in Chapter 3, care is needed in assessing changes in it. Are the fibres increased in number, thickened or fragmented (certain inherited defects of elastic tissue, Chapter 5), or decreased in size and number—even absent post-inflammatory, Chapter 6)? Are they pushed aside by a dermal infiltrate (lymphoid neoplasm) or destroyed (inflammatory infiltrate)? Are the blood vessels in the dermis normal or are they rigid-looking and tortuous (psoriasis, Chapter 6) or affected by an inflammatory process (vasculitis, Chapter 11)? Are the dermal appendages normal in quantity for the area? Are they involved in the pathological process (pemphigus (Chapter 12) often involves the epithelium of pilosebaceous follicles)?

Is there a cellular infiltrate in the dermis and, if so, what is its relationship to the other structures; i.e. is it perivascular, perifollicular or diffuse? Does it tend to occur in localised areas (in general, inflammatory) or does it insinuate itself between the collagen bundles (malignant lymphoid neoplasm)? What is the cell type of the infiltrate—are they polymorphonuclear leucocytes, lymphocytes and histiocytes, signifying inflammatory processes, or are the cells neoplastic? To what depth does the infiltrate extend in the dermis? As a rule the infiltrates of benign inflammatory dermatoses (Chapter 6) tend to be confined to the upper dermis; when they penetrate deeper to extend down along the septa of the subcutaneous fat the mind should be altered to the possibility of malignant lymphomata.

Finally we come to the subcutaneous fat. Is is involved, is there necrosis, and, if so, is there a vasculitis (nodular lesions of the legs, Chapter 10)?

This may seem a complex and time-consuming process but it is surprising how, with a little practice and self-discipline, the eye automatically registers these points and is quick to convey to the mind features which require more detailed study at higher magnification. With some experience most of these features can be assessed with the scanning lens, thus greatly reducing the time necessary to reach a diagnosis.

2
The Skin Biopsy

Instruments and material required (Fig. 2.1)

1. 2 ml disposable syringe and no. 20 needle
2. Bard–Parker scalpel handle and no. 15 blade
3. Gillies (or Kilner) hook
4. Combined needle holder and scissors
5. Size no. 26 mm reverse cutting eyeless round suture needle with no. W328 black silk
6. 1% Lignocaine without adrenaline
7. Small squares of blotting paper approx. 2.5 cm²

As in all fields of diagnostic histopathology, accurate interpretation of a skin biopsy depends primarily on the presentation of an atraumatically obtained, well-orientated specimen so that artefacts[1] which may obscure or mislead the diagnosis are reduced to a minimum. In non-neoplastic disorders, an early but developed representative lesion should be chosen. It is a useful practice to mark the outline of the proposed biopsy beforehand and to include a portion of adjacent normal skin, which acts as a natural control for comparison purposes. Bullous disorders (Chapter 12) should be biopsied within 12–18 hours of the formation of the bulla in order to prevent difficulties in interpretation due to regeneration of epithelium which could result in confusing a subepidermal bulla for an intraepidermal one. If possible the bulla (or vesicle) should be removed intact, but still with a portion of adjacent clinically normal skin.

Injection of the skin surrounding the lesion with 1% plain lignocaine makes it possible to avoid infiltration of the lesion itself, thereby preventing disruption of the collagen or an appearance indistinguishable from oedema when subsequently examined histologically. The inclusion of adrenaline in the local anaesthetic is not recommended since any advantage as far as a blood-free site is concerned is outweighed by swelling artefact of collagen.

When making the incision, the skin should be steadied between thumb and forefinger, the blade inserted perpendicular to the skin, a positive cutting movement made without a sawing effect, and the subcutaneous fat included in the biopsy.

While it is certainly true that incisional biopsy provides the best specimens, many clinicians prefer to use a punch biopsy for convenience. The specimens so obtained tend to suffer from a number of artefacts but may be useful in tumour diagnosis prior to surgery or other forms of treatment. It has also been found that a 4 mm punch biopsy will provide a satisfactory specimen for direct immunofluorescence tests.

Once the incisions have been completed, the Gillies hook is inserted at one end of the specimen and used to draw it up so that it can be separated from the deeper structures (Fig. 2.2). This use of the hook avoids the use of forceps, thus minimising trauma to the specimen.

4

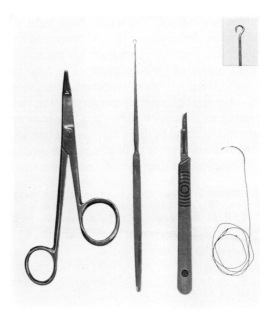

Fig. 2.1 Instruments used for skin biopsy. From left to right: combined needle holder and scissors; Gillies hook; Bard–Parker scalpel and no. 15 blade; size no. 26 mm reverse cutting eyeless round suture needle with no. W328 black silk.

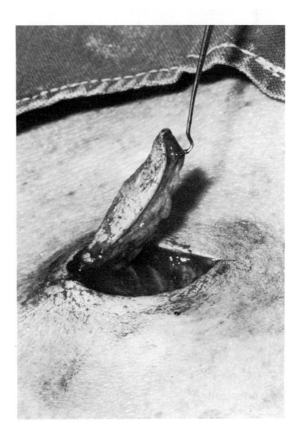

Fig. 2.2 The Gillies hook is used to control the specimen during excision, thus obviating trauma from forceps.

Small portions of skin which have been squeezed on removal by forceps cause serious diagnostic difficulties (Fig. 2.3): the collagen is crushed and cell nuclei appear pyknotic and elongated. Once the specimen has been removed, it is orientated epidermis upwards on a small square of blotting paper (Fig. 2.4), then placed in the jar of 10% neutral formalin which, being a protein coagulant, helps to stick the specimen on to the blotting paper. In this way the specimen is received in the laboratory properly orientated and not warped or twisted as it may be if blotting paper is not used. If cryostat sections are required, the specimen should be divided, one-half being snap-frozen in CO_2 snow and the other carefully orientated on a piece of blotting paper as described above.

The wound is then closed, using as many interrupted sutures as are necessary to obtain a

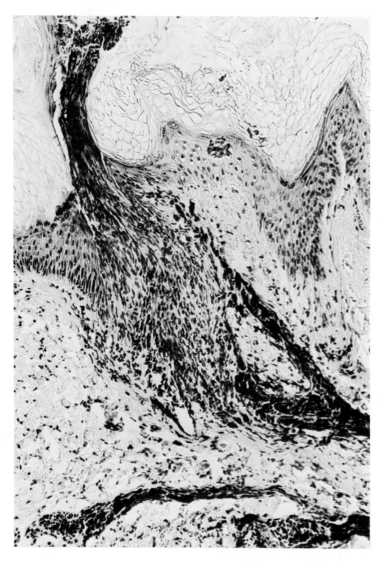

Fig. 2.3   This portion of skin has been clamped by forceps during the biopsy. Note the crushing of the collagen fibres and the elongated pyknotic cell nuclei.

good cosmetic result. It is important when suturing the wound to ensure that sutures include the corners of the wound, thus preventing any dead space and subsequent haematoma formation.

Sutures are removed from the face after 4 days, in 7 days from the trunk and upper limbs, and in 10 days from the lower limbs. With large incisions, particularly on the limbs, it is advisable to remove alternate stitches initially and to complete removal of the sutures several days later.

After approximately 12 hours' fixation the specimen is bisected at right angles to the epidermal surface with a sharp razor blade (Fig. 2.5). This small procedure is of the utmost importance in maintaining correct orientation of the tissue and helps to reduce the artefacts induced by an oblique cut (Fig. 2.6).

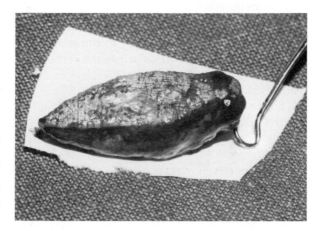

Fig. 2.4 The biopsy specimen is placed dermis downwards on a small piece of blotting paper before being placed in fixative. This is a very important step in the procedure and ensures that the specimen is received in the laboratory properly orientated.

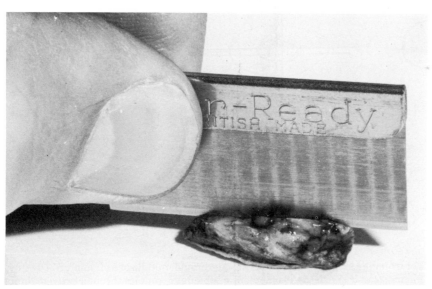

Fig. 2.5 After fixation for 12 hours the biopsy specimen is bisected at right angles to the surface with a sharp razor blade.

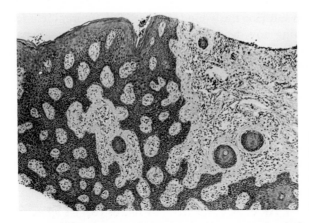

Fig. 2.6 This specimen was not orientated before fixation. Note the apparent increase in dermal papillae and 'invasion' of the dermis by the epithelial strands. These appearances are entirely due to oblique sectioning.

When the specimen submitted to the laboratory is stated to be an excision biopsy of a tumour, it is essential, particularly in the case of pigmented lesions, to ensure that blocks are taken to include the limits of excision; depending on the size of the specimen, one of the methods shown in Fig. 2.7 may be used.

The use of 10% formalin as a fixative has a number of advantages over other fixatives, the greatest being that tissue does not spoil if there is a delay in sending it to the laboratory. It also allows a wide choice of staining methods, including a number of histochemical procedures.

Other fixatives have their place in certain cases. If the tissue is unduly tough or contains a marked excess of keratin, the use of an acidic solution such as Bouin's fluid can be

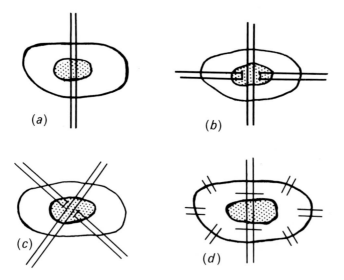

Fig. 2.7 Methods of trimming skin specimens. (*a*) One cut through middle of a circumscribed lesion (e.g. basal cell papilloma). (*b* and *c*) Alternative methods of obtaining samples through excision limits when field change may be present (e.g. squamous or basal cell carcinoma). (*d*) When dealing with a larger specimen, particularly when melanocarcinoma is suspected, several excision limit specimens should be examined.

recommended, provided that it is not allowed to remain in contact with the tissue for more than 6 hours.

The use of resin embedding and semi-thin sections has become routine in many laboratories. There is no doubt that as far as skin is concerned the improvement in cytological detail obtained by the use of this method is enormous, and it seems likely that more and more of this type of examination will be performed, particularly in the case of the cutaneous lymphomas.

In any unusual case preliminary consultation with the laboratory as to the appropriate fixative will result in the maximum information being obtained from the specimen, and in many instances obviate the necessity of subjecting the patient to a repeat biopsy. Examples of this situation are when it is proposed to perform ultrastructural studies on a portion of the tissue removed or when immunofluorescence tests are proposed, or even when tissue culture is to be performed on part of the specimen. All these three latter instances require specific procedures to be performed at the time of biopsy so as to ensure optimum results. If biopsies are intended for electron microscopy, formalin fixation is not appropriate. Small, preferably scalpel, biopsies should be transferred immediately into an initial fixative consisting of buffered glutaraldehyde and left for a period not exceeding three hours at room temperature or overnight in the refrigerator.

Reference

1. Mehregan AH, Pinkus H. Artifacts in dermal histopathology. *Arch Dermatol* 1966; **94:** 218–25.

3
The Normal Skin

One of the most difficult aspects of the interpretation of skin biopsies is the recognition of what constitutes the normal skin. There are wide regional variations in structure which are further emphasised by age, race, exposure to sunlight, prior application of topical steroids, and even occupation. The serious student of skin pathology should take every opportunity to increase his knowledge of the normal by studying sections from different anatomical sites in the various age groups. Mention has already been made in Chapter 2 of the practice of including, where possible, a portion of surrounding clinically normal skin when performing the biopsy. It is worth re-emphasising this as, apart from providing a control area, each section studied adds to the experience. The skin is a very large and complex organ. Its main component, the dermis (cutis), represents a framework of vascular connective tissue of mesodermal origin, in which are embedded the pilosebaceous units, the various secreting glands and nerve endings. The dermis is covered by an avascular multilayered epithelium of ectodermal origin, the epidermis, and cushioned by a pad of adipose tissue, the subcutaneous fat (panniculus adiposus, hypoderm).

The use of resin-embedded sections cut at $1-2\,\mu m$ is a happy compromise between the conventional paraffin-embedded sections cut at $5-6\,\mu m$ and ultrastructural examination. These thin sections allow study at high magnifications and are being used very much more frequently in dermatopathology.

The epidermis

The epidermis is a multilayered (stratified) squamous epithelium which varies in thickness from 20 or more cell layers in the palms and soles to three or four cells over the eyelids and the inner surface of the anterior forearm. In stained vertical sections its lower border, where it is in contact with the dermis, presents an undulating appearance because it has to cover the processes of the underlying dermis which project upwards like the fingers of a glove (see below). These downward projections of the epidermis are often referred to erroneously as epidermal or rete pegs because of their appearance in two-dimensional sections. A pause for reflection will make it obvious that viewed in a three-dimensional manner these are in fact ridges and their proper name should be epidermal or rete ridges. In human skin these ridges are most marked on the hands and feet, scalp and axillary regions, less pronounced on the trunk and limbs, and absent on the face. Knowledge of the regional variations of rete ridges is of more than academic importance because their absence from an area where they are normally present could signify pathological change.

It is usual to consider the microanatomy of the epidermis in terms of four distinct layers from the basal lamina (see below) upwards:

1. The basal layer, or stratum germinativum, whose lower border rests on the basal lamina which in turn is in contact with the dermis.
2. The spinous cell layer, or rete malpighii, which constitues the bulk of the epidermis.
3. The granular layer.
4. The horny layer.

While the splitting up into layers is useful from a descriptive point of view, it must be appreciated that this is highly artificial in terms of the biology of the epidermis. The progression from base to surface represents the maturation of a single cell line in the formation of the end product of epidermal differentiation, the horny layer, which forms the tough, protective, flexible outer coating of the skin. It is thus preferable to think of the great majority of epidermal cells, whatever their location in the epidermis, in terms of a unit cell, the epidermal *keratinocyte*.

The regional variations in the prominence of the epidermal layers is considerable. They are most marked in skin from the palm or sole and least marked over the eyelids. Figure 3.1

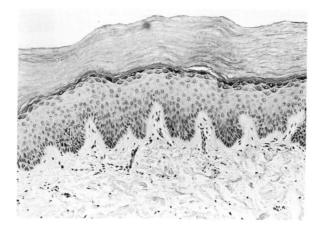

Fig. 3.1 This section shows the general structure of the human epidermis. The columnar-shaped cells of the stratum basale rest on the collagenous dermis with their long axes at right angles to the surface. Above this and constituting the bulk of the epidermis are the polygonal keratinocytes with their open vesicular nuclei. Towards the surface two or three layers of darkly staining cells comprise the stratum granulosum. A thick layer of dense, laminated anuclear keratin covers the surface. Sole of foot.

is a section, stained by haematoxylin and eosin, from the sole of a normal foot. The basal layer is seen to be composed of columnar-shaped, darkly staining cells with their long axes at right angles to the surface. In areas where the epidermis is thinner with few ridges the basal cells may appear cuboidal, or even flat. The nuclei are ovoid or round and have a strong affinity for haematoxylin and other basic dyes. The chromatin network is rather coarse and nucleoli are inconspicuous. A supranuclear cap of granules of melanin pigment is present in many cells of the basal layer, particularly in the dark-skinned races. Above the basal layer are the keratinocytes which form the spinous cell layer. These cells, larger than basal cells, are polygonal in shape and less basophilic. As already stated, this layer has considerable regional variation in thickness. As they ascend in the epidermis the keratinocytes become broader and flattened, and the cytoplasm acquires angular granules (keratohyalin granules). The granules have an avid affinity for haematoxylin, and stain dark blue with this dye. Above this level there is an abrupt change to the anucleated cells of the horny layer. In thick skin, such as that from the palms and soles, it is sometimes possible to distinguish a structureless, rather glassy-appearing zone between the granular layer and horny layer: the term 'stratum lucidum' has been applied to this area, but it is now thought to be an artefact of processing.

The horny layer in vertical sections is composed of a varying number of layers of flattened anucleated cells with dense cell walls and apparently empty interiors. Looked at from the surface and stained with haematoxylin and eosin they appear as circular or polygonal-shaped flat discs which may or may not contain the remnants of the nuclear membranes (Fig. 3.2).

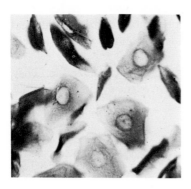

Fig. 3.2   Individual cells of the stratum corneum, showing their flattened, polygonal shape and the remnants of the nuclear membrane.

The entire cell is strongly eosinophilic. Morphologically the horny layer appears in two distinct forms. Over pressure areas such as the palms, soles and buttocks it appears in the form of dense, laminated plates (Fig. 3.3*a*), while over the flexible areas of the trunk and limbs it appears in the form of an open basket-weave (Fig. 3.3*b*). The presence of laminated horny layer in a site normally covered by basket-weave horny layer indicates either some previous pathological process or prolonged occupational trauma.

Ultrastructure of the epidermis

Electron microscopy demonstrates characteristic ultrastructural features at various levels in the skin which do not always correspond with the strata defined by light microscopy. Detailed descriptions of skin ultrastructure can be found in two atlases.[1,2]

The basement membrane zone can be resolved by electron microscopy into several structures (Fig. 3.4). The basal lamina is separated from the basal cell membrane by a less dense zone, the lamina lucida. Short striated anchoring fibrils bind the lamina lucida to the dermis.

The most characteristic feature of keratinocytes is the presence, in all strata, of tonofilaments composed of α-keratin, which progressively aggregate into tonofibrils (Fig. 3.4). Tonofibrils are attached to desmosomes (nodes of Bizzozero) (Fig. 3.5), junctional structures which are especially numerous in epidermis, ensuring the cohesive strength of the tissue. Related structures known as hemidesmosomes bind basal cells to the basal lamina (see Fig. 3.4). Tonofibril–desmosome complexes give rise to the appearance in the light microscope of 'intercellular bridges' or 'prickles', especially prominent in oedematous tissue in which non-junctional intercellular spaces have become widened.

Living keratinocytes at all levels contain the universally occurring organelles (e.g. nucleus, mitochondria, Golgi apparatus, ribosomes, endoplasmic reticulum) concerned with basic

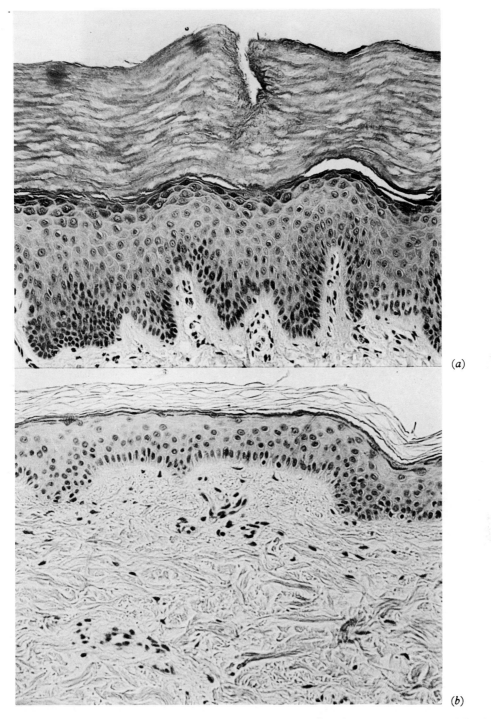

(a)

(b)

Fig. 3.3 (a) shows the dense, laminated stratum corneum found over pressure areas while (b) shows the open basket-weave type of stratum corneum found over the non-pressure areas of the skin surface. (a) Palm of hand. (b) Forearm.

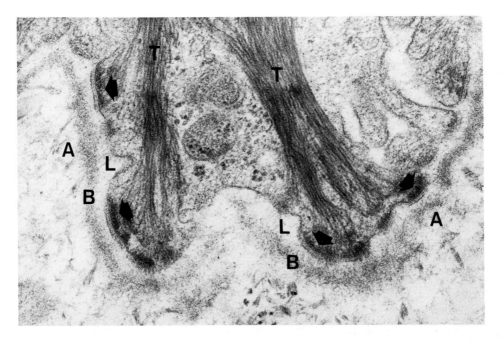

Fig. 3.4   The basement membrane zone. A, anchoring fibrils; B, basal lamina; L, lamina lucida; T, epidermal tonofilaments attached to hemidesmosomes (arrows).

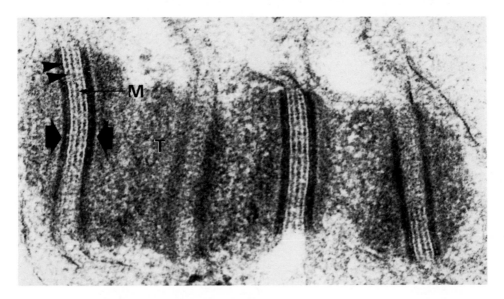

Fig. 3.5   High magnification view of four desmosomes, some in oblique section, from the spinous layer. Each contributes a dense cytoplasmic plaque (large arrows) to which tonofilaments (T), seen here in transverse section, are attached. The plaque is deposited on the cytoplasmic side of the plasma membrane which is resolved into a bilayer (small arrows). The plane of contact between the two cells is marked by a dense midline (M).

cell activities. However, other organelles are produced which are characteristic of stratifying epithelia and specific to a particular stage of differentiation (Fig. 3.6). In the upper spinous and granular layers, small ovoid bodies with lipid-rich lamellar contents (Odland bodies, membrane-coating granules) appear. The discharge of their contents into the intercellular space, which occurs in the uppermost living layers, is thought to contribute to the epidermal barrier function. At the ultrastructural level, the keratohyalin granules which characterise the granular layer are found to consist of dense material intermingled with masses of tonofilaments. This intermingling progresses through the granular layer, culminating in the 'keratin pattern' of the horny cell contents, composed of tonofilaments embedded in a dense

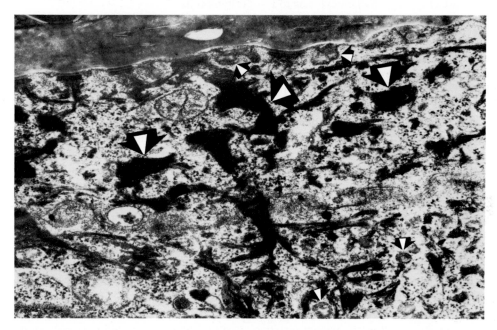

Fig. 3.6   The upper portion of epidermis, showing structures characteristic of late differentiation. Keratohyalin granules (large arrows). Odland bodies (small arrows) with internal lamellae (which are often lost during preparation) discharge their contents into the intercellular space, mainly at the horny/granular interface.

amorphous material. Most other intercellular organelles are lost during the morphologically (though not biochemically) abrupt transition between the granular and horny layers.

   The final product of epidermal differentiation, the horny layer, consists of cells, filled with the tonofilament matrix complex, surrounded by a thickened rigid and chemically resistant cell envelope, bound together by modified desmosomes and with intercellular spaces filled with lipid-rich material. The mechanical and barrier properties of the horny layer result from an interplay between all these tissue components, not simply the presence of tonofilaments. For this reason, application of the term 'keratin' both to the class of fibrous proteins to which tonofilaments belong and also as a synonym for horny layer in its entirety leads to confusion, and its use in the latter case should be abandoned.

The dendritic cells of the epidermis (epidermal symbionts)

The melanocytes and the Langerhans cells are the two major dendritic cell populations of the epidermis. As the term 'epidermal symbiont' suggests, there is some evidence to suggest a reciprocal supportive function between epidermal keratinocytes and these two populations. In addition, there is a third population, the indeterminate dendritic cell, which is identified by the *absence* on ultrastructural examination of the characteristic intracellular inclusions of the mature melanin granule or the Langerhans cell organelle. The present view regarding these cells is that they are immature dendritic cells and that they have the inherent capacity to differentiate either into melanocytes or to Langerhans cells.

The melanocyte[3]

The melanocytes or pigment-producing cells are situated mainly in the basal layer and are derived in early fetal life from the neural crest. In heematoxylin and eosin preparations of paraffin sections they are recognised easily by their rounded appearance and clear cytoplasm (Fig. 3.7). Their numbers are subject to some regional variation but they are normally present in the ratio of 1:10 to 1:5 to the epidermal basal keratinocytes. The melanocytes are endowed with a complex series of enzymes which allows them to produce the brown pigment melanin from the amino acid tyrosine. This pigment has considerable protective function in screening the dermis from the harmful effects of ultraviolet light. In this connection it is of interest to note that the total number of melanocytes per unit area is similar in matched sites from Caucasian and Negro skin. The dark colour of the Negro skin is related to the quantity and packaging of melanin pigment synthesised rather than to the numbers of melanocytes.

In order to see the true shape of the melanocytes it is necessary to stain them by means of utilising the enzymes which they contain. The method most commonly employed is to incubate fresh, unfixed, frozen sections in a buffered solution of dihydroxyphenylalanine (DOPA), when the triangular shape of the cells with their numerous fine branching processes (dendrites) is seen clearly (Fig. 3.8). Silver impregnation methods, especially in acanthotic epidermis, also will show the true shape of the melanocytes (Fig. 3.9).

The melanin is formed in the triangular-shaped cell body and extruded outwards along

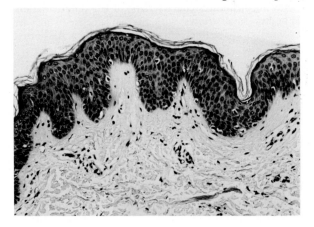

Fig. 3.7   The melanocytes are clearly recognisable by their rounded appearance, clear cytoplasm and dense pyknotic nuclei. In normal skin they are found interspersed between the cells of the stratum basale. Back of hand.

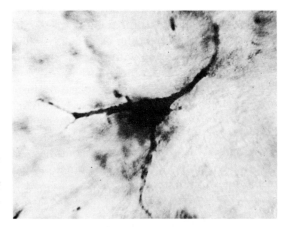

Fig. 3.8 The body of the melanocyte is triangular in shape, and from the corners fine branching processes (dendrites) can be seen. In some of the terminal dendrites granules of melanoprotein can be distinguished. Facial skin. DOPA preparation.

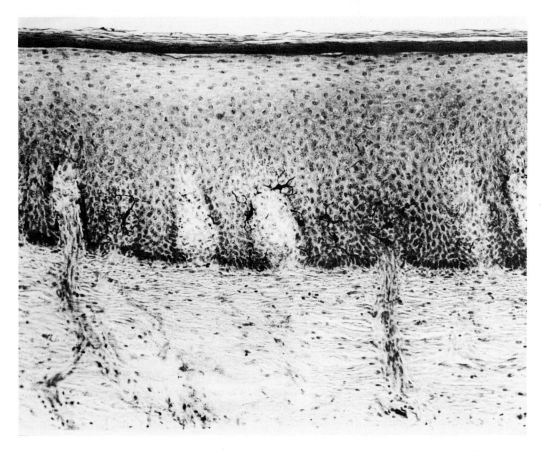

Fig. 3.9 Numerous dendritic melanocytes may be seen interspersed between the cells of the stratum basale. Normal human gingiva. Fontana silver.

the fine dendritic processes which run between the neighbouring basal cells. Recent work has indicated that basal cells receive melanin by a process of pinocytosis where the tip of a dendrite with its contained melanin is phagocytosed by the basal cell. One dendritic cell supplies the melanin requirements of a number of basal cells, and this functional unit of melanocyte and surrounding basal cells is known as the epidermal melanin unit. If normal human skin is incubated with tyrosine the melanocytes remain unstained. If, however, the skin has been irradiated previously with ultraviolet light or ionising radiation, or if the melanocytes are undergoing neoplastic transformation, the melanocytes are stained in a manner similar to staining with the DOPA technique. This indicates the presence of the enzyme tyrosinase in the cytoplasm of melanocytes in an activated state, and can be a useful procedure in the diagnosis of amelanotic melanocarcinoma provided that fresh unfixed tissue is available. It is possible that melanin has some function other than protection from the harmful effects of sunlight, as numerous basal melanocytes are found in the mucous membrane of the oral cavity.

The Langerhans cell[4]

The Langerhans cell has been the object of much interest in the past decade. These cells are situated in all the layers of the epidermis, and can be visualised at light microscopic level by the gold chloride method or by histochemical techniques using the formalin-resistant adenosine triphosphatase (ATP) reaction. Immunopathological techniques can also be used to detect these cells using the presence of Ia antigen and of an antigen shared by mature thymocytes (human thymocyte antigen, HTA) on their surface. The ultimate proof of a cell being a Langerhans cell is at the ultrastructural level by demonstration of the Birbeck granule (Fig. 3.10).

The Langerhans cell originates from the bone marrow and at present is regarded as a modified member of the monocyte/macrophage system. It carries surface receptors for the Fc component of IgG, for C_3 and for the Ia (**I**mmune-**a**ssociated) antigen. Recent work has shown it to be intimately involved in the induction of contact dermatitis.

Although recent research on the Langerhans cell has focused chiefly on its immunological role, there is evidence in smaller mammals to suggest that it may also be involved in control of keratinisation. Evidence for this in human skin is not yet forthcoming.

The basement membrane[5]

Staining with PAS or silver will reveal a linear band separating the basal cells from the underlying dermis. This is the basement membrane, and is a complex multilayered structure. When viewed at the ultrastructural level it would appear that cells can pass relatively easily from one side of the basement membrane to the other and that the notion previously held of a tough impermeable barrier is incorrect. Some knowledge of the ultrastructural components of this membrane is essential for the understanding of the bullous disorders, and in particular of the epidermolysis bullosa group of disorders. This is illustrated diagrammatically in Fig. 3.11 and ultrastructurally in Fig. 3.4. Hemidesmosomes form the areas of strongest attachment of basal cells to the underlying dermis via the basal lamina. Strong tonofilaments in the cytoplasm of the basal cells link to the attachment plaque area on the plasma membrane of the basal cell membrane. Beneath this lies the sub-basal dense zone within the lamina

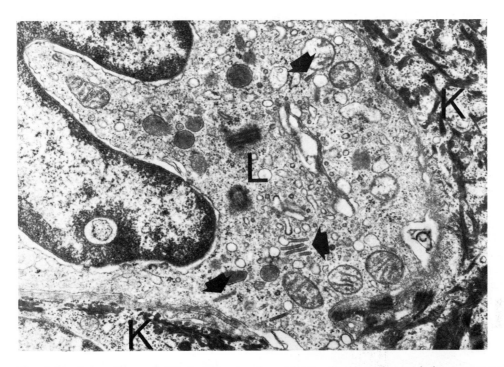

Fig. 3.10 Langerhans cell (L) showing the characteristic clear cytoplasm relative to surrounding keratinocytes (K), the deeply indented nucleus with a prominent peripheral band, and the Birbeck granules (arrows).

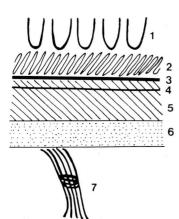

Fig. 3.11 Diagrammatic representation of the many structures that compose the basement membrane area: 1, tonofilaments; 2, attachment plaque; 3, plasma membrane; 4, subbasal dense plaque; 5, lamina lucida; 6, basal lamina; 7, anchoring fibrils.

lucida, consisting of filamentous material linking the plasma membrane and the basal lamina. Anchoring fibrils and microfibril bundles form a firm attachment between basal lamina and the dermis.

Differential distribution of molecules such as type IV collagen, bullous pemphigoid antigen, laminin and fibronectin within the basement membrane zone will permit immuno-pathological study of the site of cleavage in a variety of blistering disorders (Chapter 12).

The dermis (cutis, corium)

When the epidermis is separated from the dermis, either by putting a piece of skin dermis down on a hot-plate at 56°C for a few minutes or by trypsin digestion, a good idea of the microanatomy of the dermis is obtained. If the skin is from a region with well-marked rete ridges, such as the finger, the surface dermis resembles an egg-box composed of a number of projecting small hillocks with valleys running between them (Fig. 3.12). Each of these

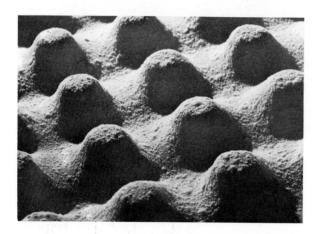

Fig. 3.12 This photograph of a model of the surface of the dermis shows the small 'hillocks' which comprise the dermal papillae and the intervening 'valleys' into which the rete ridges of the epidermis fit.

small hillocks is a finger-like projection composed of fine collagen fibres, reticulin fibres and elastic fibres, and each contains blood vessels and terminal nerves. This is the papillary dermis and the projections are known as dermal papillae. Each individual has his own characteristic arrangement of dermal papillae in the fingertips and this constitutes the morphological basis of fingerprints. In the papillary dermis the collagen bundles are fine, tend to run at right angles to the surface (Fig. 3.13) and support as a rule at least one capillary loop. The deeper part of the dermis, known as the reticular dermis, is composed of thicker, coarser bundles of collagen which form a criss-cross network with the long axis of the fibres in general tending to lie parallel with the surface (Fig. 3.14). Small extensions of the subcutaneous fat extend into the reticular dermis and in these are often found the coils of the eccrine sweat glands. Strands from the reticular dermis penetrate downwards into the subcutaneous fat, where they become continuous with the superficial fascia. The papillary dermis is most highly developed where the skin is thickest, such as on the palms and soles, and is most poorly developed where the skin is thin, for example over the face. The reticular dermis is thickest over the back of the trunk and the thighs. In the normal skin reticulin

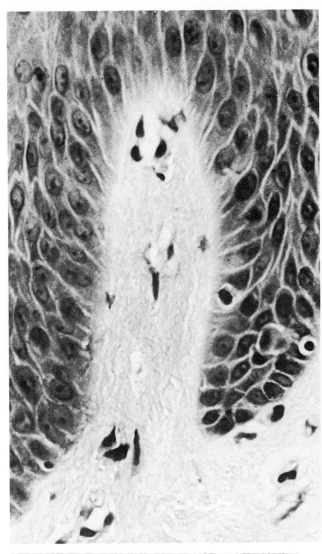

Fig. 3.13 The collagen bundles of the papillary dermis are fine and tend to run at right angles to the surface. A capillary vessel can be seen in the centre of the field. Palm of hand.

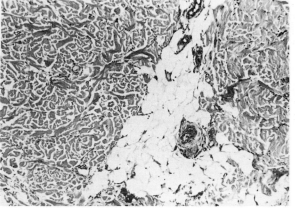

Fig. 3.14 The collagen fibres of the reticular dermis are much coarser than those of the papillary dermis. While in general their long axes run parallel with the epidermis, they form a criss-cross network and thus appear in stained sections to run in many different directions. In this section a wedge of subcutaneous fat containing a blood vessel and part of a sweat gland can be seen. Skin from back.

fibres are found only as a localised, dense band just below the epidermis corresponding in position to the basal lamina (Fig. 3.15).

The elastic tissue network (elastica) Fig. 3.16) of the dermis consists in the papillary layer of fine branching fibres running, like the collagen fibres, at right angles to the surface and ending just short of the undersurface of the epidermis. The fibres in the reticular dermis are

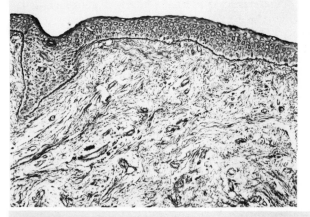

Fig. 3.15 A dense band of reticulin fibres can be seen interposed between the epidermis and dermis, corresponding to the position of the basal lamina. Skin from forearm, Gordon & Sweet's reticulin stain (Lendrum's modification).

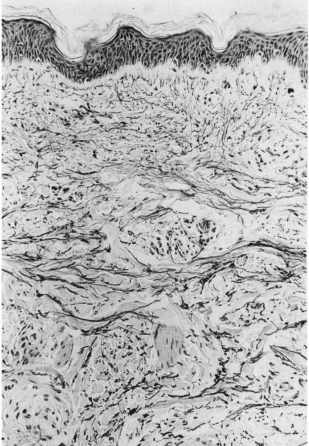

Fig. 3.16 In the papillary dermis the elastic fibres are composed of the fine branching strands which run at right angles to the surface, stopping just short of the undersurface of the epidermis. The fibres in the reticular dermis are much coarser and tend to lie parallel to the surface, but as they follow the collagen bundles they appear to run in many different directions. Skin from back. Acid orcein–methylene blue.

coarser and thicker, and again accompany the collagen feltwork, tending to run parallel with the surface. The main function of the elastic network is to prevent the dermal collagen from being overstretched. Should this happen the elastic fibres rupture, the collagen becomes overextended and damaged, and the result is a permanent scar or stria. While the arrangement of the normal elastica pattern is highly characteristic, care must be taken in basing a diagnosis solely on minor abnormalities of the elastic network. As the elastica in the reticular dermis follows the feltwork of collagen it will be cut in many different directions during the preparation of the section. This must not be interpreted as fragmentation of elastica. Small injuries or inflammatory lesions such as folliculitis may have destroyed some of the network in the past.

Blood supply of the skin

The skin has an abundant blood supply, this being greatest in areas containing numerous secreting glands; for example, the face, hands and feet. Perforating vessels from muscular arteries penetrate the fascia and run upwards in the fibrous tissue septa of the subcutaneous fat. These vessels branch and form a plexus about the middle of the dermis. From this plexus branches go to such specialised structures as hair follicles, sebaceous glands and sweat duct coils. Other branches continue upwards and unite to form a second plexus at the junction of the papillary and reticular dermis from which capillary loops run upwards to supply each dermal papilla. Figure 3.17 is a photomicrograph of a carmine gelatin injection of human

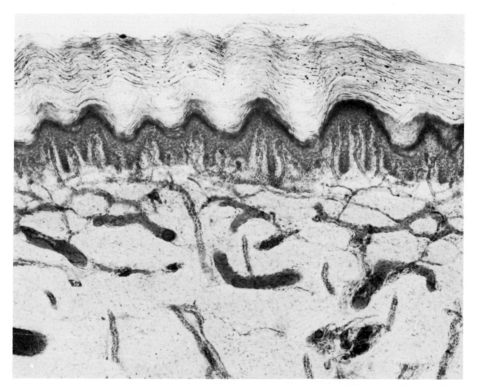

Fig. 3.17 The two vascular plexuses in the dermis and the capillary loop of each of the dermal papillae can be seen in this photomicrograph. Human skin. Carmine gelatin injection.

finger skin. The general vascular supply is clearly visible with its two networks, its papillary loops and the abundant supply to the sweat gland coils. Such injection preparations are difficult to achieve and require amputation specimens in which the vessels are often diseased. Human capillary endothelium is extremely rich in alkaline phosphate, and a very useful delineation of the capillary pattern in the skin can be obtained by using Gomori's method for demonstrating alkaline phosphatase (Fig. 3.18). This technique is suitable for small

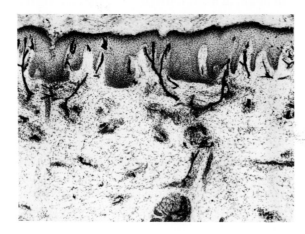

Fig. 3.18 The capillary blood supply of the skin is clearly shown in this photograph of a 75 μm thick section. Skin from dorsum of finger. Gomori's alkaline phosphatase.

blocks of tissue, which can then be embedded in paraffin and the vasculature studied in thick serial sections at leisure.

Lymphatic channels are very abundant in the dermis but are difficult to see in normal fixed tissue sections as these extremely thin-walled channels collapse when the block is fixed and dehydrated. Skin which is the seat of a chronic lymphoedema gives an idea of the richness of the dermal lymphatic network (Fig. 3.19) as the vessels appear to collapse only partially.

The pilosebaceous unit

It is logical to consider the hair follicle, the hair, the sebaceous gland, the arrectores pilorum muscle and, in certain regions, the apocrine glands as a distinct functional unit. It has been shown that about the eighth to tenth week of fetal life small groups of primitive basal epidermal cells in association with an area of condensed mesenchyme (Fig. 3.20) undergo a differentiation which commits them to form pilosebaceous complexes. The resulting hair germ grows obliquely downwards towards the developing subcutaneous fat.

Knowledge of the embryological development of the pilosebaceous unit has contributed greatly to our understanding of the biology of basal cell carcinomata and tumours derived from the epidermal appendages[6] (Chapter 15). Following the establishment of the hair germ, further growth occurs upwards towards the surface of the epidermis as well as down into the dermis. The upward growth forms the future intraepidermal hair canal (acrotrichium). Thus is formed an entire pilar follicle, including its intraepidermal portion, distinct from the surrounding surface epidermis. The establishment of this biologically separate cell line of adnexal keratinocytes (to which the name acrotrichial keratinocytes has been given) indicates that a distinct embryonic differentiation has occurred. The adnexal keratinocytes retain their

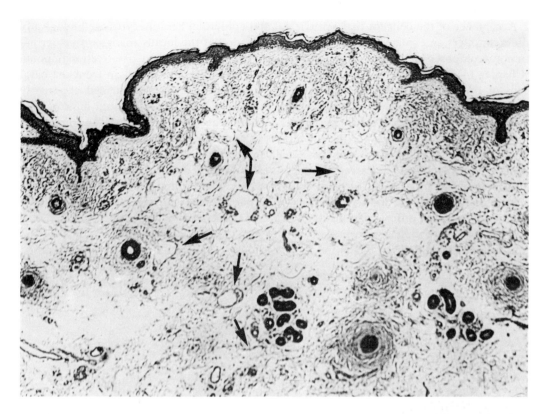

Fig. 3.19 Dilated dermal lymphatics (arrowed) can be seen in this section. Skin from lower leg (chronic lymphoedema).

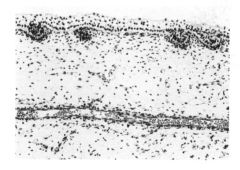

Fig. 3.20 Small foci of basal cell proliferation associated with areas of condensed mesenchyme can be seen along the stratum basale. These are the primitive hair germs. Fetal scalp, 10 weeks' gestation.

biological individuality throughout adult life. In times of severe stress, however, such as loss of surface epidermis, they can revert to their undifferentiated embryonic state and form epidermal keratinocytes until the epidermis is resurfaced. This process is relied upon daily by the plastic surgeon to heal the donor areas from which split-skin grafts have been taken. The adnexal keratinocytes of the hair canal (acrotrichial keratinocytes) cannot be distinguished in histological sections from the surrounding epidermal keratinocytes.

Acceptance of the concept that acrotrichial and epidermal keratinocytes are biologically different offers an explanation of the apparent paradox of the locally malignant epidermal tumour composed of darkly staining, basal-like cells, the so-called basal cell carcinoma (Chapter 14). The use of the term 'basal cell carcinoma' implies an origin from the basal cells of the epidermis, and indeed many photographs have been published apparently indicating such an origin. If epidermal basal cell origin is accepted it would indicate that such a tumour would be equal to or perhaps even more aggressive than a squamous carcinoma as the basal epidermal cells are the precursors of squamous cells. Experience has shown, however, that this is untrue. While 'basal cell carcinomata' exhibit local invasion, recorded instances of metastases are extremely rare. It is to be hoped that further study either by electron microscopy or by histochemistry will clarify the essential differences between the acrotrichial keratinocyte and the epidermal keratinocyte. At present the view that a definite embryological act of differentiation has given rise to the acrotrichial keratinocyte, which may be a cell type much less aggressive should it become neoplastic, certainly accounts for the paradox of the basal cell carcinoma and explains the many variations in structure encountered in these tumours.

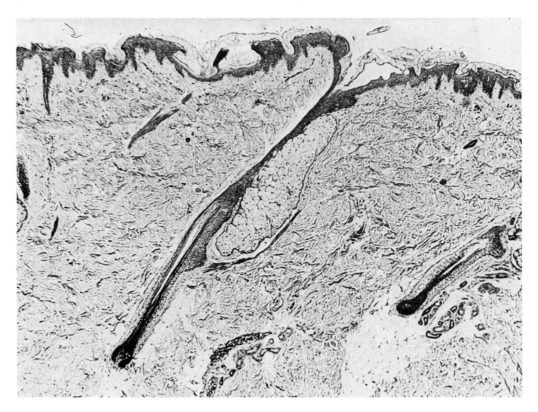

Fig. 3.21   This picture shows an entire pilosebaceous unit. The hair follicle runs obliquely downwards and to the left, terminating in the claw-shaped hair bulb. The arrectores pilorum muscle is inserted into a bulge at the junction of the lower one-third with the upper two-thirds of the hair follicle. A sebaceous gland lobule is visible occupying the space on the right between the upper part of the follicle and the arrectores pilorum muscle. Skin from chest.

In post-fetal life the hair follicles are found at different levels in the dermis. The coarse terminal hairs of the scalp, beard and pubic regions usually extend into the subcutaneous fat while the finer body hairs go to mid or lower dermis and the fine vellus hairs commonly found on the face lie in the superficial dermis. Figure 3.21 shows the general arrangement of a hair and its follicle, with its root near the subcutaneous tissue, its obliquely inserted arrectores pilorum muscle and the sebaceous gland lobule in the angle subtended by the follicle and the undersurface of the epidermis.

The lower part of the hair consists of a claw-like expansion, the hair bulb, which encloses an area of highly vascular connective tissue (hair papilla) (Fig. 3.22) and is the most active

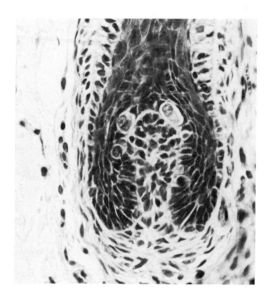

Fig. 3.22   Hair papilla. The claw-like expansion (hair bulb) of the lower part of the hair can be seen enclosing a finger-like process (hair papilla) of highly vascular cellular connective tissue. Note the numerous melanocytes in the 'stratum basale' of the hair bulb. Skin from scalp.

growth area of the hair. As can be seen from the photomicrograph, it contains large numbers of melanocytes. The fine structure of the growing part of the hair is very complex, and for details of this and the phases of hair growth the reader is referred to an excellent account of the subject.[7] Figure 3.23 is a transverse section of a hair just above the hair bulb which gives some idea of the complexity of its structure.

The lower part of the hair is the seat of growth and differentiation. About half way up the follicle it becomes a keratinised structure devoid of living cells. The junction of these two zones (Adamson's fringe) is the level at which growth of the keratinophilic fungi which infect the non-living part of hair ceases. As the actual living part of the hair is not therefore affected by these fungi no permanent hair loss follows ringworm infection of the scalp. Should secondary pyogenic infection occur, however, the resulting suppuration may cause permanent loss of hair follicles.

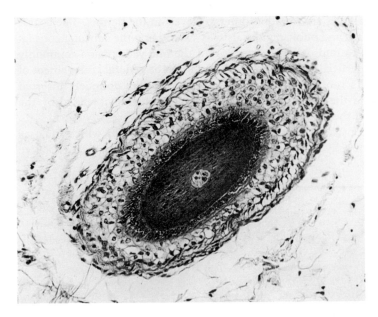

Fig. 3.23   Slightly oblique section of hair follicle just above the region of the hair bulb to show the complex structure of the growing hair. Skin from scalp.

Sebaceous glands

The sebaceous glands are an integral part of the pilosebaceous unit and are found over the entire body surface, with the exception of the palms and soles. The gland itself consists of several lobules separated by highly vascular connective tissue. These lobules all empty into a short duct which enters the upper part of the hair follicle (Fig. 3.24). More than one sebaceous gland unit may be associated with a hair follicle and thus more than one sebaceous duct may enter the upper part of the hair follicle. The structure of a sebaceous gland lobule is illustrated in Fig. 3.25. The periphery of the gland is composed of flattened, darkly staining cells (basal cells). From the basal layer inwards the cells increase in size and become foamy in appearance in haematoxylin and eosin stained sections. This is due to their contained lipid being dissolved out during processing. Towards the centres of the lobules the cells disintegrate completely (holocrine secretion) and the resulting lipid mass with cell debris (sebum) enters the duct, finally finding its way into the upper part of the hair follicle. Sebaceous glands are found occasionally in the mucous membranes of the lips and cheeks. They open directly on to the surface through a short, keratinised duct (Fig 3.26). This is due to a developmental displacement of sebaceous glands and is known as Fordyce's disease. A similar heterotopia of sebaceous glands is occasionally seen in the stratified squamous epithelium of the vagina and vaginal portion of the cervix.

Apocrine glands

In certain anatomical sites in man the pilosebaceous units are associated with secreting glands with a distinctive structure, the apocrine glands. These were originally called apocrine

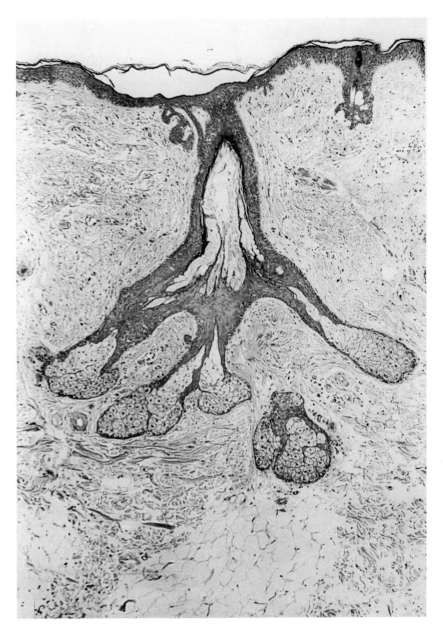

Fig. 3.24 Upper part of pilosebaceous follicle with its related sebaceous gland lobule. Each lobule empties into the follicle through a short duct. Skin from chest.

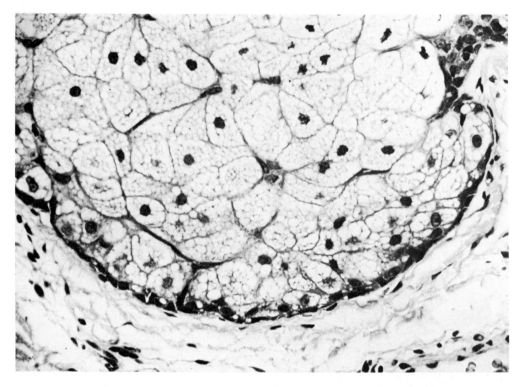

Fig. 3.25   Part of a sebaceous gland lobule, showing the darkly staining small basal cells around the periphery and the large, foamy cells which increase in size towards the centre. Human facial skin.

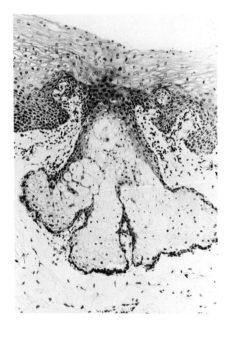

Fig. 3.26 Heterotopic sebaceous gland opening directly on to buccal mucosa (Fordyce's disease). Oral mucosa, buccal aspect. (Section by courtesy of Professor D.K. Mason, Glasgow.)

because of their supposed mode of secretion by 'decapitation' of cells. It is now known that this was a histological artefact. Normally these are found in the axillae, the pubic and perineal regions, the labia minora, the prepuce and scrotum, the areola and nipple of the mammary gland, the eyelids and the external auditory meatus. Occasionally, ectopic glands are found on the scalp, forehead and around the umbilicus. The glands are simple coiled tubes which lie deep in the dermis or upper part of the subcutaneous fat. The secreting coils are lined by a single layer of rather eosinophilic cells, each containing a single nucleus at the base. The cells vary in height from low cuboidal to high columnar with a definite constriction at their tips (Fig. 3.27). This variation in height is suggestive of a cyclical function of the epithelium. Interposed between the secreting cells and the basal lamina are darkly staining, elongated, myoepithelial cells. In some acini brownish granules which stain blue with the Prussian blue stain for ferric salts are seen. The apocrine gland duct has a double-layer structure similar to the eccrine sweat duct (see below) but is shorter and, instead of opening on to the surface, empties into the pilosebaceous follicle above the sebaceous duct.

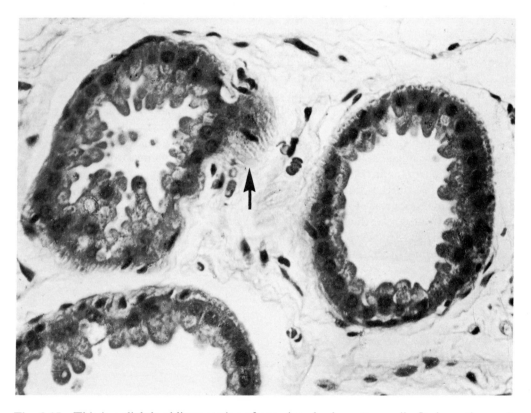

Fig. 3.27 This is a slightly oblique section of apocrine gland secretory coils. It shows the varying height of the columnar epithelium and the constriction of the tips of some of the cells. The darkly staining elongated nuclei seen round the outside of the secretory coils belong to the myoepithelial cells. These can be seen more easily when sectioned obliquely (arrow). Axillary skin.

The eccrine sweat glands

The true sweat glands of man are universal over the body surface, with the exception of the vermilion borders of the lips. They are most numerous on the hands and feet and decrease in number on the head, trunk and extremities. The eccrine sweat gland unit is composed of a single tubular duct which extends from the epidermis to mid dermis where it becomes coiled on itself, forming the secreting portions. In tissue sections the secreting coils are found about the middle of the dermis, usually lying in a small finger-like pad of fat which extends from the subcutaneous tissue. In structure they consist of a single layer of cells, the luminal borders of which are rather irregular (Fig. 3.29). Two types of secreting cell are found and these vary in proportion in different regions of the body. There is a small, superficial, darkly staining cell with basophilic cytoplasm and a deeper, clear cell with a definitely acidophilic cytoplasm. The functional significance of these two types of cell or of their regional variations is not clear. Along the base of the secreting cells and running parallel to their lumen are the rather inconspicuous myoepithelial cells. There is an abrupt transition to the excretory duct which is lined by a double layer of darkly staining cuboidal cells. Where these abut on the lumen they are bounded by a rather hyaline, PAS-positive cuticle. The duct (acrosyringium) passes relatively straight upwards to the undersurface of the epidermis. It enters the epidermis and pursues its spiral course through it (Fig. 3.30), the number of coils of the spiral being inversely related to the thickness of the epidermis. During its intraepidermal course the duct retains its own distinct lining, which can be distinguished clearly from the surrounding epidermal keratinocytes (Fig. 3.31). The acrosyringial keratinocytes, as they are called, are paler and smaller than epidermal keratinocytes and have pale-staining, round nuclei. They are devoid of melanin granules but keratohyalin granules may be seen in the cells forming the lower part of the duct.

The eccrine sweat glands, like the pilosebaceous follicles but distinct from them, are seen first about the fourth month of fetal life as condensations of small groups of primitive basal cells (Fig. 3.28). As in the differentiation of the hair germ, further growth occurs both upwards towards the surface to form the intraepidermal part of the sweat duct (acrosyringium) and downwards as a straight cord, which becomes canalised about the seventh month of fetal life, to become the excretory duct. From the lower portion of this, by a process of growth and infolding, the coils of the secretory portion of the gland arise. Like its counterpart

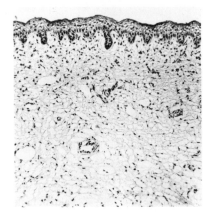

Fig. 3.28 Small cords of condensed basal cells grow downwards from the primitive basal layer to form the eccrine sweat glands. Fetal palm of hand (approx. 16 weeks' gestation.)

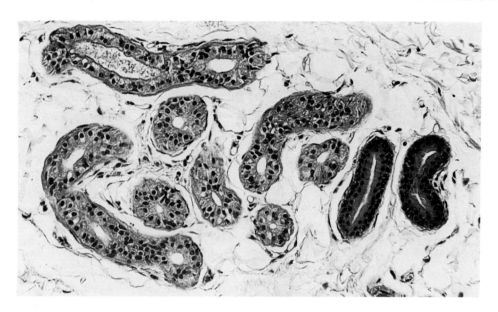

Fig. 3.29   Secretory coils of eccrine sweat gland lying in a prolongation of the subcutaneous fat. The coils are composed of a single layer of small, dark cells intermixed with larger, clearer cells. In some of the coils the oblique plane of section gives the appearance of more than one layer. The darker-staining tubules lines by a double layer of epithelium to the right of the picture are portions of the excretory duct. Palm of hand.

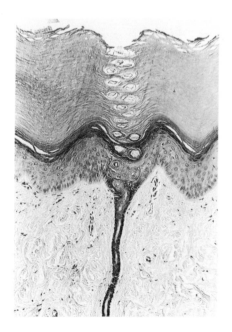

Fig. 3.30   The sweat duct (acrosyringium) can be seen running straight up through the dermis. It becomes coiled on entering the epidermis and maintains this configuration until it opens on to the surface. Palm of hand.

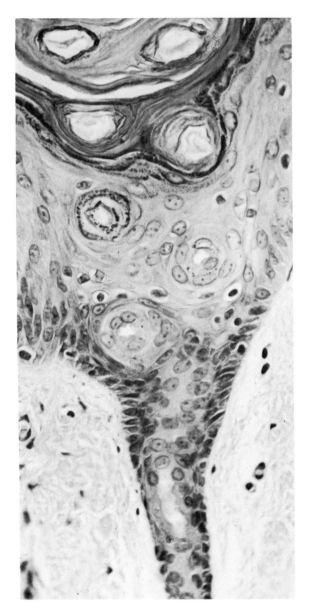

Fig. 3.31 Intraepidermal portion of sweat duct which clearly shows the difference between the acrosyringal keratinocytes and the surrounding epidermal keratinocytes. Palm of hand.

the acrotrichial keratinocyte, the acrosyringial keratinocyte retains its separate biological identity throughout life, reverting to its early embryonic state only after such severe stimuli as loss of the surface epithelium, when it may contribute to the resurfacing. The rather striking morphological differences between the secretory coils, the intradermal excretory duct and the intraepidermal portion of the excretory duct of the eccrine sweat apparatus tend to be maintained in tumours arising from the sweat apparatus (Chapter 15).

Nerve supply

The skin is abundantly supplied with sensory nerve fibres, and thus can provide us with a large amount of sensory information. The fine, terminal nerve fibres require special silver impregnation to demonstrate them (Fig. 3.32), although in routine stained sections the end organs such as the Vater–Pacini corpuscle (Fig. 3.33) are recognised easily in those areas where they occur. Small nerve trunks also are recognised easily in routine haematoxylin and eosin sections by the characteristic pattern of the Schwann cell nuclei (Fig. 3.34). It is sometimes difficult to distinguish between portions of nerve trunk and portions of the

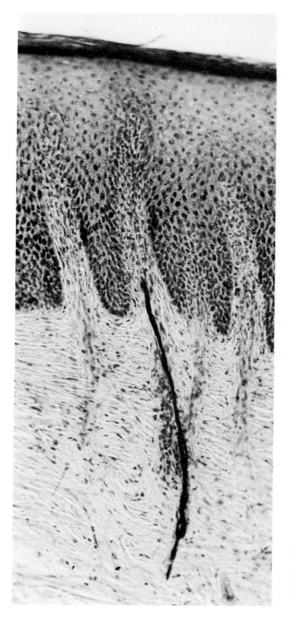

Fig. 3.32 A terminal nerve fibre is seen running upwards towards the epidermis, ending just short of a papilla. To determine the precise course of such fibres it is necessary to study them in serial sections. Skin from areola. Richardson's silver impregnation technique.

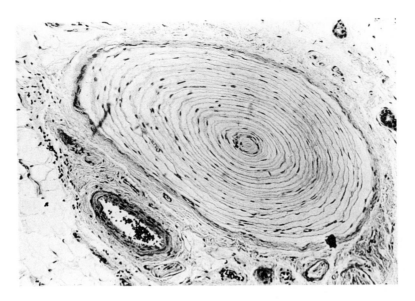

Fig. 3.33   A Vater–Pacini corpuscle seen in the dermis of a biopsy from finger skin.

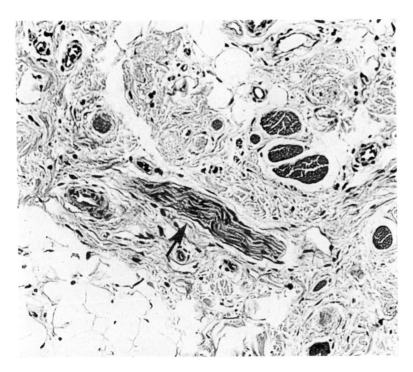

Fig. 3.34   Small cutaneous nerve in longitudinal section (arrowed), showing the characteristic wavy pattern produced by the Schwann cell nuclei. Facial skin.

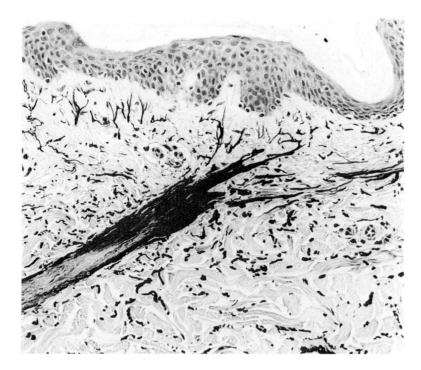

Fig. 3.35 Terminal portion of an arrector pili muscle, showing the abundant elastic fibres. Facial skin. Orcein-methylene blue.

arrectores pilorum muscle. Should doubt exist, an elastic tissue stain such as synthetic orcein will demonstrate the presence of elastic fibres in the terminal portion of the latter (Fig. 3.35).

Normal anatomy of mucous membranes

Oral and vaginal mucous membranes are frequently involved in disease processes (e.g. lichen planus) which also involve the skin, and it is therefore important to understand the normal histological appearances in these sites. The mucosa of the oral cavity is divided broadly into two types: one in which keratinisation is proceeding, and which therefore has a differentiation

Table 3.1 Keratinisation pattern in oral mucosa

'Physiological parakeratosis' (no stratum granulosum)	Anuclear keratinisation (with stratum granulosum)
Lip	Free gingiva
Cheek	Attached gingiva
Soft palate	Hard palate
Crevicular epithelium	Dorsum of tongue
Alveolar mucosa	
Sublingual mucosa	

pattern very similar to skin; and areas in which anuclear keratinisation does not occur, characterised by retention of nucleated cells in the outermost layers and the absence of a stratum granulosum. Table 3.1 indicates the sites in which these two patterns may be seen, and emphasises the necessity of knowing the exact site from which an oral biopsy is taken. In some diseases involving the oral mucosa both the distribution and appearance are related to the varying epithelial patterns (Fig. 3.36).

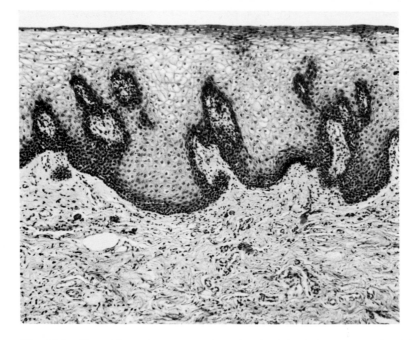

Fig. 3.36   Normal buccal mucosa to show the physiological parakeratosis which occurs in some parts of the oral cavity. There is no stratum granulosum. The cells of the stratum corneum are vacuolated and contain small, round pyknotic nuclei. Sublingual mucosa. (Section by courtesy of Professor D.K. Mason.)

In the vulva the inner surfaces of the labia majora and the medial surface of the labia minora are normally composed of keratinising epithelium with a granular layer and anuclear cornified outer layer. The mucocutaneous junction (Fig. 3.37) illustrates the abrupt transition from this pattern to the non-keratinising mucosal surface characterised by the presence of nucleated cells in the upper layers and absence of any granular layer.

Ageing of skin

The rate of ageing of human skin is a complex process dependent on many factors. Race apart, genetic influences such as skin coloration, exposure to the elements (in particular, sunlight), nutritional deficiencies and concomitant disease, as well as skin diseases such as lupus erythematosus, can accelerate the rate of ageing. The morphological changes produced by age are often subtle and not readily apparent to the casual observer. In general the thickness of the epidermis decreases with the passage of time and this is often associated with an apparent increase in the horny layer. The basal layer of the epidermis becomes

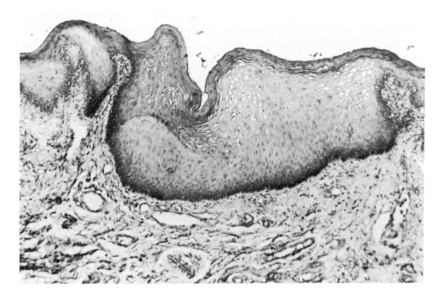

Fig. 3.37 Section through the mucocutaneous junction of the oral cavity to show the abrupt transition fron anuclear keratin with a stratum granulosum to the physiological parakeratosis of the mucosa. Oral mucosa.

rather disorganised and lacks the orderly alignment at right angles to the basal lamina seen in the young. Melanocytes become larger and their distribution irregular. In areas of the skin where there has been excessive exposure to sunlight the melanocytes may show focal increase associated with some cellular atypia. There is loss of dermal papillae and consequently the epidermis loses its 'ridges' (Fig. 3.38). Sweat glands are reduced in total number.

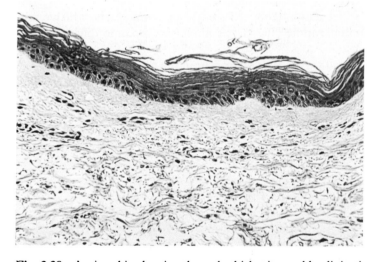

Fig. 3.38 Ageing skin showing the early thickening and hyalinization of the individual elastic fibres in the upper and mid dermis. The epidermis is atrophic and there is hyperkeratosis. There is a loss of rete ridges and dermal papillae. The collagen fibres of the reticular dermis are atrophic. Dorsum of hand.

The epithelium of the secreting ducts tends to shrink, increasing its normal uneven appearance and causing the lumen of the gland to appear larger. Pigment granules appear in both the clear and the dark cells, this pigment being apparently similar to the so-called wear and tear pigment which occurs in other organs. The flattening out of the papillary dermis is usually most pronounced in light-exposed areas (Fig. 3.39). In these areas it is often asso-

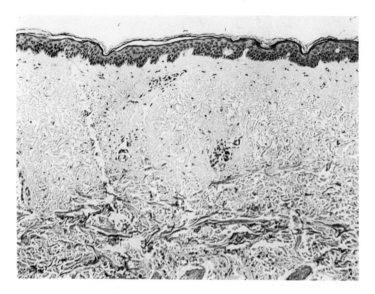

Fig. 3.39   Ageing skin showing extensive actinic changes in the upper part of the dermis. The collagen and elastic fibres are thickened and have a refractile appearance. In some areas they have fused together to give areas of rather homogeneous appearance. Skin from side of neck.

ciated with changes in the tinctorial staining properties of the dermal collagen which tends to become more basophilic. Initially individual elastic fibres may become thickened and hyalinised (Figs 3.40 and 3.41).

In order to emphasise the regional variations which occur in the normal subject, Fig. 3.42 shows sections from representative areas of the body surface.

References

1. Zelickson AS. *Ultrastructure of Normal and Abnormal Skin*. London: Kimpton, 1967.
2. Breathnach AS. *An Atlas of the Ultrastructure of Human Skin*. London: Churchill, 1971.
3. Hu F. Melanocyte cytology in normal skin. In: Ackerman AB, ed. *Masson Monographs in Dermatopathology—I*. New York: Masson, 1981: pp. 1–22.
4. Rowden G. The Langerhans cell. *CRC Crit Rev Immunol* 1982; **3:** 95–179.
5. Briggaman RA. Biochemical composition of the epidermal–dermal junction and other basement membrane. *J Invest Dermatol* 1982; **78,** 1–6.
6. Pinkus H. Adnexal tumours. Benign, not so benign and malignant. In: Montagna W, Dobson RL, eds. *Carcinogenesis*. Oxford: Pergamon, 1966: pp. 255–87.
7. Montagna W, Dobson RL. *Hair Growth*. Advances in Biology of Skin, vol. 9. Oxford: Pergamon, 1969.

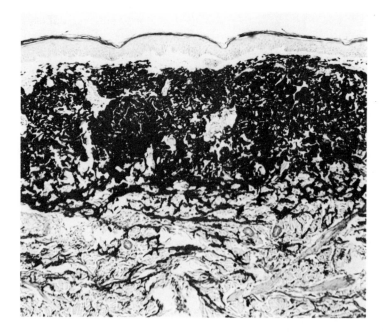

Fig. 3.40 Further section from skin illustrated in Fig. 3.39 to show the cushion-like mass of 'elastica' in the upper dermis. Skin from side of neck. Orcein–methylene blue.

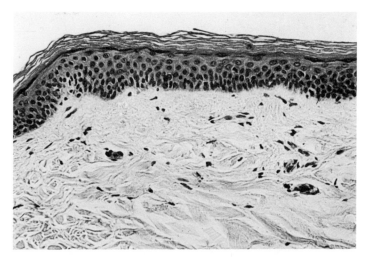

Fig. 3.41 Aged skin from covered area of the body. The atrophy of the collagen bundles is most noticeable in the lower part of the dermis. Anterior aspect, male lower limb.

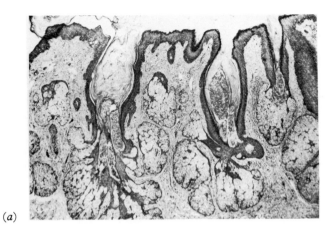

(a)

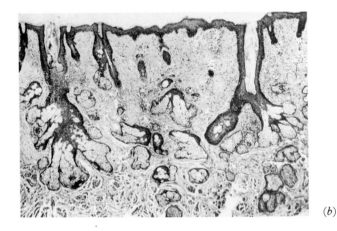

(b)

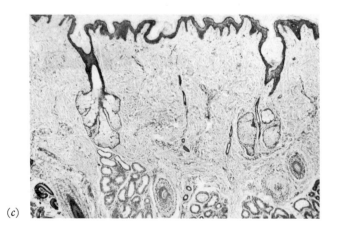

(c)

Fig. 3.42 (*a–f*)   These sections from different areas of the normal skin in a similar age group emphasize the wide regional variations: (*a*) face; (*b*) scalp; (*c*) axilla.

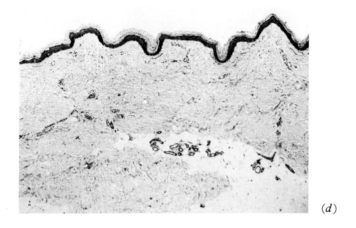

(d)

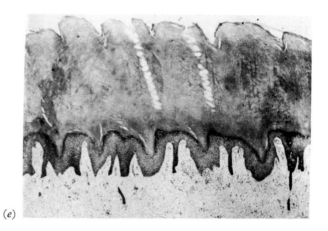

(e)

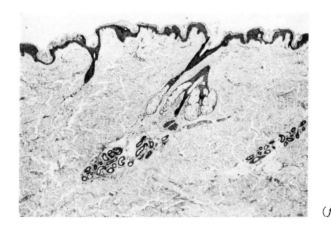

(f)

Fig. 3.42 *cont.*   (d) Forearm; (e) palm of hand; (f) back.

4

Descriptive Terms used in Cutaneous Pathology

In describing the pathological changes in diseased skin a number of terms are used, most of which have no counterpart in general pathology.

Acantholysis

This refers to loss of cohesion between neighbouring epidermal cells subsequent to damage

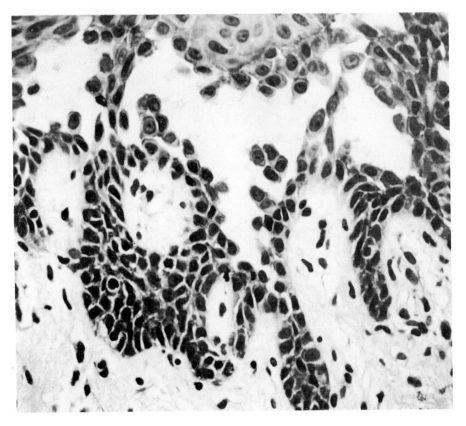

Fig. 4.1 Acantholysis (benign) in pemphigus vulgaris. Above the basal layer the cells are separating from each other and some lie free in the blister cavity. The separated cells and their nuclei become 'rounded off'.

in the region of their desmosomes. It is customary to recognise two types of acantholysis: (1) a benign type and (2) a malignant type.

The benign type occurs mainly in the serious group of blistering disorders, pemphigus. In these diseases the individual keratinocytes become rounded off and separate from each other forming an intraepidermal blister, commencing as a rule just above the basal layer (Fig. 4.1). The cells eventually undergo degenerative changes and finally die. Benign acantholysis is also seen in the genodermatoses, Darier's disease and benign familial pemphigus (Chapter 5). Minor degrees of acantholysis may be seen in conditions such as impetigo contagiosa and subcorneal pustular dermatosis (Chapters 6 and 12) in which a high content of polymorphonuclear leucocytes and their proteolytic enzymes are trapped within the epidermis.

Malignant acantholysis is seen in some types of neoplasia of squamous epithelium, in particular carcinoma in situ arising in actinic keratosis (Chapter 14). In addition to the rounding-off and separation of the squamous cells, there are cytological features of neoplasia such as loss of polarity, nuclear pleomorphism and hyperchromatism (Fig. 4.2), and aberrant mitoses.

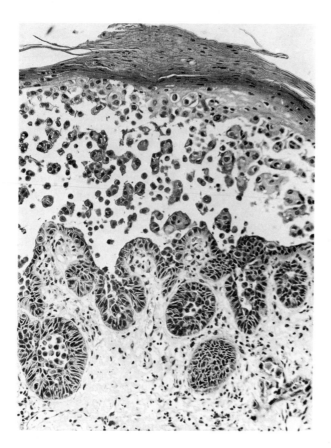

Fig. 4.2   Acantholysis (malignant) in squamous carcinoma in situ arising in an actinic keratosis. The separation between the cells produces an adenomatous appearance and the free acantholytic cells are seen in the blister cavity. In addition, dysplastic changes can be seen in the epidermal cells.

Acanthosis

This term is used to describe benign localised increase in thickness of the spinous layer. It is a common reaction pattern of the skin to a number of differing stimuli. The type of acanthosis varies to a certain extent with the causative agent. One of the most common, which may be designated reactive acanthosis, is a diffuse thickening over a limited area, this type being most commonly seen in chronic dermatitis (Chapter 6); it is related to the duration of the disease process and to the degree of itching and subsequent scratching. In many instances acanthosis of this type is associated with hyperkeratosis (Fig. 4.3) and hypertrophy

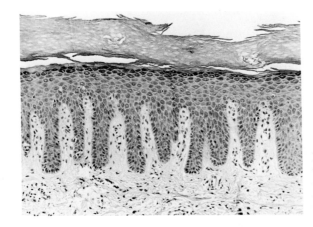

Fig. 4.3 Acanthosis in lichenfied dermatitis of forearm. There is a generalised thickening of the spinous layer associated with a hypertrophied granular layer and hyperkeratosis.

of the granular layer. Another variety of acanthosis is seen in the chronic skin disease, psoriasis (Chapter 7). In this disorder there is marked elongation of the rete ridges with a tendency for adjacent ridges to fuse together (Fig. 4.4). The dermal papillae are also elongated and the part of the epidermis overlying the tips of the papillae is reduced to one or two cells in thickness. In contrast to reactive acanthosis, in psoriasis the granular layer is absent and there is parakeratosis of the horny layer. Invasion of the epidermis by some viruses also produces acanthosis. In the common wart (Chapter 8) this is characteristically associated with inclusions in the epidermal cells and the overlying stratum corneum. The area of acanthosis is sharply delineated by claw-like rete ridges which tend to underline and delineate the area of epithelial thickening (Fig. 4.5). Invasion of the epidermis by the virus of molluscum contagiosum (Chapter 8) produces a characteristic tumour-like acanthosis. The affected rete ridges become bulbous, compressing the connective tissue of the dermal papillae into thin thread-like strands (Fig. 4.6).

Dyskeratosis

This implies premature or abnormal keratinisation of individual epidermal cells. Both benign and malignant types of dyskeratosis occur. The benign type is seen in such conditions as Darier's disease and benign familial pemphigus (Chapter 5), in both of which a low-grade type of acantholysis occurs. The dyskeratotic cells are larger than normal and the cytoplasm homogeneous and strongly eosinophilic in haematoxylin and eosin preparations (Fig. 4.7). Nuclear remnants may or may not be seen. Malignant dyskeratosis is seen in Bowen's disease (Chapter 14) (Fig. 4.8) and in poorly differentiated squamous carcinoma (Chapter 14) (Fig.

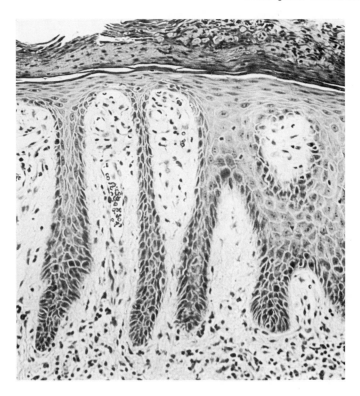

Fig. 4.4 Acanthosis in psoriasis. There is a marked elongation of the rete ridges associated with narrowing of the suprapapillary part of the epidermis. Note the parakeratosis and absent granular layer.

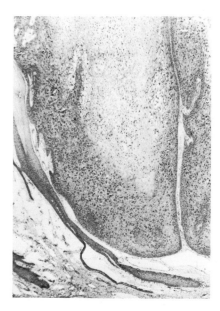

Fig. 4.5 Acanthosis in verruca vulgaris. The sharply demarcated thickening of the stratum spinosum is underlined in a claw-like fashion by a stretched rete ridge.

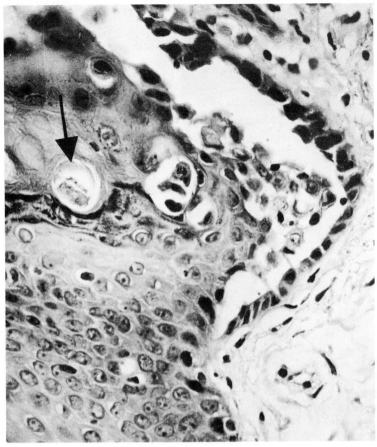

Fig. 4.7 Dyskeratosis (benign), in Darier's disease. A large, prematurely keratinised cell is indicated by the arrow.

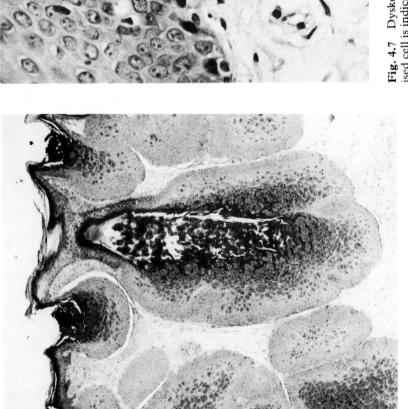

Fig. 4.6 Acanthosis in molluscum contagiosum showing tumour-like acanthosis, with the thickened bulbous rete ridges appearing to invade the epidermis.

4.9). In these conditions, in addition to the individual cell keratinisation, there are cytological features of malignancy such as nuclear pleomorphism and aberrant mitosis.

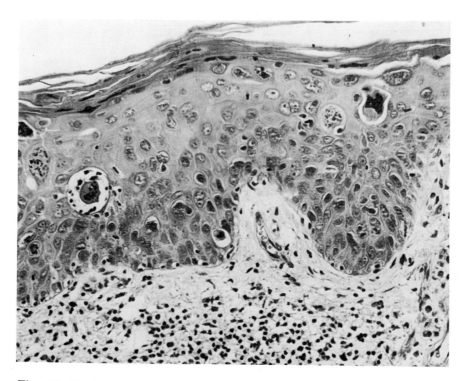

Fig. 4.8 Dyskeratosis (malignant) in Bowen's disease. Large prematurely keratinised cells with aberrant hyperchromatic nuclei are seen at different levels in the epidermis.

Dysplasia

Dysplasia literally means disordered growth. The term as generally used describes not only loss of the normal arrangement and maturation of the cells (i.e. loss of polarity) but also cellular atypia.

Cellular atypia includes the following features: pleomorphism of the cells and their nuclei which are irregular in size and shape; an increase in the nuclear/cytoplasmic ratio; and hyperchromatism (increase in staining) of the nuclei. There is often an increase in the number of mitotic figures and these may be seen above the basal layer.

Dysplastic changes may be seen as a result of chronic irritation (Fig. 4.10) but are also seen in premalignant conditions such as actinic keratosis (Fig. 4.11), and it is not always possible to differentiate between the two.

Hamartoma

'Hamartoma' is a term used to describe a group of tumour-like lesions which result from a localised disproportionate overgrowth of one or more of the elements of normal tissue. While

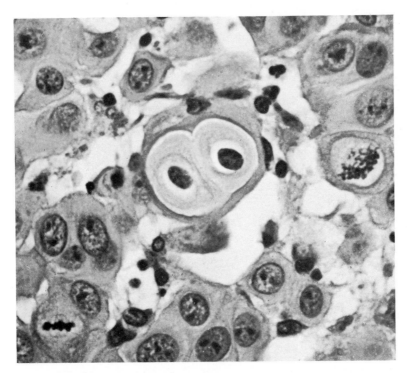

Fig. 4.9 Dyskeratosis (malignant) in poorly differentiated squamous carcinoma. Two large prematurely keratinised cells are seen in the centre.

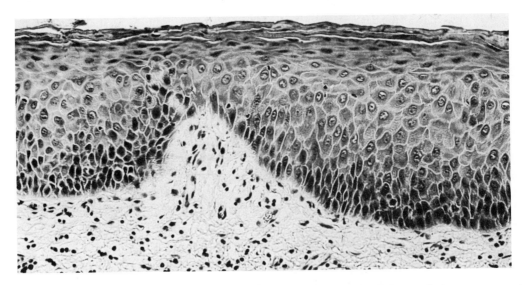

Fig. 4.10 Dysplasia in clinical leucoplakia. Note on the left the loss of the regular arrangement of cells along the basal layer, the loss of polarity of the lower layers of the epithelium, and the cellular atypia with nuclear hyperchromatism and increase in the nuclear/cytoplasmic ratio. While this degree of dysplasia could be premalignant, it is also seen in relation to chronic infection and irritation.

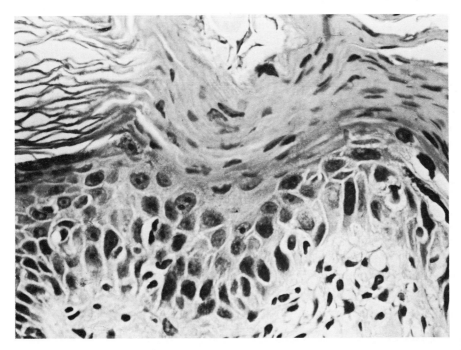

Fig. 4.11 Dysplasia in actinic keratosis. Note the more obvious disordered growth, cellular atypia and lack of maturation of the cells with replacement of the horny layer by nucleated keratin.

they enlarge with growth of the individual, they do not have the properties of unrestricted growth characteristic of neoplasia. They are frequently congenital.

Hyperkeratosis

This term is self-explanatory, and refers to an increase in thickness or density of the stratum corneum. Hyperkeratosis is usually associated with hypertrophy of the granular layer with the exception of autosomal dominant ichthyosis where the hyperkeratosis is associated with a diminished or absent granular layer. It should be recalled that the structure of the horny layer differs in different parts of the body. Over pressure areas such as the palms, soles and buttocks this cornified layer has a dense, laminated appearance, while over the flexible areas, such as the limbs and the trunk, it is looser and resembles a basket-weave in appearance. It should be emphasised that a laminated layer in the limbs or trunk indicates hyperkeratosis and is abnormal.

Hyperkeratosis is a feature of many chronic skin diseases, and may be associated with acanthosis in chronic dermatitis (see Fig. 4.3). It also occurs in relation to repeated trauma such as is seen in occupational callosities and those which occur with badly fitting or unsuitable footwear. Hyperkeratosis is a constant feature of lichen planus (Chapter 7), where it is associated with focal wedge-shaped areas of hypertrophy of the granular layer. In some disorders such as chronic discoid lupus erythematosus (Chapter 11) the hyperkeratosis may be predominantly follicular and associated with epidermal atrophy (Fig. 4.12). Epidermal

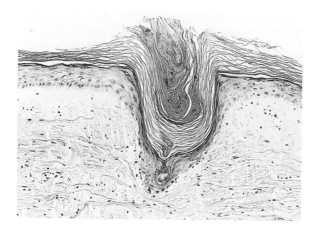

Fig. 4.12 Hyperkeratosis (follicular) in chronic discoid lupus erythematosus. A plug of laminated keratin is present in the dilated follicular opening.

atrophy associated with hyperkeratosis is also seen in chronic actinic skin damage and certain rare hyperkeratotic diseases of the lower limbs such as Kyrle's disease.

Individual cell necrosis

An appearance not unlike dyskeratosis is seen when epidermal cells have undergone necrosis. This is not unexpected since with cell death the intermediate filaments of the maturing keratinocyte condense in a fashion similar to that of keratinisation. This individual cell

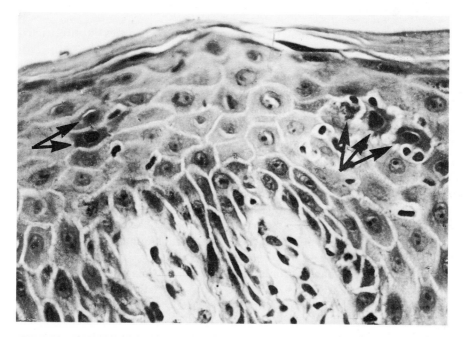

Fig. 4.13   Individual cell necrosis in a patient treated with cyclophosphamide. A number of keratinocytes undergoing premature cell death are indicated by the arrows. They have pyknotic nuclei and deeply staining eosinophilic cytoplasm.

necrosis is seen following sun-burning, radiation, treatment with cytotoxic drugs, in the graft versus host reaction, and in lichenoid reactions, particularly those related to drugs (Fig. 4.13).

Liquefaction degeneration

This change in the basal layer of the epidermis is characteristically seen in chronic discoid lupus erythematosus (Chapter 11). The cells of the basal layer become swollen and lose their staining affinities, becoming clear in appearance. Eventually there is disintegration of the cell walls and in advanced cases the basal cells may disappear (Fig. 4.14).

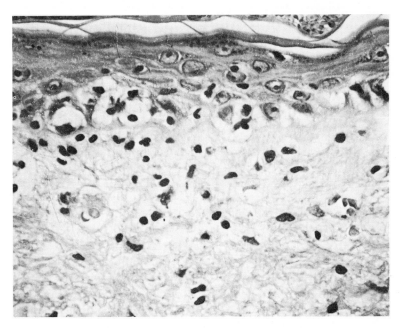

Fig. 4.14 Liquefaction degeneration in chronic discoid lupus erythematosus. The basal cells are swollen and contain shrunken, pyknotic nuclei. In a few areas the basal cells have disappeared.

Liquefaction degeneration of the basal layer is also seen in acute lupus erythematosus, in lichen planus (Chapter 7) in the poikiloderma associated with dermatomyositis (Chapter 11), and in some cases of mycosis fungoides (Chapter 13). In all of these conditions the dermo-epidermal junction is breached by either an inflammatory or a neoplastic cellular infiltrate and the basal lamina may be lost.

Parakeratosis

Parakeratosis is the name given to the formation of a keratin layer which retains its nuclei. It is seen in a number of inflammatory skin conditions. It is not diagnostic *per se* of any condition and merely indicates that the epidermis has recently been the seat of a pathological process which has upset the metabolism of the keratinocytes. Parakeratosis is recognised by the fact that the cells of the horny layer retain somewhat elongated, haematoxylinophilic

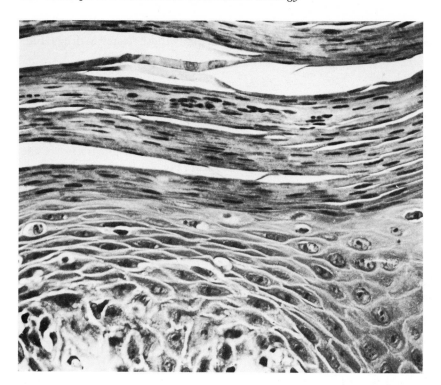

Fig. 4.15 Parakeratosis in psoriasis. The horny layer contains darkly staining elongated nuclei. The granular layer is absent. Note the separation of the layers of the abnormal stratum corneum.

nuclei (Fig. 4.15). Nucleated horny layer is less cohesive than the normal anucleated variety and therefore it tends to split, with the formation of air spaces. This splitting accounts for two well-known dermatological clinical signs: (1) the scaling which occurs in many chronic inflammatory skin diseases; and (2) the fact that such scales are often silvery in appearance. The silvery appearance of the scales is caused by the *in vivo* splitting of this parakeratotic keratin and air spaces forming between the layers.

Invariably associated with parakeratosis is the absence of the granular layer. In a healing lesion one may see a column or a layer of parakeratosis and underneath it normal anucleated keratin with a well-marked granular layer. Such a lesion is usually too old for diagnostic purposes (Fig. 4.16).

Chronic actinic damage of the epidermis is characterised by alternating columns of parakeratosis and hyperkeratosis. These features are so constant that they may be regarded as the hallmark of chronic actinic damage to the skin (Chapter 14). Even when such lesions undergo malignant change this hallmark remains on the surface of the skin and can enable one to recognise squamous carcinoma which has arisen on the basis of actinic skin damage.

In certain mucosal sites, such as the non-masticatory surfaces inside the mouth and the inner part of the labia minora, a nucleated superficial layer is normal and this physiological parakeratosis should not be misinterpreted as early malignancy.

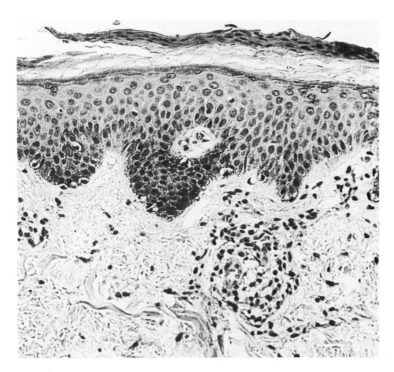

Fig. 4.16 Parakeratosis. Healing lesion of acute dermatitis. The superficial part of the stratum corneum is composed of a parakeratotic layer overlying a normal anucleated layer. This appearance is seen in a healing lesion and has no diagnostic significance.

Pseudoepitheliomatous hyperplasia

In the majority of skin disorders in which there is hyperplasia of the epidermis, the process occurs in a regular manner with a well-defined lower edge contained by a basement membrane. However, there is a group of diseases of widely varying aetiology in which the acanthotic epidermis has an irregular growth pattern and appears to invade the dermis, in the manner of a malignant tumour. It is usually associated with some features of dysplasia, loss of cell polarity and cellular atypia, and is referred to as pseudoepitheliomatous hyperplasia.

Disorders regularly associated with pseudoepitheliomatous hyperplasia include persistent insect bite (Chapter 6), granular cell myoblastoma (Chapter 17) and Spitz naevus (Chapter 16). It is common at the edge of long-standing ulcers (e.g. stasis ulcers and old sinus tracks), and may also at times be seen in association with certain fungal and viral infections, tuberculosis and syphilis (Chapter 9).

It may be extremely difficult to distinguish between pseudoepitheliomatous hyperplasia and invasive squamous carcinoma. In both, the dermis may seem to be invaded by strands or finger-like processes of epithelium. In pseudoepitheliomatous hyperplasia this 'invasion' tends to be restricted to the dermis above the level of the sweat glands. While some cellular atypia, and mitoses, may be seen, the cells composing the epithelial processes of pseudoepitheliomatous hyperplasia lack the pronounced hyperchromatism and loss of nuclear polarity seen in infiltrating squamous carcinoma. In pseudoepitheliomatous hyperplasia the epithelial strands are almost invariably infiltrated by inflammatory cells; this seldom happens in invasive squamous carcinoma unless there is superimposed acute pyogenic infection or the tumour is arising in a moist area, such as a mucous membrane.

While the recognition of one of the associated disorders such as granular cell myoblastoma or Spitz naevus may help to clarify the true nature of an epithelial hyperplasia, there are instances—in particular when it is associated with a chronic ulcer—when it is not possible on histological grounds to exclude squamous carcinoma with complete confidence. In this context it should be remembered that oblique sectioning can simulate dermal invasion, and thus great care should be taken to orientate biopsies taken from the edge of chronic ulcers or sinus tracks.

If an individual cell or a column of cells is seen breaking out from one of the cords or finger-like processes and invading between individual collagen bundles, the lesion is a squamous carcinoma and not pseudoepitheliomatous hyperplasia.

Reticular degeneration

This results in a peculiar type of intraepidermal blister which is characteristic of some viral infections of the skin (Chapter 8). The infected keratinocytes become grossly enlarged due to nuclear and cytoplasmic swelling (balloon degeneration) and eventually rupture. The cell walls, however, tend to remain intact and to adhere to each other so that the blister cavity is traversed by strands of cell walls, giving a multilocular blister (Fig. 4.17). It is to this appearance that the term 'reticular degeneration' is applied.

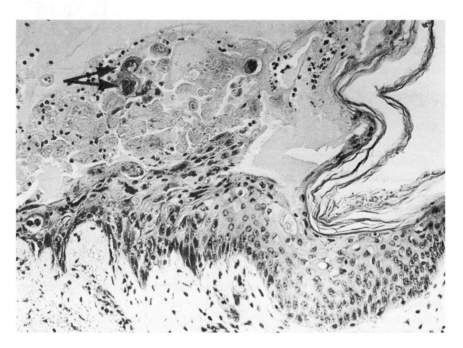

Fig. 4.17 Reticular degeneration in varicella. Strands of degenerate cell walls traverse the blister cavity causing it to be multilocular. Two keratinocytes showing balloon degeneration are indicated by the arrows.

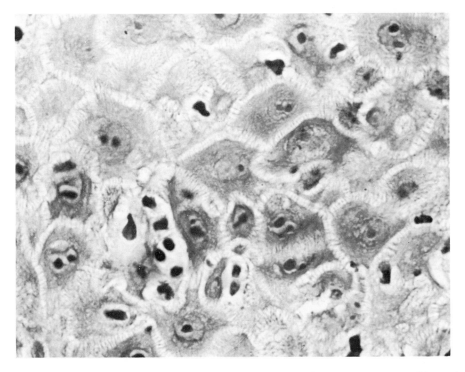

Fig. 4.18 Spongiosis in early acute dermatitis. The keratinocytes are separated by oedema fluid and their points of adhesion are stretched out. A few of the keratinocyte nuclei are pyknotic and lymphocytes may be seen in some of the widened intracellular spaces.

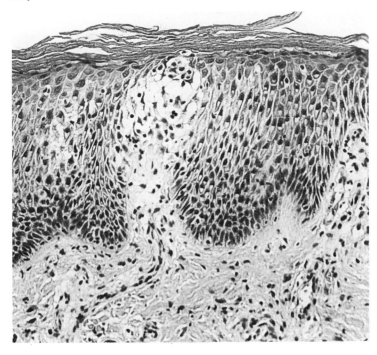

Fig. 4.19 Spongiotic vesicle in acute dermatitis. An early spongiotic vesicle is seen in the epidermis above the dermal papilla in the centre of the field.

Spongiosis

This term is used to describe intercellular oedema of the epidermis, which is most commonly seen in the dermatitis reaction (Chapter 6). In the early stages the individual keratinocytes are separated by oedema fluid and their points of contact become stretched out (Fig. 4.18). Eventually some of the cells separate completely and small vesicles (spongiotic vesicles) are formed (Fig. 4.19).

5
Congenital and Inherited Disease of the Skin

In considering this group under one heading it must be appreciated that the only logic in so doing is because they are present at birth, or tend to have a familial incidence or are considered to show a definite genetic inheritance pattern. The pathological processes involved vary from disturbances in keratinisation, blister formation, pigmentary disturbances, maldevelopment of elastic fibres and benign abnormal proliferation of mast cells to genetically determined invasive epithelial malignancy.

This is a vast subject and in the present account only those conditions which are relatively common or have distinctive diagnostic histopathology will be considered.

Ichthyosis[1]

A proper understanding of ichthyosis, or fish skin disease, has been hampered for many years by a proliferation of descriptive names, often coined to 'name' minor clinical variations of the same disorder. Recent work, however, has put the classification of ichthyosis on a firm genetic basis and has done much to bring order out of chaos.

Sex-linked ichthyosis—Recessive inheritance

This condition is confined to males and is characterised by the presence of large, dark, adherent scales which are shed infrequently. A recent exciting development is the identification of a steroid sulphatase deficiency in these patients.[2] Histological examination reveals a marked hyperkeratosis associated with hypertrophy of the stratum granulosum and acanthosis of the epidermis (Fig. 5.1). Sebaceous and sweat glands are present in normal numbers. In the dermis there are focal aggregations of lymphocytes and histiocytes grouped around the vessels of the upper dermis.

Autosomal dominant ichthyosis (ichthyosis vulgaris, ichthyosis simplex, xeroderma, hyperkeratosis congenita)

This is the type of ichthyosis most often encountered in practice. In contrast to the sex-linked variety, which is usually present at birth, this variety normally appears at about the age of 3 months. The type of scaling differs also, consisting of small scales, white in colour, which are shed continuously. Histological examination reveals a mild hyperkeratosis of laminated type associated with absence or diminution of the stratum granulosum (Fig. 5.2). The epidermis itself is otherwise normal. Sebaceous glands and, to a lesser extent, sweat

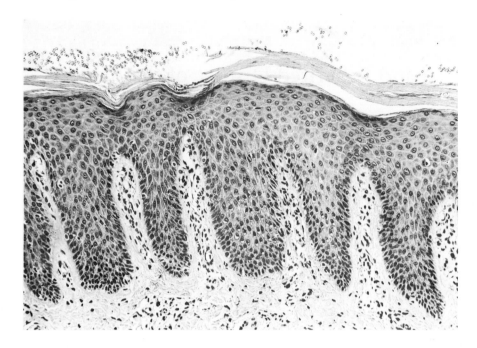

Fig. 5.1 Ichthyosis (sex-linked), showing the marked hyperkeratosis associated with hypertrophy of the stratum granulosum and acanthosis of the epidermis. There is a mild perivascular lymphocytic histiocytic infiltrate in the upper dermis.

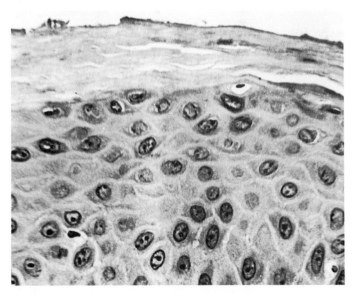

Fig. 5.2 Ichthyosis (autosomal dominant). There is a mild hyperkeratosis of the dense, laminated type associated with an absence of the stratum granulosum.

glands are diminished in numbers. Dermal inflammatory infiltrate is minimal. Some 45 per cent of individuals with autosomal dominant ichthyosis exhibit also one or more features of the atopic state. The histological features described above thus may be complicated by various stages of a superimposed dermatitis reaction (see Chapter 6).

Epidermolytic hyperkeratosis (Bullous congenital ichthyosiform erythroderma)

This condition is inherited by autosomal dominant transmission and presents at or shortly after birth with large yellow or brown scales and in some cases bullae. The striking histological feature is the presence within the mid portion of the epidermis of gross intracellular oedema leading to balloon degeneration, predominantly of the cells of the mid portion of the stratum spinosum but at times extending further towards the surface (Fig. 5.3). The swollen cells rupture, giving rise to microvesicles. These microvesicles may coalesce, forming a multilocular bulla in the mid portion of the epidermis. This oedema may involve the stratum granulosum, which is thickened, but more often the granular cells are swollen and show a well-marked perinuclear halo. There is an associated hyperkeratosis and when the cells of the stratum granulosum are disrupted, parakeratosis. The dermis shows a varying amount of perivascular lymphocytic and histiocytic infiltrate. In sections taken from non-bullous areas the changes are often non-specific and consist of acanthosis, hypertrophy or absence of the stratum granulosum, hyperkeratosis and patchy parakeratosis. Careful search through

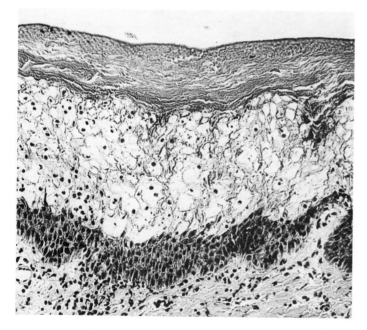

Fig. 5.3 Epidermolytic hyperkeratosis. This section shows the gross intracellular oedema of the keratinocytes in the mid and upper portions of the stratum spinosum. In some areas the cell walls have ruptured, to give rise to microvesicles. Hyperkeratosis is marked. (Section by courtesy of Dr J.M. Beare, Belfast.)

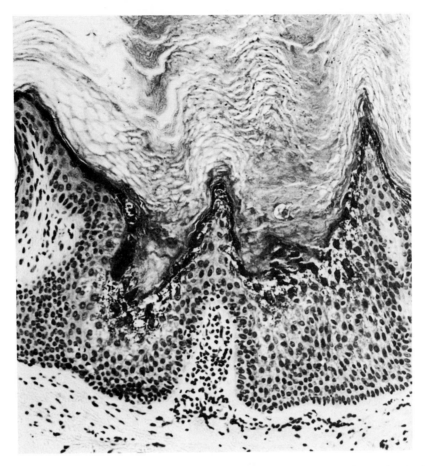

Fig. 5.4   Epidermolytic hyperkeratosis. There is a gross degree of hyperkeratosis and parakeratosis. The epidermis is acanthotic. In the region of the stratum granulosum the cells are swollen and show the characteristic perinuclear pallor. (Section by courtesy of Dr J. Rogers, Dundee.)

the material, however, may reveal small areas of intracellular oedema with microvesicle formation or the swollen granular cells with the characteristic perinuclear halo (Fig. 5.4).

Lamellar ichthyosis (Non-bullous congenital ichthyosiform erythroderma)

This condition is inherited by autosomal recessive transmission. In very severe cases the child is encased in armour-plate-like scales (harlequin fetus) and is usually still-born or dies shortly after birth. In milder cases a congenital erythroderma persists throughout life or gradually clears. The pathological findings are non-specific with laminated hyperkeratosis, a thickened granular layer, acanthosis, and a mild chronic dermal infiltrate.

Darier's disease (keratosis follicularis)

This familial disorder, of dominant inheritance, consists of warty, somewhat greasy papules which affect the skin to a greater or lesser degree, and is in some instances associated with similar lesions in the buccal and genital mucosa.[3] Its histological features are sufficiently characteristic that taken together with the clinical history they will allow a firm diagnosis to be made.

In the early stages the striking feature is the presence of suprabasilar clefts in the epidermis. These are caused by acantholysis. Overlying these clefts there is a thick layer of abnormally keratinised cells. Closer examination will reveal a number of other features. Within the epidermis above the cleft are seen small, shrunken-looking keratinocytes, some of which show premature keratinisation (benign dyskeratosis—see Chapter 4). High in the epidermis,

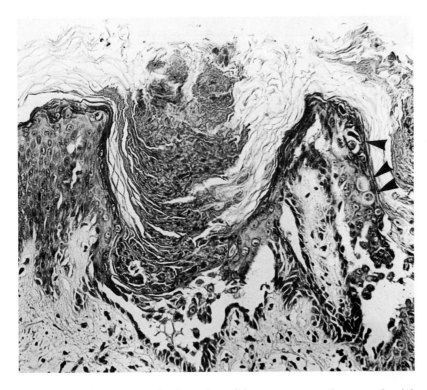

Fig. 5.5 Darier's disease. In the region of the stratum granulosum to the right of the picture are the enlarged keratinocytes which have undergone premature keratinisation (arrowed). These are the corps ronds of Darier.

often within the stratum granulosum, can be seen large cells of varying number. These are two to three times the size of normal keratinocytes with eosinophilic hyalinised keratinised cytoplasm and large, circular, deeply basophilic nuclei (Fig. 5.5). The cell wall is sharply delineated so that these cells stand out from the surrounding cells. These are the corps ronds of Darier. In the hyperkeratotic centre of the lesion are areas of a peculiar type of parakeratosis. This is characterised by the stratum corneum cells retaining small, often pointed, darkly staining nuclei, more prominent than the usual parakeratotic nuclei. These peculiar parakeratotic cells are known as grains (Fig. 5.6), because they resemble grains of rice. In more florid lesions, in addition to the features described above there would seem to be an increase in the number of dermal papillae. The dermal papillae are lengthened. The apparent increase in their number is an artefact due to oblique sections of the convoluted epidermis.

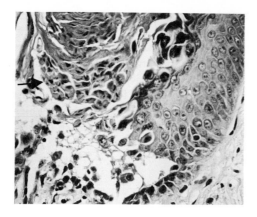

Fig. 5.6 Darier's disease. This picture from the centre of a lesion shows the characteristic grain-like parakeratosis (arrowed) of the stratum corneum. These constitute the grains of Darier. In addition, the suprabasilar clefting, the rounded-off acantholytic cells and the corps ronds can be seen clearly.

The pathological changes which occur in the epidermis in Darier's disease are not confined solely to the follicular epidermis, hence the synonym 'keratosis follicularis' is not really appropriate. If an area of skin is involved by very numerous small lesions a number of these will involve the skin of the pilosebaceous follicles or sweat duct openings by chance. Some of the clinical dermatologists' follicular eruptions are explainable on this basis. Occasionally, biopsy of such a 'follicular eruption' will reveal very small, isolated foci of Darier's disease (Fig. 5.7) scattered throughout the epidermis. Inflammatory infiltrate in the dermis is so

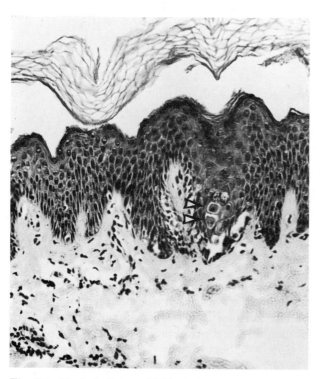

Fig. 5.7 Darier's disease. 'Follicular' type. There is a small suprabasal acantholytic cleft at the tip of one rete ridge. Just above this are the enlarged prematurely keratinised corps ronds (arrowed).

variable as to have no diagnostic significance. Large solitary lesions of Darier's disease are encountered occasionally. These lesions have the same histological features as the more common type. The term 'warty dyskeratoma' is sometimes used to describe these lesions.

In the differential histological diagnosis of Darier's disease conditions such as benign familial pemphigus (see below) and the pemphigus group of disorders (Chapter 12) must be considered. The superficial hidradenoma, naevus syringocystadenomatosus papilliferus (Chapter 14), may sometimes cause confusion with solitary lesions of Darier's disease. However, examination of the villous projections seen in the former condition shows them to be lined by a double layer of epithelium, the more superficial one being tall columnar in type. Plasma cell infiltration of the stroma is a constant feature and dyskeratosis is not seen.

Benign familial chronic pemphigus (Hailey-Hailey disease)[4]

This rare, autosomal dominantly inherited disorder is characterised by an eruption of vesicles and bullae which by peripheral extension and central healing produce circinate

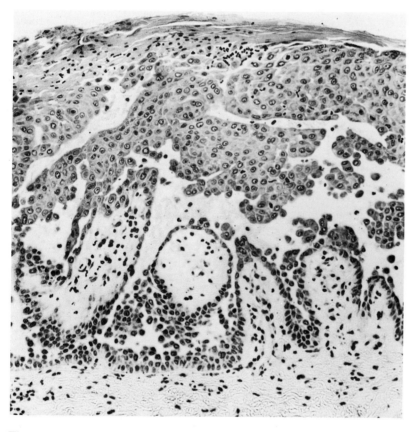

Fig. 5.8 Benign familial chronic pemphigus. There is extensive acantholysis with suprabasilar cleft formation and a bulla containing numerous well-stained, 'rounded-off', acantholytic cells. No dyskeratotic cells comparable to corps ronds are seen, but on the surface there is a grain-like area of parakeratosis. The dermal papillae are prominent and appear increased in number.

lesions. The sites most commonly affected are the sides of the neck, the axillae, groins and natal cleft.

Histologically the features are in many ways similar to those of Darier's disease. There are extensive suprabasal clefts due to acantholysis but there is also extension upwards of this process into the overlying epidermis, giving much more widespread acantholysis than is usually seen in Darier's disease. The acantholytic cells are plumper, more rounded in appearance and contain well-stained nuclei (Fig. 5.8), and they lack the shrunken appearance with nuclear pyknosis of the acantholytic cells of Darier's disease. Dyskeratosis with corps ronds and grain formation may occur, but is much less prominent than in Darier's disease. These differences, however, lessen as the lesions age, until it may be impossible on histological grounds to differentiate between benign familial chronic pemphigus and Darier's disease or even pemphigus vulgaris. Indeed, to confirm or exclude the latter it may be necessary to use immunological techniques (Chapter 12).

Porokeratosis

Two well-recognised clinical presentations of porokeratosis have identical pathological features, and separation of the two varieties must therefore depend on clinical features. *Porokeratosis of Mibelli*[5] is usually inherited by autosomal dominant transmission and lesions tend to develop in childhood, predominantly on the limbs. The lesions may be single or multiple and begin as a papule which extends slowly to form a plaque with a raised palpable edge and an atrophic centre. The second variety, *disseminated superficial actinic porokeratosis*,[6] also appears to be inherited by autosomal dominant transmission. Lesions develop later in life than in the Mibelli variety and are found on sun-exposed sites of white-skinned individuals. It is postulated that the underlying mechanism in both varieties is a localised clone of abnormal epidermal cells.

The histological changes are diagnostic. Sections through the advancing edge of a lesion show that the hyperkeratotic ring consists of a feather-like plug of parakeratotic keratin (the cornoid lamella) (Fig. 5.9). Under the lamella the stratum granulosum is absent and the epidermal cells are vacuolated (Fig. 5.10). They may contain irregular basophilic granules. The epidermis in the centre of the lesion is atrophic and usually hyperkeratotic. A moderate chronic inflammatory infiltrate of lymphocytes and histiocytes is seen in the upper dermis,

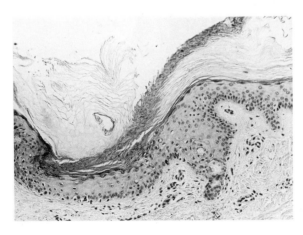

Fig. 5.9 Porokeratosis of Mibelli. This section through the hyperkeratotic margin of a lesion shows the feather-like plug of parakeratosis (cornoid lamella). (Section by courtesy of Dr A. Tay, Epsom.)

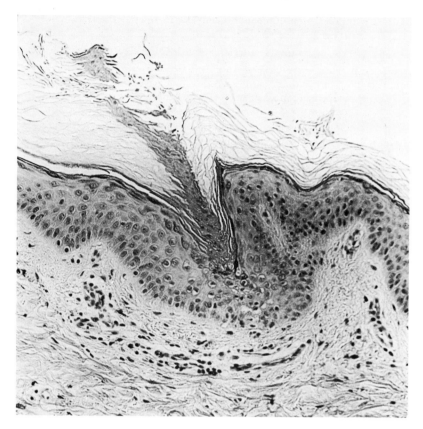

Fig. 5.10 Porokeratosis of Mibelli. This is another section from the lesion illustrated in Fig. 5.9. Note the absence of the stratum granulosum and vacuolation of the keratinocytes under the cornoid lamella. (Section by courtesy of Dr A. Tay, Epsom.)

mainly underneath the cornoid lamella but extending inwards under the atrophic epithelium. This may be followed by dermal atrophy with loss of dermal appendages.

Epidermolysis bullosa

This group of genetically determined blistering disorders presents as a number of variants with differing clinical features, prognosis and mode of inheritance. Sixteen different clinical entities, many of extreme rarity, have been described.[7] For the purposes of genetic counselling, electron microscopy is used to classify epidermolysis bullosa into four main groups, according to the site of onset of the split (Table 5.1, Fig. 5.11).

In *epidermolysis bullosa simplex*, a remarkably localized split appears, following rarefaction in the subnuclear cytoplasm of the basal cell, leaving the basal cell membrane and fragments of cytoplasm still attached by hemidesmosomes to the blister floor. Initially, the split in *junctional epidermolysis bullosa* clearly separates epidermis from dermis through the lamina lucida. Hemidesmosome hypoplasia is observed both in the lesion and in adjacent areas. In older lesions, the loss of basal cell material attached to the blister floor in epidermolysis bullosa simplex and the gradual lysis of the blister roof in junctional epidermolysis bullosa

Table 5.1 Clinical and ultrastructural features of the four main varieties of epidermolysis bullosa

Name	Ultrastructural features	Clinical features
Epidermolysis bullosa simplex (autosomal dominant)	Split in subnuclear basal cell cytoplasm: mechanism unknown	Onset at 1–2 years. Tense blisters on hands and feet. Pigmentation but no scarring
Junctional epidermolysis bullosa (autosomal recessive)	Split between basal cell and basal lamina: hemidesmosome hypoplasia	Onset early infancy. Severe extensive blister formation. Shedding of nails. Webbing between fingers
Dystrophic epidermolysis bullosa (autosomal dominant)	Split between basal lamina and dermis: anchoring fibril defect with abnormal glycosaminoglycan production	Onset early infancy. Blisters on limbs. Heal with atrophic scars and milia
Dystrophic epidermolysis bullosa (autosomal recessive)	Split in upper dermis with dissolution of anchoring fibrils and collagen: possibly due to increased amounts of an abnormal collagenase	Onset early infancy. Large haemorrhagic bullae, mucosal involvement. Hair, teeth and nails also defective

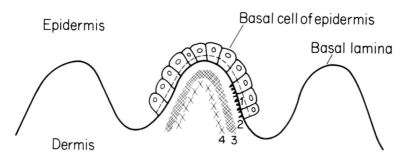

Fig. 5.11 Diagrammatic representation of the sites of split in the major subdivisions of epidermolysis bullosa (EB). (1) Site of split in EB simplex is through the cytoplasm of the epidermal basal cells. (2) Site of split in junctional EB is between basal cells and the basal lamina, within the lamina lucida. Hemidesmosome hypoplasia is thought to be the cause of the pathological lesion. (3) Site of split in autosomal dominant variety of dystrophic EB is between the basal lamina and the dermis. It is thought to be due to an anchoring fibril defect. (4) Site of split in autosomal recessive variety of dystrophic EB. The ultrastructure is similar to autosomal dominant dystrophic EB but in addition degenerate collagen is seen in the upper dermis. Biochemical assays have demonstrated a net increase in abnormal collagenase activity.

can lead to confusion between these types. Similar problems are encountered in distinguishing between the *dominant* and *recessive forms of dystrophic epidermolysis bullosa.* In the dominant form anchoring fibril formation is defective, giving a split immediately below the basal lamina. In the recessive form, the defect is more pronounced, with additional dermolytic changes in the uppermost collagen fibrils. The distinction between these forms thus depends on a quantitative assessment of defects in anchoring and collagen fibrils, which can be obscured as the lesion ages. These points emphasize the absolute requirement for a biopsy consisting of a fresh lesion and perilesional skin, and for adequate sampling of the specimen, if ultrastructural diagnosis is to be accurate.

Incontinentia pigmenti (Bloch–Sulzberger disease)

This condition is found very much more frequently in female than in male infants, giving rise to the suggestion that the condition is transmitted either by autosomal dominant inheritance and is lethal in the male, or is via a sex-linked gene on the X chromosome.[8] Affected infants present at or shortly after birth with multiple blisters, often in a linear arrangement arising on inflamed skin. These lesions may be widespread. As the blisters heal, a gross and striking verrucous hyperkeratosis develops on the sites of previous blister formation. In time this is succeeded by macular hyperpigmentation in a whorling or frond-like pattern. These changes generally occur within the first few months of life so that after

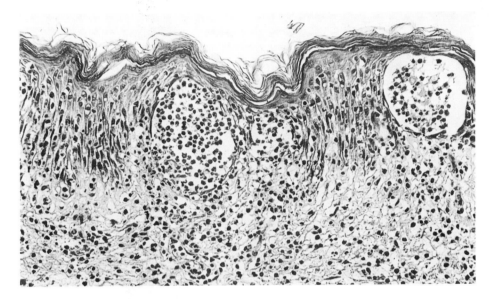

Fig. 5.12 Incontinentia pigmenti (vesicular phase). A number of spongiotic vesicles can be seen in the epidermis. These contain numerous eosinophil leucocytes. The papillary dermis is oedematous and heavily infiltrated with eosinophil leucocytes.

the age of 1 year only minor macular pigmentary abnormalities of the epidermis persist. Other organs are, however, frequently involved.

From the clinical evaluation of the lesions it will be seen that the histological picture will depend on the timing of the biopsy. In the early vesicular phase the epidermis is the seat of an acute dermatitis reaction with the formation of vesicles (Chapter 6), which in this condition are packed with eosinophil leucocytes (Fig. 5.12). There is vascular engorgement and oedema of the dermis with an extensive inflammatory infiltrate in which eosinophils predominate. Taken in conjunction with the clinical history and age of the child this lesion is diagnostic. Once the vesicular phase is past and the hyperkeratosis supervenes the histological picture is no longer pathognomic. There is now a varying amount of acanthosis and hyperkeratosis of the epidermis (Fig. 5.13). A constant feature is the presence of melanin-containing histiocytes in the papillary dermis, and there may be an associated patchy chronic inflammatory cell infiltrate. In some cases, but not all, the basal cells are vacuolated and depleted of melanin (hence the term 'incontinentia').

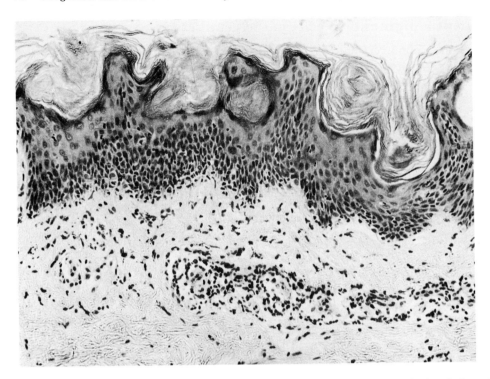

Fig. 5.13 Incontinentia pigmenti (late stage). There is a moderate acanthosis of the epidermis associated with hyperkeratosis. Many of the cells of the stratum basale are vacuolated. In the papillary dermis there are a number of melanin-containing histiocytes. There is also a patchy perivascular lymphocytic histiocytic infiltrate.

Pseudoxanthoma elasticum

The skin changes which occur in this inherited generalised disturbance of connective tissue are patchy in distribution and vary considerably in extent. The common sites of cutaneous involvement are the sides of the neck, the axillae and the groins.[9] The skin lesions may be overshadowed by progressive visual disturbance (angioid streaks on the retina), subarachnoid haemorrhage from involvement of meningeal vessels, or haematemesis or melaena from involvement of the vessels of the gut. Sections from an involved area of skin stained with haematoxylin and eosin reveal a zone of swollen basophilic 'collagen' fibres in the mid zone of the dermis (Fig. 5.14). Elastic tissue stains show the elastic fibres in the papillary dermis to be relatively normal whereas those in the adjacent zone of the reticular dermis are broken up, thickened and often curled up into skein-like clumps (Fig. 5.15). These fibres have an increased calcium content, as can be demonstrated by the von Kossa stain. Irregular areas of calcification surrounded by foreign body granulomata may subsequently develop. The vascular accidents in the other bodily systems are caused by similar changes in the elastica of their vessels.

The changes in pseudoxanthoma elasticum are easily differentiated from the juvenile elastoma, which shows a marked increase in morphologically normal elastic fibres in the dermis, and from the generalised cutis laxa, in which all the elastic fibres in the dermis (papillary and reticular) are fragmented.

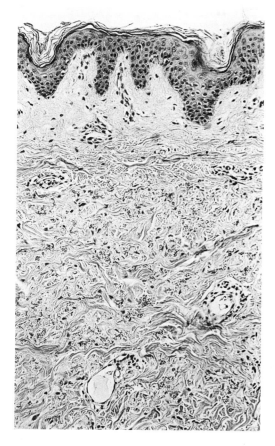

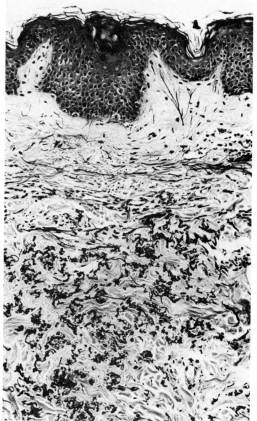

Fig. 5.14 Pseudoxanthoma elasticum. The collagen fibres in the mid dermis are swollen, and have a somewhat refractile appearance. They are also more basophilic than normal. (Section by courtesy of Dr C.E. Stuart, Wakefield.)

Fig. 5.15 Pseudoxanthoma elasticum. In this further section from the case illustrated in Fig. 5.14 the elastic tissue pattern in the papillary dermis is normal, but in the mid dermis the elastic fibres are broken up, thickened and curled up into skein-like clumps. Orcein–methylene blue. (Section by courtesy of Dr C.E. Stuart, Wakefield.)

Ehlers–Danlos syndrome

A condition which is associated in about 50 per cent of cases with pseudoxanthoma elasticum is the Ehlers–Danlos syndrome (cutis hyperelastica). At least eight different genetic varieties have been recognised, and the condition clinically presents as loose areas of hyperextensile skin which scars easily and forms ugly pseudotumours over sites of friction such as the Achilles tendon area. Other organs are also involved.

The histological features of the cutaneous lesions are not specific although there is an impression of fragmentation of collagen bundles and increased numbers of blood vessels[10] (Fig. 5.16). The condition is best diagnosed by fibroblast culture and biochemical identification of the enzyme defect. This is worthwhile as the biochemical variants have very different prognoses.

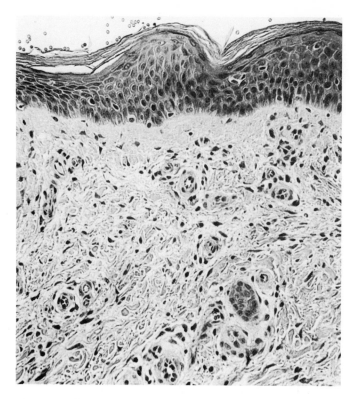

Fig. 5.16 Ehlers–Danlos syndrome. This biopsy from the forearm shows fragmentation of the collagen bundles of the reticular dermis. The dermis is more vascular than normal, containing many bundles of thick-walled capillary vessels.

Tuberous sclerosis (adenoma sebaceum, Bourneville's disease, Pringle's disease, epiloia)

This condition is inherited by autosomal dominant transmission. The skin manifestations consist of yellowish, soft tumours on the malar regions and nasolabial folds, shagreen-like patches of skin (usually in the lumbar region), and periungual fibromata. Despite the name 'adenoma sebaceum' the facial lesions have nothing whatsoever to do with sebaceous glands. They are in fact angiofibromata for the most part derived from the adventitiae of dermal vessels (Fig. 5.17 opposite) or from the fibrous sheath of hair follicles. The shagreen patches, despite their striking clinical appearances, fail to show any recognisable histological abnormality, while the periungual fibromata have the features of a benign fibroma of varying degrees of cellularity.

Xeroderma pigmentosum

This condition is inherited by autosomal recessive transmission. The underlying aetiology appears to be related to defective or absent mechanisms for repairing damage to DNA induced by exposure to sunlight.[11] The defect is specific and DNA repair after ionising radiation proceeds normally. At present at least eight different complementation groups are

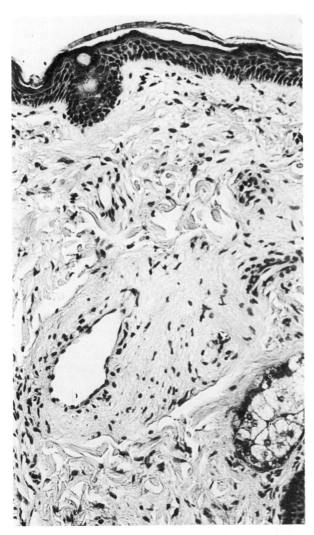

Fig. 5.17 Tuberous sclerosis. This section shows a small angiofibroma arising from the adventitia of a small facial venule. Masson's trichrome.

recognised associated with varying degrees of severity of epidermal damage and in some cases with associated central nervous system defects—the de Sanctis-Cacchione syndrome.

Affected children present at the age of 2-5 years with freckling, poikiloderma and atrophy of light-exposed shin which has the aged appearance of a normal individual in the sixth or seventh decade of life. If effective sun-screening is not introduced they proceed to development of actinic keratoses, basal cell carcinoma, squamous carcinoma and malignant melanoma. Prior to the introduction of stringent sun avoidance, death from cutaneous malignancy before the third decade was a common occurrence.

If a biopsy is taken in the atrophic stage, most of the changes of actinic or solar keratosis (Chapter 14) may be seen, including cellular atypia in the epidermis. At a later stage there is some thickening of the epidermis with hyperkeratosis. The basal layer loses its regular outlines, the cells become irregular with loss of nuclear polarity and the individual basal cell nuclei show hyperchromasia of varying degree (Fig. 5.18). There may be focal areas where basal melanocytes are hyperplastic and individual melanocytes are often aberrant (Fig. 5.19).

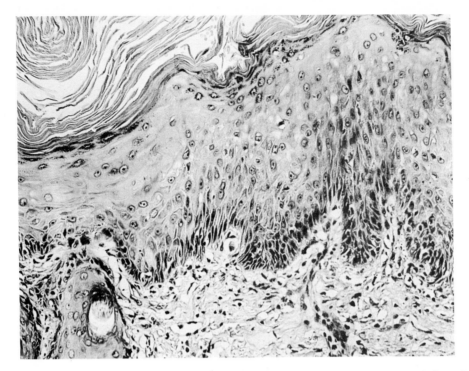

Fig. 5.18 Xeroderma pigmentosum. This biopsy from the face of a child 7 years of age shows marked acanthosis of the epidermis associated with hyperkeratosis and some parakeratosis. The cells of the stratum basale show loss of polarity and varying degrees of nuclear hyperchromatism. The child eventually developed an infiltrating squamous carcinoma.

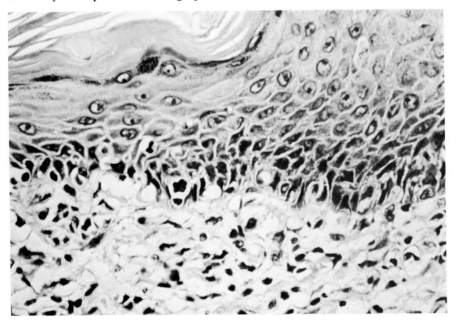

Fig. 5.19 Xeroderma pigmentosum. This is another area of the specimen illustrated in Fig. 5.18. The basal melanocytes are increased in size and number. Some show aberrant hyperchromatic nuclei.

While none of these changes is specific they should be interpreted in conjunction with the clinical history and age of the patient. Fibroblast culture for DNA repair studies will confirm the diagnosis.

Urticaria pigmentosa (mastocytosis)

Urticaria pigmentosa is relatively rare but is the commonest of the disorders which result from mast cell proliferation. The only justification for including it in this chapter is the fact that a small number of cases have been recorded in cousins, a fact which can be taken as presumptive evidence of a genetic factor. In the majority of cases and in the other manifestations of mast cell proliferation no genetic factors are evident.

Most cases of urticaria pigmentosa begin in early infancy, although the disease may not appear till adult life. In infancy histological examination reveals the upper dermis to be packed with round or oval-shaped cells with rather pale vesicular nuclei (Fig. 5.20). In haematoxylin and eosin stained preparations the cytoplasm appears agranular and faintly eosinophilic. A polychromatic stain such as polychrome methylene blue or toluidine blue, however, will reveal that the cytoplasm is packed with reddish-blue granules (Fig. 5.21), characteristic of mast cells. If a lesion from a child is biopsied in the urticated phase there may be a separation by oedema fluid at the dermo-epidermal junction. A grosser subepidermal bulla may be seen in the rare instances where the disease presents as blisters.

In the type of urticaria pigmentosa which begins in adult life, mast cells are much less numerous and tend to be located just around the dermal vessels (Fig. 5.22). In childhood

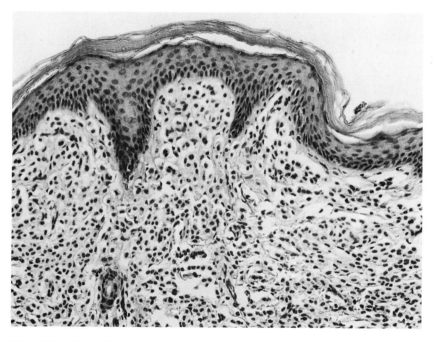

Fig. 5.20 Urticaria pigmentosa (mastocytosis). In this section from the infantile type the upper dermis is packed with rounded or oval-shaped cells with pale eosinophilic cytoplasm (mast cells).

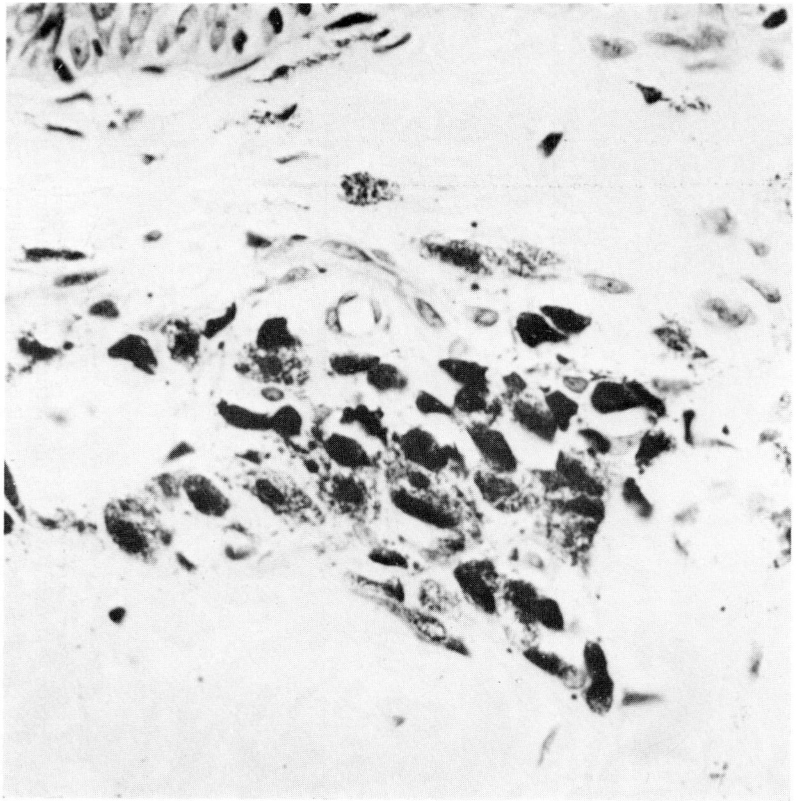

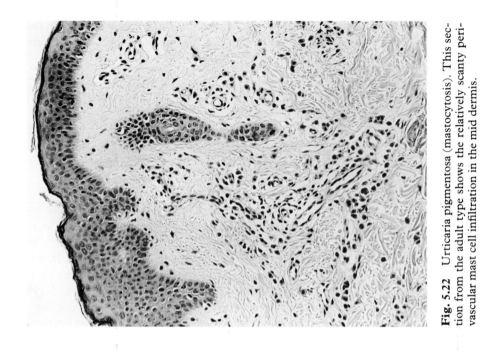

Fig. 5.22 Urticaria pigmentosa (mastocytosis). This section from the adult type shows the relatively scanty perivascular mast cell infiltration in the mid dermis.

Fig. 5.21 Urticaria pigmentosa (mastocytosis). This field from the edge of the lesion illustrated in Fig. 5.20 shows the characteristic granules of the mast cells revealed by staining with a polychromatic dye. Polychrome methylene blue.

and adult cases the brown colour of the macular lesions is due to an increased melanin pigmentation of the basal cells of the epidermis. Care must be taken to avoid undue trauma in performing the biopsy in cases of suspected urticaria pigmentosa as this may cause discharge of the mast cell granules. This particularly important in the adult variety, where mast cells may be scanty. In the childhood type of urticaria pigmentosa there is extensive infiltration by mast cells of the sinusoids of superficial lymph nodes as well as the portal tracts of the liver and splenic sinusoids. Despite these extensive deposits of mast cells, systemic effects are rarely encountered.

Solitary benign mast cell tumours (mast cell naevi) have been described in both children and adults. Histologically these lesions are indistinguishable from the childhood type of urticaria pigmentosa. A diffuse erythroderma due to mast cell infiltration, associated with flushing, palpitations and transient hypertension has been recorded in the adult.

The histological features of urticaria pigmentosa in children may easily be mistaken for Letterer–Siwe disease. Use of a polychromatic stain, and the fact that in urticaria pigmentosa there is no invasion of the epidermis by the dermal infiltrate, should allow easy separation.

Focal dermal hypoplasia (Goltz syndrome)

This genodermatosis is inherited by autosomal dominant transmission, and to date the vast majority of reported cases have been female.[12] Affected infants present at birth with areas of

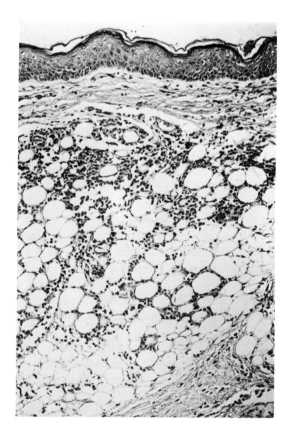

Fig. 5.23 Biopsy from an infant with focal dermal hypoplasia taken at 72 hours after birth. Note the relatively normal epidermis, the absence of any significant area of dermis and fat cells with an infiltrate in the dermal space. A high proportion of cells in this infiltrate are eosinophils.

raw denuded skin and areas with a very thin membranous epidermis overlying areas of subcutaneous fat. Fat herniation may occur, giving a striking picture. Other associated abnormalities may include retinal colobomata, skeletal defects, cobblestone papules on the oral mucosa and mental retardation.

The histological picture is diagnostic (Fig. 5.23). Under a relatively normal epidermis there is little or no dermis and a striking picture of fat cells abutting on the basal layer. In one reported case a dense eosinophilic infiltrate has been observed in this inappropriately situated fat pad.

Basal cell naevus syndrome (Gorlin's syndrome)

This condition is inherited by autosomal dominant gene transmission and has multiple and variable forms of expression.[13] The commonest presentation to the dermatologist is of multiple basal cell carcinomata presenting in the second decade in the absence of other cutaneous malignancies. Skeletal malformations are extremely common and include bifid ribs and odontogenic or keratinous cysts of the maxilla and mandible.[14]

The histology of the basal cell carcinomata is similar to that seen in the classic, non-genetically determined lesions but a high proportion of the lesions are of the morphoeic type and show a very striking pattern of small whorls of dark basiloid cells embedded in a very abundant stroma. This picture may also resemble a desmoplastic trichoepithelioma (p. 273).

Multiple self-healing epithelioma (Ferguson-Smith disease)[15]

Although this condition is in some texts confused with multiple keratoacanthoma, it is a distinct clinical and pathological entity inherited by autosomal dominant transmission. Two large pedigrees are traced in the West of Scotland[16] and it is clearly possible that new mutations may arise.

Patients usually present in early adult life with a lesion or lesions, commonly on the face, which has grown rapidly into a large hyperkeratotic mass. Untreated, the natural course of these lesions is slow regression over a period of months to leave a scar with a striking and extremely characteristic crenellated edge. Local excision or shaving of the lesion will give a better cosmetic result. Lesions tend to recur in crops.

Histological examination of these lesions shows a clearly demarcated lesion with features very similar to those of an invasive squamous carcinoma. There is epidermal hyperplasia and isolated islands of epithelial cells are seen invading the dermis. An inflammatory infiltrate is frequently seen around these areas, and on occasion apparent perineural invasion may be present (Figs. 5.24 and 5.25).

In contrast to a classic keratoacanthoma, the well-defined edge or 'shoulder' is not usually present and the lesion may appear to be invasive at several points along the epidermis (Figs. 5.26 and 5.27).

It can be seen from the above that diagnosis of this extremely rare condition will depend on a history of multiple lesions and a positive family history rather than on specific histological features. Recognition of a new mutant would obviously require perspicacity and an awareness of the condition.

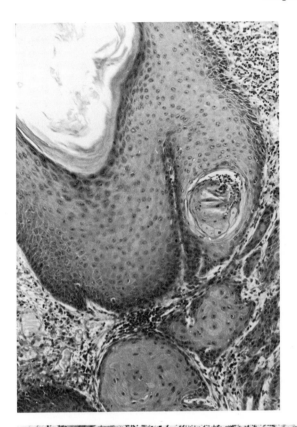

Fig. 5.24 Familial self-healing epithelioma (early lesion). This biopsy from the margin of a recent lesion, shows the infiltration of the dermis by strands of keratinocytes, some of which are forming 'epithelial pearls'. Note the absence of any shoulder to the lesion (cf. keratoacanthoma, Fig. 14.8).

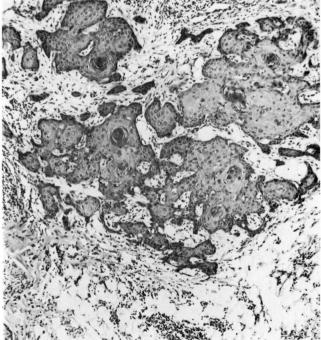

Fig. 5.25 Familial self-healing epithelioma (fully formed lesion). Strands of atypical keratinocytes, some of which contain 'epithelial pearls', are beginning to infiltrate the subcutaneous fat. This is much deeper than is seen in keratoacanthoma.

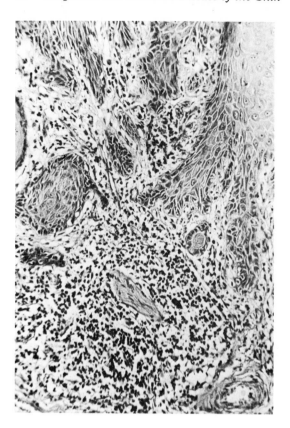

Fig. 5.26 Familial self-healing epithelioma. Biopsy specimen taken 8 weeks after the start of the lesion. Note the presence of isolated strands of keratinocytes within the dermis and the presence of a lymphocytic infiltrate around these strands.

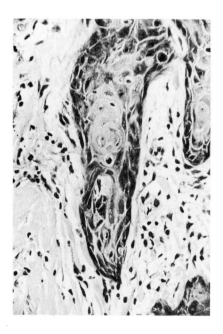

Fig. 5.27 Familial self-healing epithelioma (late lesion). This finger-like process composed of aberrant keratinocytes (including an abnormal mitosis) is in the reticular dermis. Note that in contrast to keratoacanthoma there is no invasion of the epithelium by inflammatory cells.

References

1. Marks R, Dykes PJ, eds. *The Ichthyoses*. Lancaster: MTP Press, 1978.
2. Shapiro LJ, Weiss R, Buxman MM, Vidgoff J, Dimond RL. Enzymatic basis of typical X-linked ichthyosis. *Lancet* 1978; **2:** 756-7.
3. Gottlieb SK, Lutzner MA. Darier's disease. *Arch Dermatol* 1973; **107:** 225-30.
4. Lever WF. *Pemphigus and Pemphigoid*. Springfield, Illinois: Charles C Thomas, 1964; p. 127.
5. Reed RJ, Leone P. Porokeratosis—a mutant clonal keratosis of the epidermis. *Arch Dermatol* 1970; **101:** 340-7.
6. Chernosky ME, Freeman RG. Disseminated superficial actinic porokeratosis. *Arch Dermatol* 1961; **96:** 611-24.
7. Gedde-Dahl T. Sixteen types of epidermolysis bullosa. *Acta Derm Venereol (Stockh)* 1981; Suppl. **95:** 74-87.
8. Carney RG. Incontinentia pigmenti. A world statistical analysis. *Arch Dermatol* 1976; **112:** 535-42.
9. Pope FM. A study of pseudoxanthoma elasticum in England and Wales. Cardiff, Wales: University of Wales, 1973. MD thesis.
10. Sulica VI, Cooper PH, Pope FM, Hambrick GW, Gerson BM, McKusick VA. Cutaneous histologic features in Ehlers–Danlos syndrome. *Arch Dermatol* 1979; **115:** 40-3.
11. Cleaver JE. DNA damage and repair in light sensitive human skin disease. *J Invest Dermatol* 1970; **54:** 181-95.
12. Goltz RW, Henderson RR, Hitch JM, Ott JE. Focal dermal hypoplasia syndrome. *Arch Dermatol* 1970; **101:** 1-11.
13. Gorlin RJ, Goltz RW. Multiple naevoid basal-cell epithelioma, jaw cysts and bifid rib. A syndrome. *N Engl J Med* 1970; **262:** 908-12.
14. Clendenning WE, Bloch JB, Rodde IC. Basal cell naevus syndrome. *Arch Dermatol* 1964; **90:** 38-54.
15. Currie AR, Ferguson-Smith J. Multiple primary spontaneous-healing squamous cell carcinomata of the skin. *J Pathol Bacteriol* 1952; **64:** 827-31.
16. Ferguson-Smith MA, Wallace D, James Z, Renwick J. Multiple self-healing squamous epithelioma. *Birth Defects* 1971; **7:** 157-63.

6

Dermatitis and Inflammatory Disorders of the Pilosebaceous Follicle

The dermatitis reaction

There is as yet no general agreement amongst dermatologists as to the precise usage of the terms 'dermatitis' and 'eczema'. While many use them interchangeably, others consider the term 'dermatitis' as a more general one, embracing many inflammatory diseases of which eczema is one. In this account both terms are considered synonymous, and the name dermatitis preferred. For accurate interpretation of a biopsy from a lesion of dermatitis it is essential to have a good understanding of the chronological development of these lesions.

The initial lesion of the *acute dermatitis reaction* is an erythema which is followed by the development of vesicles (vesicular phase). If the epidermis is thin, these vesicles rupture and serous exudate escapes from the surface (weeping phase). As the *subacute dermatitis reaction* develops, the serous exudate dries up (crusted phase) and the lesion becomes scaly (scaling phase) before returning to normality. Not every case of dermatitis, of course, goes through all these phases. If the causal factor is removed, or appropriate therapy instituted, the lesions may subside at any stage. Should, however, the lesion be untreated, overtreated, or the causal factor continue to operate, resolution may not occur and the *chronic dermatitis reaction* is produced. The picture may also be complicated further by superimposed pyogenic infection.

Thus the histological picture is dependent not on the aetiological agent responsible but on the clinical phase of the reaction at which the biopsy was taken.

This brief explanation provides a framework for interpretation of these lesions. In the report, therefore, all the histologist can do is to describe the changes and interpret the lesion as an acute, subacute or chronic dermatitis reaction. The use of the terms 'acute' or 'subacute' is somewhat arbitrary and will obviously depend to a large extent on the observer. Table 6.1 suggests a workable clinicopathological correlation.

Table 6.1 Dermatitis reaction

Histological grading	Clinical phase
Acute	Erythematous
	Vesicular
Subacute	Weeping
	Crusted
	Scaling
Chronic	Lichenified

Clinical varieties of dermatitis

For the clinician, two of the major divisions of the many varieties of dermatitis are those in which a specific allergen has induced sensitisation—allergic contact dermatitis—and those in which a substance which causes irritation to all skins on first contact is involved—primary irritant dermatitis. Work by Silberberg and her colleagues[1] has clearly established the role of the epidermal Langerhans cell in the induction phase of sensitisation in the former of those two conditions. Ultrastructural studies show contact of the Langerhans cells with passenger lymphocytes and subsequent apparent damage to Langerhans cell membranes. At present, however, there are few absolute points of differentiation at light microscopic level between allergic contact and primary irritant dermatitis, and acute, subacute and chronic phases of both conditions exist. The allergic form tends to show less damage to high-level epidermal cells, more eosinophils in the infiltrate, and more intercellular oedema (Fig. 6.1). These are, however, relative pointers, and patch-testing to possible allergens is the definitive method of differentiating between the two.

Other recognised clinical varieties of dermatitis include nummular dermatitis, neurodermatitis and atopic dermatitis. In each case the pathological picture will be of an acute, subacute or chronic dermatitis reaction, and liaison with clinical colleagues will be needed to establish the clinical variety.

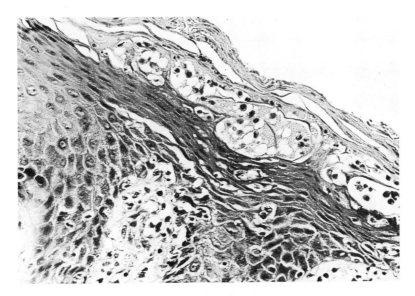

Fig. 6.1 Patch test from a patient with known allergic contact dermatitis biopsied 72 hours after application of sensitiser. Note the obvious infiltrate of lymphocytic cells, some of them with large nuclei, in the epidermis and the presence of serous exudate in the higher parts of the epidermis.

Acute dermatitis reaction

The earliest recognisable histological changes consist of vascular dilatation of the papillary vessels associated with early intercellular oedema (spongiosis) resulting in elongation and slight separation of the epidermal cells with a stretching of the 'epidermal bridges' (Fig. 6.2).

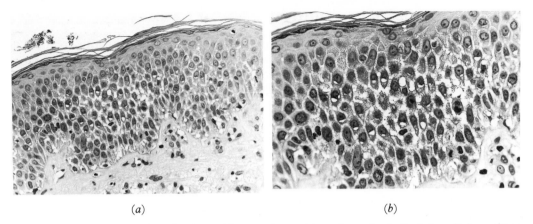

(a)   (b)

Fig. 6.2 Thin (1 μm) section of patient with acute dermatitis to show clearly the intracellular oedema which is straining connections between individual epidermal cells. A variety of cell types can be easily identified in the underlying papillary dermis.

As the oedema increases, some of the bridges rupture and microvesicles form in the epidermis (Fig. 6.3), containing serous exudate and occasional inflammatory cells. The epidermis bordering the vesicles shows spongiosis and the cells are characteristically elongated and bowed outwards. At a later stage the vesicles may contain a considerable number of inflam-

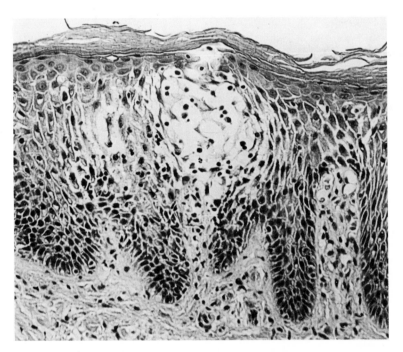

Fig. 6.3 Acute dermatitis reaction. This shows the formation of an early vesicle. In the centre of the field some of the 'epidermal bridges' have ruptured and the keratinocytes are separated from each other, leaving a space within the epidermis containing serous exudate and some lymphocytes. A mild lympho-histiocytic infiltrate is seen in the upper dermis.

matory cells as well as disintegrating epidermal cells. Inflammatory reaction in the dermis takes the form of a mixed lympho-histiocytic perivascular infiltrate confined to the papillary dermis and varies in quantity with the age of the lesion. Differing degrees of oedema of the papillary dermis are seen.

Subacute dermatitis

The acute phase passes imperceptibly into the subacute phase. Where the skin is thin, such as on the forearm, the vesicles quickly rupture, allowing the escape of serous exudate to the surface. The histological picture at this stage is variable. If the biopsy is taken from an actively 'weeping' area some acanthosis of the epidermis is seen. Overlying some dermal papillae the epidermis is deficient or absent and the dilated capillary vessel in the papilla is exposed to the surface (Fig. 6.4). This lesion is known as the dermatitis pit. In cases where

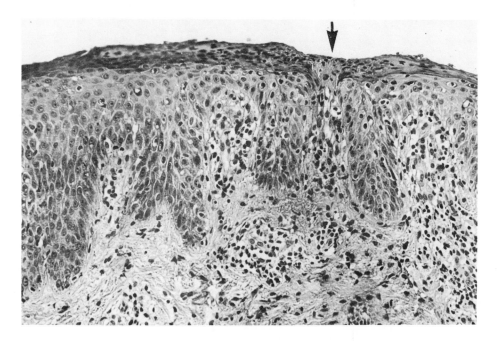

Fig. 6.4 Subacute dermatitis reaction (weeping phase). The surface of the epidermis is covered for the most part by parakeratotic keratin. About the centre of the field the epidermis is deficient (arrowed) and the underlying dermal papilla is covered by a blob of serous exudate containing inflammatory cells. The lympho-histiocytic infiltrate of the dermis is more pronounced than in the acute phase.

the exudate has coagulated (crusted phase) a discrete mass of serous exudate can be seen on the surface (Fig. 6.5). In both the weeping and crusted phases there is usually acanthosis, and areas of spongiosis may also be found which sometimes progress to vesicle formation. The disturbance of epidermal nutrition leads to the absence of the stratum granulosum and parakeratosis of the stratum corneum. The clinical phase of scaling is a further step in the process towards healing. The epidermis is still acanthotic and covered by a thicker, para-

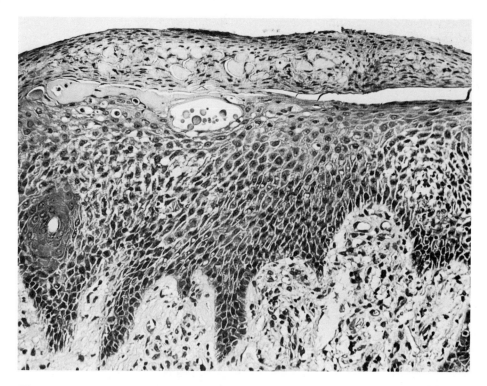

Fig. 6.5 Subacute dermatitis reaction (crusted phase). A layer of serous exudate intermingled with parakeratotic keratin covers the surface. The underlying acanthotic epidermis contains a small vesicle and there are foci of spongiosis. The papillary vessels are dilated and there is a moderate degree of lympho-histiocytic infiltrate.

keratotic scale and the stratum granulosum is absent (Fig. 6.6). Parakeratotic horny layer does not have normal cohesiveness, and so splits or air spaces are often seen. This type of horny layer is often lost during processing, even if care is taken when cutting the specimen.

The dermal infiltrate is heavier than in the acute stage, although still confined to the papillary dermis. It consists predominantly of lymphocytes and histiocytes with occasional eosinophil leucocytes. This and the degree of acanthosis and parakeratosis indicate that the disease process has been present for some time, justifying the term 'subacute'.

Chronic dermatitis

This may result as a direct sequel of an acute dermatitis failing to resolve or may arise as a result of prolonged scratching or rubbing of the skin (localised neurodermatitis or lichen simplex chronicus). Clinically the skin is thickened with exaggerated surface markings (likened to the bark of a tree overgrown with lichen—hence the term 'lichenified') and often shows increased pigmentation. Sections show a marked acanthosis, with lengthening and broadening of the rete ridges. There is a well-marked stratum granulosum and hyperkeratosis (Fig. 6.7). This latter is usually of the dense laminated type, which in healthy skin is associated with pressure areas. The vessels in the dermal papillae are dilated with a rather prominent endothelial lining. A patchy cellular inflammatory infiltrate composed of lym-

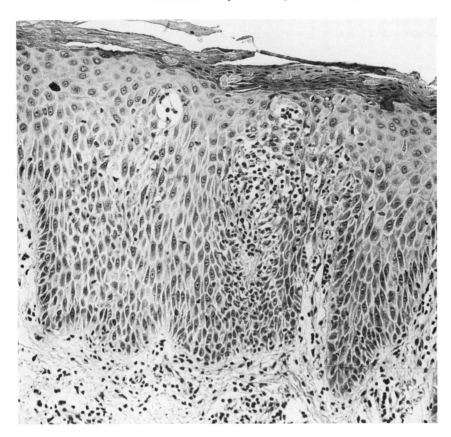

Fig. 6.6 Subacute dermatitis reaction (scaling phase). There is considerable acanthosis of the epidermis with areas of spongiosis and microvesicle formation. On the left of the picture the stratum corneum is normal and the stratum granulosum can be seen. On the right the stratum granulosum is absent and the stratum corneum is parakeratotic.

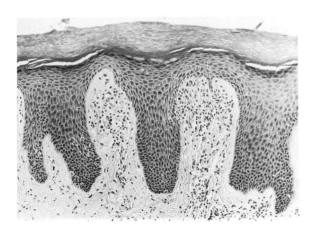

Fig. 6.7 Chromatic dermatitis reaction (lichenified phase). The epidermis is acanthotic with lengthening of the rete ridges. There is a well-marked stratum granulosum associated with a marked hyperkeratosis of the dense, laminated type. The capillaries in the dermis have a prominent endothelial lining, and are surrounded by a lympho-histiocytic infiltrate.

phocytes, histiocytes and eosinophil leucocytes is present in the upper and mid dermis. Mitotic figures may be seen in some mononuclear cells.

As the lesions of chronic dermatitis are usually very itchy, small superficial foci of spongiosis or even vesicle formation may be seen when the lesion has been vigorously scratched just before the biopsy. It is surprising just how much damage the fingernails can do to even a normal skin. Figure 6.8 is from a patient with primary biliary cirrhosis and shows that a portion of superficial epidermis has been dug out by the patient's fingernail and the space is now filled with serous exudate. The surrounding epidermis shows spongiosis and a parakeratotic stratum corneum.

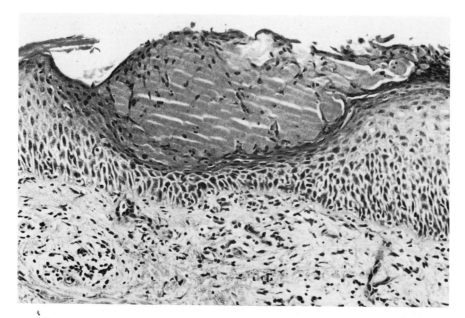

Fig. 6.8   Scratch mark (patient with primary biliary cirrhosis). A superficial portion of the surface epidermis has been removed and the resulting gap filled with serous exudate. There is mild spongiosis of the surrounding epidermis. A few lymphocytes are seen around the dermal capillaries.

Clinical conditions with the histological picture of a dermatitis reaction

Pityriasis rosea

This striking, self-limiting clinical entity with its oval scaly patches on the trunk is rarely biopsied as there is usually no doubt about the clinical diagnosis. Sections from the active border of the fully formed lesion show an area of acute dermatitis with spongiosis and microvesicle formation, this area being covered by a parakeratotic scale (Fig. 6.9). There is a moderate perivascular cellular infiltrate composed mainly of lymphocytes. Should an earlier lesion be biopsied the changes are more diffuse and consist of marked oedema of the papillary dermis with a diffuse lymphocytic infiltrate. This infiltrate invades the epidermis which shows spongiosis, and tiny vesicles filled with lymphocytes may be seen (Fig. 6.10).

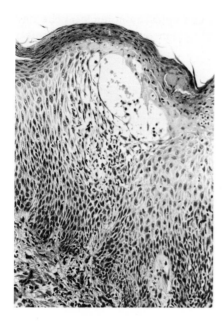

Fig. 6.9 Pityriasis rosea (advancing margin of lesion). There is an area of spongiosis and microvesicle formation in the upper epidermis covered by a layer of parakeratotic keratin.

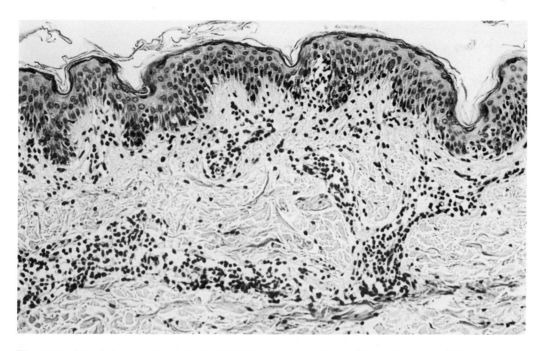

Fig. 6.10 Pityriasis rosea (early lesion). Mild patchy spongiosis of the epidermis, which in one area has progressed to microvesicle formation, can be seen. This vesicle contains lymphocytes. The papillary dermis is oedematous and is diffusely infiltrated by lymphocytes which in places invade the dermo-epidermal junction. There is also a moderate perivascular lymphocytic infiltrate of the vessels in the mid dermis.

Occasionally the quality of the lymphoid infiltrate with large atypical mononuclear cells may cause problems in differentiating the lesion from an early cutaneous lymphoma. Clinical consultation should rapidly resolve this problem.

Seborrhoeic dermatitis

Histological examination of this condition reveals essentially a subacute dermatitis reaction with spongiosis and even vesicle formation (Fig. 6.11). There is also considerable acanthosis,

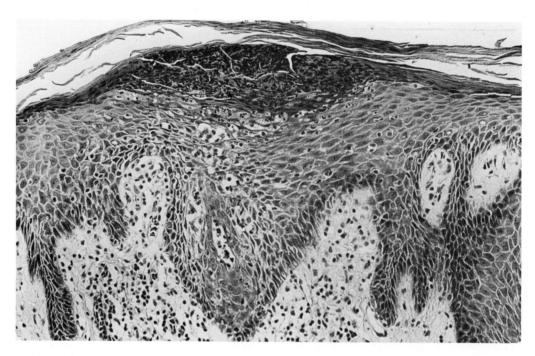

Fig. 6.11   Seborrhoeic dermatitis. The epidermis is acanthotic and there is some branching of the rete ridges. Areas of spongiosis and microvesicle formation can be seen in the ridge in the centre of the photograph. Some degenerate leucocytes can be seen just under the central parakeratotic scale.

with elongation and clubbing of the rete ridges, and there may be some thinning of the suprapapillary part of the epidermis. These features may cause difficulty in differentiating the condition from psoriasis (Chapter 7). Uncomplicated psoriasis does not show spongiosis or vesicle formation, although it may do so if irritated by strong local applications. Seborrhoeic dermatitis lacks the rigid-looking dilated dermal capillaries of psoriasis.

Pinkus has described the 'squirting papillae' as the hallmark of seborrhoeic dermatitis.[2] This term describes the common and characteristic picture of a dermal papilla with a dilated capillary directly underlying an area of epidermal infiltration with polymorphs (Fig. 6.12). The interpretation of this picture is that small aggregates of polymorphs and lymphocytes are regularly extruded from the underlying vessel and make their way through the epidermis. In some cases of nummular dermatitis a similar but less well-developed picture is seen.

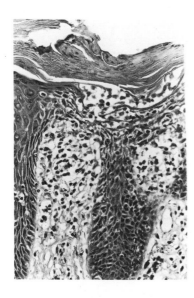

Fig. 6.12   Biopsy from a patient with seborrhoeic dermatitis to illustrate what has been described as a 'squirting' papilla. Note the lymphoid cells passing through the epidermis immediately above a dermal papilla in which there is evidence of distended blood vessels and a lymphocytic infiltrate.

Dyshidrotic dermatitis (cheiropompholyx and podopompholyx)

Despite the name 'dyshidrotic', the pathology of this condition has nothing to do with sweat glands, although it is most commonly seen in association with hyperhidrosis of the hands and feet. It is essentially an acute vesicular dermatitis occurring in the thick skin of the palms or soles. The thick stratum corneum in these sites prevents the vesicles from rupturing, so they tend to persist as 'sago grains' until the contents are absorbed. The older view that these lesions represented occlusion and distension of the intraepidermal area of the sweat duct is no longer tenable. Figure 6.13, from a case of cheiropompholyx, shows an acute dermatitis reaction, with spongiosis and vesicle formation covered by a thick stratum corneum. For comparison, Fig. 6.14 shows an occluded and distended sweat duct within the epidermis. The sweat duct lining can be clearly seen, and although the surrounding epidermis shows a mild spongiosis the two conditions are obviously different.

Here it must be stressed once more that some skin diseases which eventually have diagnostic histological features, in very early stages show only a dermatitis reaction. This is why, except in the case of blisters, time must be allowed for a lesion to develop fully before being subjected to biopsy.

Exfoliative dermatitis (erythroderma)

Generalised redness of the skin which may be associated with extensive scaling and desquamation is known as erythroderma or exfoliative dermatitis.

Histological examination in these cases shows a subacute, low-grade dermatitis: surprisingly little, in fact, considering the striking clinical picture. This should not deter the clinician from repeating biopsies at intervals, as a small proportion of cutaneous lymphomas present initially as exfoliative dermatitis.

Overvigorous treatment of psoriasis, seborrhoeic dermatitis or atopic dermatitis may result in exfoliative dermatitis. Where this occurs the histopathology remains that of the primary disease.

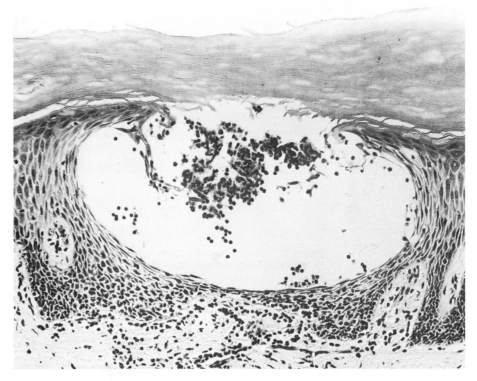

Fig. 6.13 Dyshydrotic dermatitis (cheiropompholyx). This lesion, from the lateral aspect of the finger, shows an acute dermatitis reaction with spongiosis and microvesicle formation. Note the thick stratum corneum which is normal for this site.

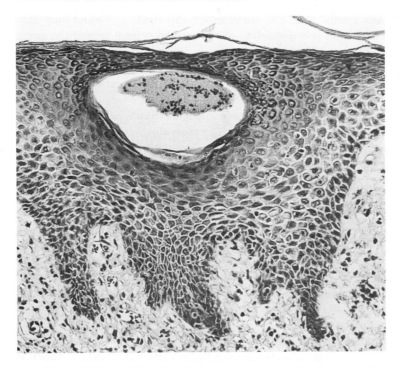

Fig. 6.14 Miliaria. This microphotograph shows a dilated intraepidermal sweat duct containing serous exudate and inflammatory cells. The lining of the duct can be clearly seen, and although the surrounding epidermis shows a mild spongiosis the condition is clearly different from dyshydrotic dermatitis (cf. Fig. 6.13).

The most difficult diagnostic type is that associated with cutaneous lymphoma (Chapter 13). In the premycotic stages the histology may be that of a low-grade, subacute dermatitis and may in fact remain so for a period of years. Eventually, however, the dermal infiltrate begins to change in character and finally declares itself. Sequential biopsies may be needed before definite proof of a lymphoma is obtained. This fact must always be kept in mind when reporting biopsies from cases of exfoliative dermatitis. Unless the changes are clearly recognisable as, say, those of psoriasis, a repeat biopsy in 3–6 months' time should always be considered if the clinical condition persists.

Radiodermatitis[3]

Ionising radiation produces permanent damage to the skin. The extent of the damage depends on multiple factors, amongst which total dosage is one of the most important. Large doses produce an almost immediate reaction in the skin, while the effects of small doses may not be evident until many years later. It is important to realise that the damage done to the skin by irradiation is permanent and progressive. The acute changes which may be seen, for example, following radiotherapy to a basal cell carcinoma appear to subside in a relatively short time. The tissue changes, however, progress relentlessly, to cause some 10–15 years later an area of atrophy, pigmentation and telangiectasia, and even necrosis and indolent

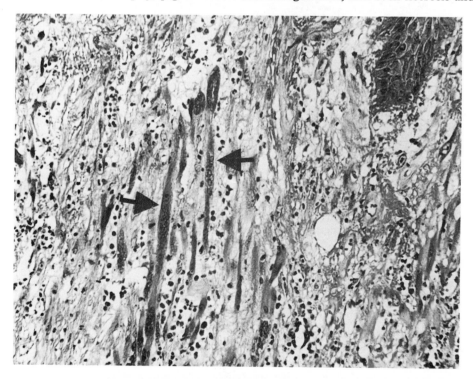

Fig. 6.15 Radiodermatitis. This photograph shows the profound changes which have occurred in the dermis a few weeks after a therapeutic dose for a basal cell carcinoma. There is intense oedema, vascular engorgement and inflammatory cell infiltrate. The most striking feature is the change in the dermal fibroblasts (arrowed). These are enlarged, strap-like in shape and contain large basophilic nuclei, so pronounced as to suggest sarcomatous change.

ulceration. Fortunately, today, with the strict control of radiotherapy, late radiodermatitis is rarely seen.

It is obvious that histological changes of radiodermatitis will vary with the interval between therapy and biopsy. A few weeks after a moderate therapeutic dose they can be quite alarming. There is considerable vascular engorgement with oedema and free haemorrhage, and profound changes in dermal fibroblasts (Fig. 6.15). These are markedly enlarged, strap-like and contain large basophilic nuclei, all of which strongly suggest sarcomatous change. After a time the picture changes. Figure 6.16 is from the skin surrounding a basal

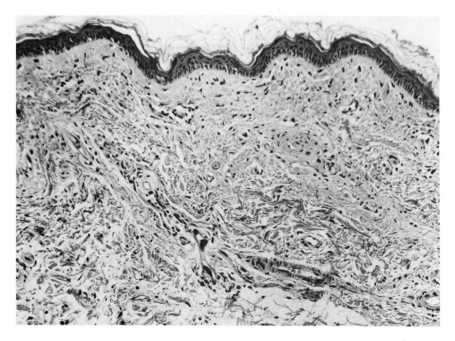

Fig. 6.16 Radiodermatitis. There is a mild hyperkeratosis and an increase in melanocytes of the stratum basale of the epidermis. The dermal fibroblasts are increased in number and have prominent nuclei, some of which are triangular in shape. The capillary endothelium is swollen and hyperchromatic. Some of the vessels in the mid dermis show an obliterative endarteritis.

cell carcinoma which was successfully treated by radiotherapy some five years previously. There is a mild hyperkeratosis with an increase of melanocytes in the basal layer of the epidermis. There is now swelling of the capillary endothelium and obliterative thickening of the larger vessels. The dermis shows an increased cellularity due to a large number of fibroblasts with prominent triangular nuclei (see below). Late chronic radiodermatitis is nowadays rarely seen, but an occasional case can still be encountered, a reminder of the overenthusiastic irradiation of 40 years ago. Figure 6.17 shows a section from the dorsum of the hand of a young woman. Twenty years previously, when still a child, she had a wart treated by a radium mould. There is now atrophy of the epidermis: the dermis, its appendages and the small dermal capillaries have been destroyed and replaced by acellular fibrous tissue containing large telangiectatic vessels. In some areas the collagen is beginning to show necrosis (Fig. 6.18). Surrounding this area are numerous triangular-shaped fibroblasts.

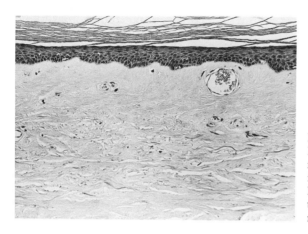

Fig. 6.17 Radiodermatitis (late). There is hyperkeratosis and atrophy of the epidermis with loss of rete ridges. The dermis and its appendages have been replaced by acellular fibrous tissue containing a large, telangiectatic vessel visible in the upper right-hand portion of the field.

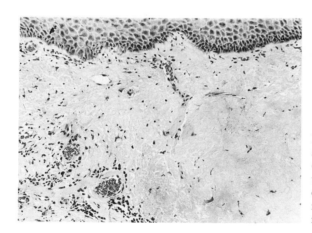

Fig. 6.18 Radiodermatitis (late). This is a further section from the patient in Fig. 6.17. In addition to the telangiectasia and the triangular-shaped fibroblasts (at the left of the picture), the dermal collagen (at the right of the picture) shows incipient necrosis.

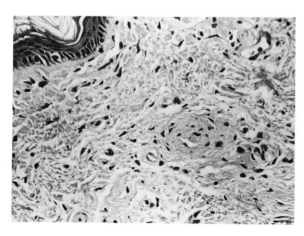

Fig. 6.19 Chronic radiodermatitis. The fibroblast nuclei are swollen and basophilic, and many are triangular in shape. These changes in the fibroblasts are the hallmark of previous ionising radiation.

These changes may end in the complete breakdown of the collagen and epithelium with the formation of an indolent ulcer.

It is now clear that although the whole skin undergoes progressive irreversible damage as a result of ionising radiation, it is the change in the fibroblasts and their prominent nuclei that appears almost immediately after the irradiation and persists throughout the years. The nuclei are swollen, basophilic, and triangular in shape (Fig. 6.19), and are a veritable hallmark of previous irradiation. With the exception of the central portion of some keloid scars (Chapter 14) fibroblasts of this type appear to be confined to radiodermatitis.

Inflammatory disorders of the pilosebaceous follicle

Acne vulgaris[4]

The initial lesion in this distressing disorder of adolescence is the blocking of a pilosebaceous follicle by a keratinous plug, the comedo or blackhead (Fig. 6.20). Some cases do not progress

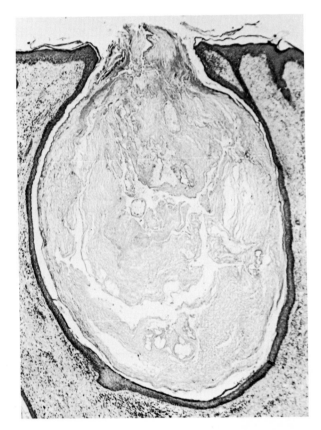

Fig. 6.20 Acne vulgaris. The upper portion of a pilosebaceous follicle is distended by a keratinous plug (comedo).

beyond this. In the majority of cases, however, sebum secretion continues and becomes dammed up behind this plug. If the follicular wall remains intact this results in a cystic cavity lined by squamous epithelium and containing keratinous debris (Fig. 6.21). Should the follicular wall rupture (Fig. 6.22), the contents prove to be extremely irritating to the

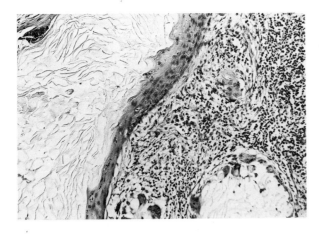

Fig. 6.21 Acne vulgaris (cystic type). To the left of the picture is a keratin-filled cyst lined by the intact squamous epithelium. To the right of the picture small foreign body granulomata and foci of lympho-histiocytic infiltration can be seen.

surrounding tissue and inflammatory changes (Fig. 6.23) rapidly ensue. Foreign body granulomata may form around the released keratin and portion of hair shaft. The degree of inflammatory response varies and the lesion heals by granulation tissue formation with its inevitable scarring.

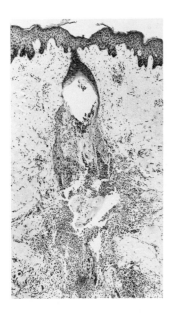

Fig. 6.22 Acne vulgaris. The upper part of the pilosebaceous follicle is distended. Below this the follicular wall has disintegrated and an acute inflammatory response has developed around the discharged contents of the follicle.

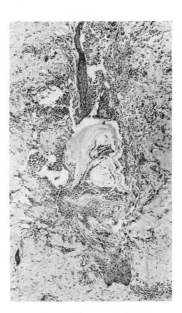

Fig. 6.23 Acne vulgaris. In the upper and lower parts of the field portions of pilosebaceous follicular epithelium remain. In the centre the discharged keratinous material heavily infiltrated by neutrophil leucocytes can be clearly seen.

Rosacea (acne rosacea)[5]

This eruption mainly affects the central part of the face in adults. It is more common in women. The histological changes seen in early rosacea may be similar to those seen in mild acne vulgaris. There is a fairly dense lymphocytic infiltrate around the neck of the follicle and some prominent dilated thin-walled capillaries (telangiectasia). The inflammatory infiltrate eventually destroys the pilosebaceous follicle. When the glands are destroyed, the lymphocytic infiltrate is replaced by a rather poorly defined follicular granuloma composed largely of epithelioid cells with an occasional foreign body giant cell (Fig. 6.24). This lesion

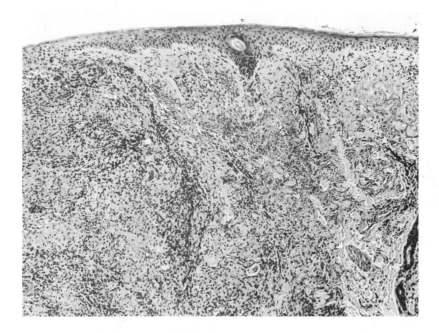

Fig. 6.24   Papular rosacea. The dermis is occupied by follicular aggregates of epithelioid cells with an occasional giant cell and a few lymphocytes. Such a granulomatous lesion must be distinguished from other follicular granulomata (see Chapter 9).

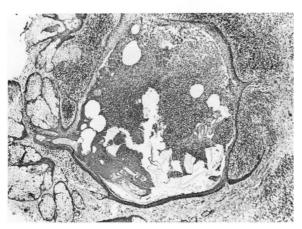

Fig. 6.25   Rhinophyma. A large, dilated, pilosebaceous follicle is filled with keratinous debris and inflammatory cells. In the dermis are patches of dense lympho-histiocytic infiltrate.

is referred to as papular rosacea, and has in the past been confused with a tuberculide. Papular rosacea must be distinguished from other follicular granulomata (Chapter 9). Some cases of rosacea, particularly in men, are associated with a bulbous hypertrophy of the nose which is called rhinophyma. Sections show extensive comedo formation associated with gross sebaceous gland hyperplasia and keratin-filled epidermal cysts (Fig. 6.25). There is also a patchy, non-specific, chronic inflammatory infiltration.

Acne necrotica[6]

This condition, despite its name, is not connected with acne vulgaris. It occurs in adults and consists of small, necrotic, haemorrhagic lesions which heal by scarring. The disorder is confined to the hair margin and the scalp. Histologically (Fig. 6.26) there is acute necrosis of the upper part of the wall of the hair follicle, the adjacent epidermis and dermis and an associated intense lymphocytic infiltrate. The dermal necrosis is responsible for the subsequent scarring.

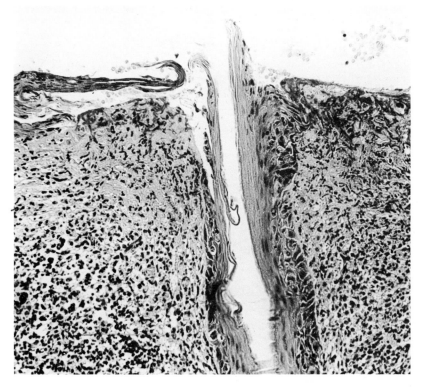

Fig. 6.26 Acne necrotica. There is necrosis of the surface epidermis and the upper portion of the pilosebaceous follicle together with the surrounding dermis. Associated with these changes and surrounding them is an intense lymphocytic infiltrate.

References

1. Silberberg I, Baer RL, Rosenthal SA. The role of Langerhans cells in allergic contact hypersensitivity. A review of findings in man and guinea pigs. *J Invest Dermatol* 1976; **66:** 210–17.
2. Pinkus H, Mehregan AH. The primary histologic lesion of seborrhoeic dermatitis and psorasis. *J Invest Dermatol* 1966; **46:** 109–16.
3. Van Scott EJ, Reinertson RP. Detection of radiation effects on hair root of the human scalp. *J Invest Dermatol* 1957; **29:** 205–12.
4. Strauss JS, Kligman AM. The pathologic dynamics of acne vulgaris. *Arch Dermatol* 1960; **82:** 779–90.
5. Søbye P. Aetiology and pathogenesis of rosacea. *Acta Derm Vener* (Stockh) 1950; **30:** 137–58.
6. Montgomery H. Acne necrotica miliaris of the scalp. *Arch Dermatol* 1937; **36:** 40–4.

7

Psoriasis and Lichenoid Tissue Reactions

Psoriasis

The manifestations of this disorder, which affects some 2 per cent of the population, vary from a few scaly patches on the knees and elbows to a socially and economically crippling eruption which affects almost the entire skin surface, including the nails. Sometimes the disease is associated with a severe arthropathy. Although the aetiology is not known, it is well established that there is an increase in transit time of cells through the epidermis.[1,2] This accelerated epidermal passage explains many of the histological features detailed in this chapter.

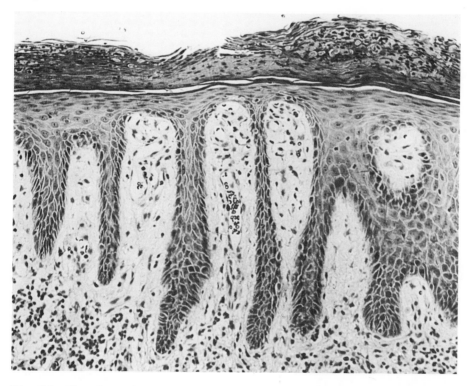

Fig. 7.1 Chronic psoriasis. The surface is covered by a parakeratotic stratum corneum and the stratum granulosum is absent. The rete ridges of the epidermis are elongated and there is some clubbing of their tips. The dermal papillae, which are slightly oedematous, contain prominent dilated capillaries. The epidermis overlying the papillae is reduced in thickness.

The classic histological changes of chronic psoriasis are:

1. Parakeratosis with absence of the stratum granulosum.
2. Small collections of polymorphonuclear leucocytes (Munro microabscesses) within or just below the stratum corneum.
3. Thinning of the epidermis overlying the dermal papillae.
4. Acanthosis of the rete ridges of the epidermis in the form of marked elongation with clubbing of their tips.
5. Dilatation and tortuosity of the dermal capillary loops.

The general features of psoriasis are illustrated in Fig. 7.1.

Parakeratosis   This, of course, is not specific for psoriasis, occurring as it does in any situation where normal differentiation is disturbed. The amount of parakeratotic scale varies

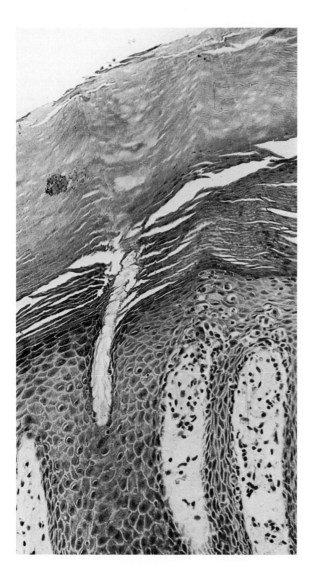

Fig. 7.2 Chronic psoriasis (edge of patch). To the left of the sweat duct opening there is a well-marked stratum granulosum with a normal stratum corneum. To the right the stratum granulosum is absent and the stratum corneum is parakeratotic.

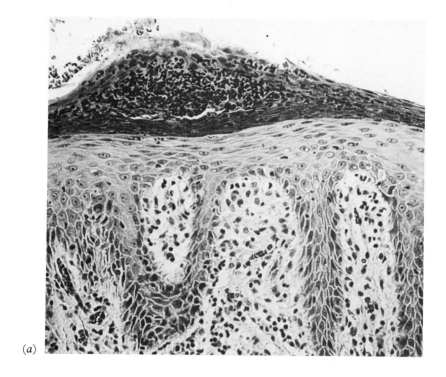

(a)

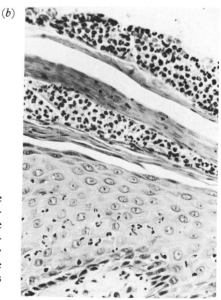

(b)

Fig. 7.3 Chronic psoriasis. (*a*) A collection of degenerate polymorphs with shrunken pyknotic nuclei (Munro microabscesses) is seen within the parakeratotic keratin. (*b*) The localised collections of degenerate polymorphs with pyknotic nuclei (Munro microabscesses) are seen more clearly at this higher magnification. Note also the absence of the stratum granulosum and the migration of polymorphs through the epidermis.

considerably from case to case. As has already been mentioned, parakeratotic keratin does not have the cohesive properties of normal keratin so that splits in it appear even *in vivo*, allowing the formation of air spaces. This is largely responsible for the silvery appearance of the psoriatic scale which is so noticeable on clinical examination. It is thought that the bubbles of air trapped in the scale reflect light in a way similar to that of air bubbles trapped on the sides of a glass when it is rapidly filled with water. While in most cases the involved epidermis is covered by a parakeratotic scale, this may be patchy and associated with areas of hyperkeratosis. This should not be confused with the regular alternating columns of hyperkeratosis and parakeratosis seen in actinic keratosis. In very long-standing cases of psoriasis the hyperkeratosis may be much more in evidence than the parakeratosis. As always, where there is parakeratosis the granular layer is absent. The psoriatic patch is usually sharply demarcated from surrounding normal skin. Figure 7.2, taken from the edge of a lesion, shows normal keratinisation with a stratum granulosum at one side of a sweat duct opening with the abrupt change of parakeratosis with absent stratum granulosum at the other side.

Microabscesses (Munro)   These consist of small collections of polymorphonuclear leucocytes either in the stratum corneum or just beneath it where the stratum granulosum would normally be. The polymorphs are usually degenerate with shrunken pyknotic nuclei

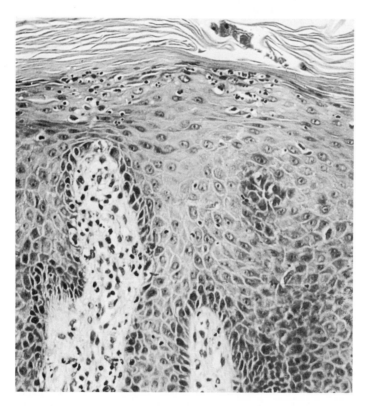

Fig. 7.4   Acute psoriasis. A few polymorphs may be seen migrating through the epidermis and forming loose collections (Munro microabscesses) in the region of the stratum granulosum. Some of the cells of the stratum granulosum are empty and have a vacuolated appearance. Parakeratotic keratin is evident on the right of the picture.

and are closely packed together (Fig. 7.3). In more acute lesions polymorphonuclear leucocytes may be seen migrating through the epidermis and early Munro microabscesses are seen as loose collections of polymorphs collected in and around empty vacuolated cells in the upper epidermis just below the stratum corneum (Fig. 7.4). Such lesions are very like a miniature edition of the spongiform pustle of Kogoj seen in pustular psoriasis; in fact the two are probably the same, differing only in extent.

Thinning of the suprapapillary epidermis   This is often a striking feature of psoriasis, the epidermis over the tips of the papillae being reduced to two or three cells thick (Fig. 7.5). This epidermal thinning is the basis of a useful clinical diagnostic aid in psoriasis.

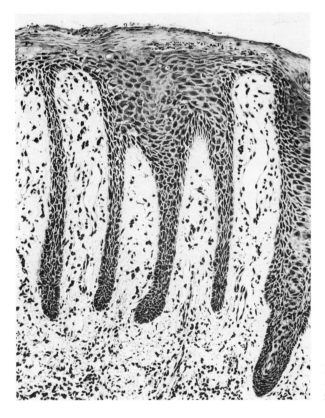

Fig. 7.5   Chronic psoriasis. The epidermis overlying the papillae is markedly reduced in thickness.

If the scale is removed by a curette or the fingernail, further gentle scraping will result in the appearance of tiny bleeding points (Auspitz's sign). As can be seen from Fig. 7.5, the removal of two to three layers of epidermal cells will expose the dilated tortuous capillary and damage its endothelium, causing the bleeding point.

Acanthosis of the epidermal ridges   This is a constant feature of psoriasis. In its most characteristic form it consists of test-tube-like lengthening of the ridges, the tip of the ridge being slightly bulbous (see Fig. 7.1). It is more common, however, to see a more complex picture with apparent branching and fusion of some of the ridges to form more solid areas of acanthosis (Fig. 7.6). It is debatable if this is true branching of the ridges; it is probable that this picture is the result of oblique sectioning of thickened ridges. As the epidermal turnover

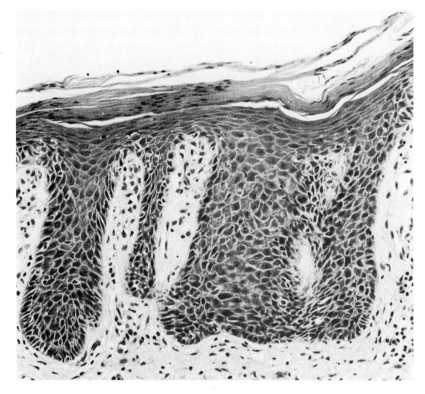

Fig. 7.6   Chronic psoriasis. In addition to the elongation and bulbous thickening of the tips of the rete ridges there is a more solid area of acanthosis (to the right of the photograph) formed by fusion of adjacent ridges.

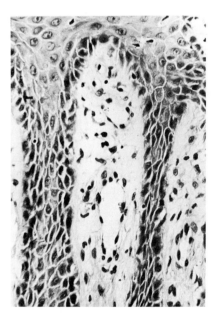

Fig. 7.7   Chronic psoriasis. The capillary loop in this papilla is dilated and lined by flattened endothelium. It has been cut in several different planes, indicating a degree of tortuosity. The capillaries have a fixed, rigid look.

time in psoriasis is greatly accelerated, mitotic figures in the epidermal cells are increased (up to tenfold) compared with the normal epidermis.

The papillary vessels The capillaries in the dermal papillae are dilated and on routine haematoxylin and eosin sections appear cut in several places, indicating tortuosity. The cells of the capillary endothelium appear elongated and somewhat flattened and the vessel has a rather 'rigid' look about it (Fig. 7.7). This dilatation and tortuosity can easily be confirmed by thick sections stained by the alkaline phosphatase technique (Fig. 7.8).

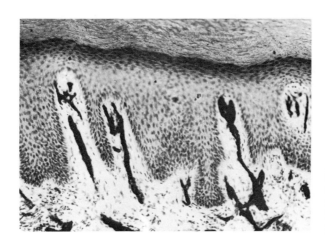

Fig. 7.8 Chronic psoriasis. Photomicrograph of a thick section to show the dilated and tortuous dermal capillaries in psoriasis. Gomori's alkaline phosphatase.

The dermal papillae These show a mild oedema and the tips tend to be dilated or spatulate in shape. The basal lamina over the tips of the papillae may be thinned or even absent (Fig. 7.9). Sparse lymphocytic infiltration is seen in the papillae and in the dermis immediately underlying them. If the dermal infiltrate is heavy, serious doubt must be cast on the diagnosis of psoriasis.

In the classic case of psoriasis there should be no difficulty in establishing a histological diagnosis. However, the classic cases do not present any clinical diagnostic problems and are thus rarely biopsied. Those which are biopsied are the atypical ones and, as could be expected, these are often also histologically atypical. In assessing the histology of these cases the most constant and helpful diagnostic features are the dilated tortuous capillaries, the narrowing of the suprapapillary epidermis, the microabscesses and parakeratosis, in that order.[3] Psoriasis can be difficult to differentiate from seborrhoeic dermatitis, as already mentioned, and from long-standing chronic dermatitis which may develop a psoriasiform type of acanthosis. These differ from psoriasis by areas of spongiosis, and even microvesiculation can be found if looked for. In addition, the dermal inflammatory infiltrate in both these conditions is much more extensive than in psoriasis. Spongiosis in the epidermis practically excludes a histological diagnosis of psoriasis, unless of course there has been a superimposed contact dermatitis from the therapy employed. The topical application of potent corticosteroids can modify considerably the histological picture of psoriasis, and for that matter any other inflammatory conditions. It is worth re-emphasising that in some instances it may be necessary to withhold treatment for a period before a diagnostic biopsy is obtained.

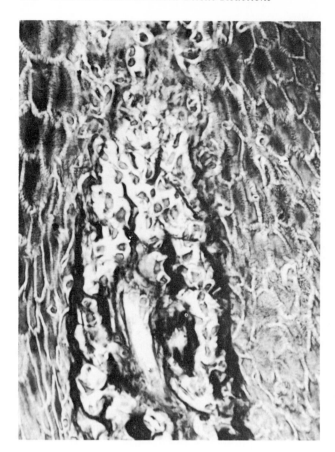

Fig. 7.9 Chronic psoriasis. The basal lamina at the tip of this dermal papilla is absent. (JSDB 109.)

Pustular psoriasis

Occasionally during the course of an ordinary chronic psoriasis the disease enters a more acute phase, and becomes widespread and pustular in character.[4] These pustules begin as discrete subcorneal lesions which enlarge slowly and by coalescence with neighbouring lesions may form quite large superficial lakes of pus. Bacteriological examination of this pus, either by direct examination or by culture, fails to reveal micro-organisms. Histological examination of such a lesion shows a large collection of polymorphonuclear leucocytes under the stratum corneum. These lie in and between the empty remains of epidermal cells, giving the pustule a spongiform appearance (spongiform pustule of Kogoj; Fig. 7.10). In pustular psoriasis all or some of the features of psoriasis are detectable; in Fig. 7.10 the dilated capillaries and the elongation of the rete ridges can be clearly seen.

In the so-called pustular psoriasis of the palms and soles, spongiform pustules also occur. Some of these do occur in patients with chronic psoriasis and the biopsis will show, in addition to the spongiform pustule, some or all of the features of psoriasis. In other cases none of the features of psoriasis is recognisable in the biopsy and the non-committal name of palmoplantar pustulosis is appropriate.

Other conditions in which spongiform pustules occur   The appearance of a spongiform pustule within the epidermis is not diagnostic of pustular psoriasis and other features of psoriasis must be sought on the section as supportive evidence. Other conditions in which spongiform pustules may be observed include the acute phase of seborrhoeic dermatitis, Reiter's disease,[5] so-called impetigo herpetiformis and geographic tongue. In the case of seborrhoeic dermatitis obvious spongiosis and the presence of 'squirting' papillae are both helpful additional evidence. Reiter's disease is characterised by the combination of pustular bodies and gross hyperkeratosis on the palms and soles—keratoderma blennorrhagica. Ocular symptoms, urethritis and arthropathy are additional clinical features. In some cases gastrointestinal symptoms are also observed. The epidermis adjacent to the spongiform

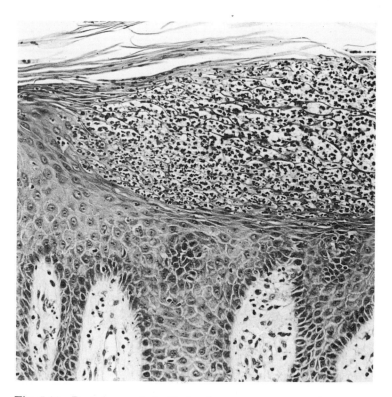

Fig. 7.10 Pustular psoriasis. Under the stratum corneum there is a collection of neutrophils lying in and between the empty remains of epidermal cells which gives the lesion a spongiform appearance (spongiform pustule of Kogoj). The rete ridges are elongated and the dermal capillaries dilated and rigid-looking.

pustule of Reiter's disease is frequently oedematous with spongiosis but the squirting papillae of seborrhoeic dermatitis are lacking. In impetigo herpetiformis an acute superficial sterile pustular eruption develops during pregnancy or the puerperium. Many reported cases have low levels of serum calcium and some have a strong family history of psoriasis. The diagnosis of the spongiform pustule of geographic tongue is facilitated by knowledge of the site of biopsy.

It must be stressed that the differential diagnosis of the spongiform pustule is eventually a clinical rather than a pathological exercise. Good collaboration between clinician and pathologist and a good history will in most cases clarify the situation.

Psoriasis and psoriasiform drug reactions

A number of fairly commonly used drugs may give rise to a psoriasiform drug eruption in susceptible individuals, and another group of drugs may apparently aggravate pre-existing psoriasis. It is therefore important to have a complete history of recently ingested drugs listed on the biopsy request form.

Causes of psoriasiform drug eruptions include diuretics and antihypertensives such as methyldopa.[6] Drugs which appear to aggravate pre-existing psoriasis include lithium[7] and the beta-blocker group of drugs.[8] In the case of lithium, this observation has led to research into the mode of action of lithium on epidermal keratinocytes[9] in the hope that this may act as a model to throw light on underlying mechanisms in psoriasis.

Parapsoriasis

This term has for many years given rise to confusion and its use is not recommended. It has previously been used in two quite distinct and prognostically very different situations: parapsoriasis en plaque and guttate parapsoriasis. The former has been used to describe psoriasiform pruritic plaques which may be an early precursor phase of the cutaneous lymphoma, mycosis fungoides (Chapter 13). In this group of disorders the alternative term 'premycotic eruption' is less confusing and more accurate. Although clinically the lesions may bear some slight superficial resemblance to plaques of psoriasis and thus explain the origin of the term, there is little histological similarity between the two. In premycotic plaques the picture is essentially that of a lymphocytic infiltrate invading the papillary dermis and, on occasion, individual cell infiltration of the overlying epidermis. High-power examination of the individual cells comprising this infiltrate will reveal the presence of a high nuclear/cytoplasmic ratio and possibly some abnormal mitotic figures.

The term 'guttate parapsoriasis' is synonymous with pityriasis lichenoides chronica, and this latter term is preferred although recent studies cast doubt on the clear division between the acute and chronic forms of pityriasis lichenoides. They are therefore discussed together in Chapter 10.

Lichenoid tissue reactions

Lichen planus

This intensely pruritic eruption is characterised by crops of lilac-coloured, polygonal-shaped papules occurring mainly on the flexor surfaces of the body. The mouth is also frequently involved, and the condition tends to remit spontaneously after a period of months. This relatively rare condition has many histological features in common with the acute phase of cutaneous graft versus host reaction and may therefore be regarded as an interesting naturally occurring model of this important and topical problem (p. 114). The individual papules will be seen to be covered by a criss-cross network of white lines (Wickham's striae).

The disorder may begin in mucous membranes and remain localised to these sites for some considerable time before the skin lesions appear. On mucous membranes the lesions appear as white patches or streaks, and may be confused clinically and histologically with other causes of white patches on mucosal surfaces.

In a fully developed lesion the histological picture is characteristic[10] (Fig. 7.11):

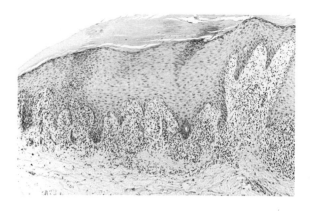

Fig. 7.11 Lichen planus. There is a marked hyperkeratosis which is associated with wedge-shaped areas of hyperplasia of the stratum granulosum. The epidermis is acanthotic and its lower border has a jagged, saw-tooth appearance. The dermal papillae are broadened and dome-shaped, and there is a dense band of lympho-histiocytic infiltrate which forms an almost straight line at the junction of the papillary and reticular dermis.

1. There is a moderate to marked hyperkeratosis. As the lesions occur predominantly on flexor surfaces the normal basket-weave keratin is replaced by the dense, laminated type.

2. The stratum granulosum shows focal wedge-shaped areas of hyperplasia. These areas of focal thickening of the stratum granulosum, like the epithelial ridges, will run as ridges or lines when viewed three-dimensionally.

3. A characteristic type of acanthosis of the epidermis is seen in which the lower border of the thickened epidermis has a rather jagged, pointed appearance. This is due to the rete ridges being stretched over broadened dermal papillae and has been aptly likened to the teeth of a saw.

4. The dermal papillae are broadened and there is, in the early stages, a dense band of lymphocytes and histiocytes in the upper dermis which crosses and obliterates the epidermo-dermal junction, and is often associated with liquefaction degeneration of the basal layer. The lower border of this infiltrate forms an almost straight line at the junction of the papillary and reticular layers of the dermis.

In the mucous membranes the histological changes are similar (Fig. 7.12). In children and adults with very acute lesions there may be, in addition, separation at the dermo-epidermal junction by serous fluid (bullous lichen planus). The changes described above represent the fully developed lesion of lichen planus. As the lesion ages the dermal infiltrate decreases considerably in quantity, tending to become patchy. In addition to the lymphocytes and histiocytes there are now a number of mast cells. As the infiltrate clears, the liquefaction degeneration of the basal layer and the increased vascularity of the papillary dermis become clearly visible. The hyperkeratosis, focal increase in the stratum granulosum and the saw-tooth acanthosis remain unchanged (Fig. 7.13). At this stage round hyaline or colloid bodies (Civatte bodies), which stain a homogeneous pink with eosin, may be found in the upper dermis in the region of the dermo-epidermal junction (Fig. 7.14). These bodies are probably derived from epidermal cells which have undergone hyaline degeneration.[11] These are not a constant feature of lichen planus, although when evident are usually present in large numbers. They may also be seen in the more acute stages but tend to be masked by the inflammatory infiltrate. While their presence, especially if abundant, tends to favour a diagnosis of lichen planus they cannot be regarded as specific for this disease. Occasional similar hyaline bodies may be seen in chronic discoid lupus erythematosus and in poikiloderma which sometimes accompanies dermatomyositis (Chapter 11).

Further resolution of the lesion is marked by an accumulation of melanin-containing

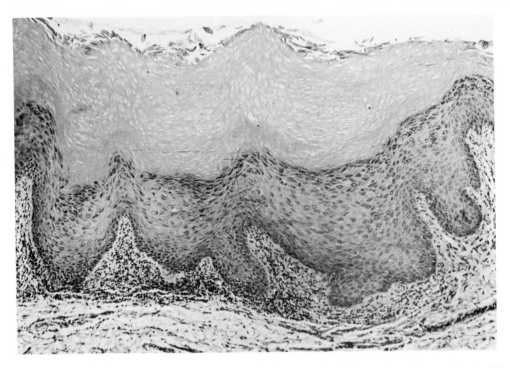

Fig. 7.12 Lichen planus (buccal mucosa). There is a marked hyperkeratosis associated with the characteristic wedge-shaped areas of hyperplasia of the stratum granulosum. The epithelium is acanthotic although in this particular example it lacks the saw-tooth appearance of its lower border. There is a band-like infiltrate of lymphocytes and histiocytes confined to the upper part of the subepithelial connective tissue.

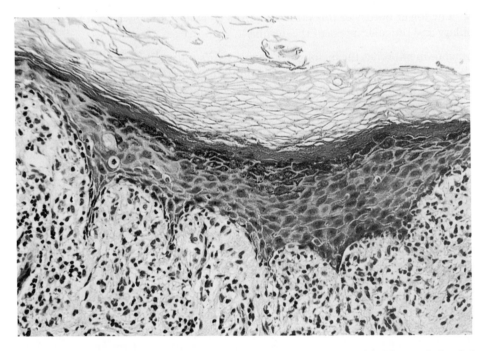

Fig. 7.13 Lichen planus (involuting lesion). The hyperkeratosis, focal hyperplasia of the stratum granulosum and the saw-tooth appearance of the lower border of the epidermis are still clearly visible. Foci of liquefaction degeneration of the basal layer are seen. The dermal infiltrate is reduced in quantity and patchy in distribution.

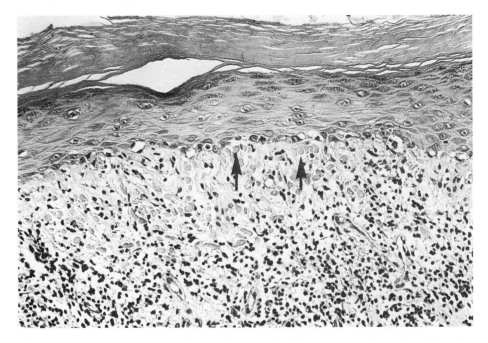

Fig. 7.14 Lichen planus (involuting lesion). Hyperkeratosis and focal hyperplasia of the stratum granulosum can still be seen although in this example the dermo-epidermal junction has become flattened. Numerous rounded hyalinised bodies (Civatte bodies) (arrowed) can be seen in the upper dermis.

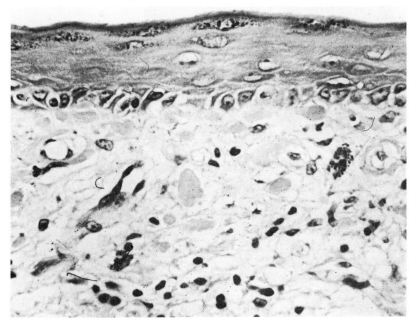

Fig. 7.15 Lichen planus (late lesion). The epidermis is rather atrophic but the stratum granulosum is prominent. There is some liquefaction degeneration of the stratum basale. Civatte bodies are prominent, and macrophages containing melanin granules can be seen in the upper dermis.

macrophages in the upper part of the dermis (Fig. 7.15). This presumably results from phagocytosis of the melanin granules released by the basal cells disrupted by liquefaction degeneration. Again this is not specific for lichen planus and can occur with the other conditions associated with liquefaction degeneration of the basal layer, such as lupus erythematosus. Even at this late stage of lichen planus the hyperkeratosis and focal hyperplasia of the stratum granulosum are still recognisable. The epidermis is usually thinned but in places still retains its saw-tooth appearance. Drug eruptions due to the antimalarial drugs, or following the use of photographic colour developers, produce a lichen-planus-like eruption which is histologically indistinguishable from true lichen planus.

While the histological diagnosis of lichen planus may be relatively straightforward in the fully developed lesion, it may be extremely difficult to distinguish an involuting one from discoid lupus erythematosus. Both conditions exhibit hyperkeratosis and while this is usually

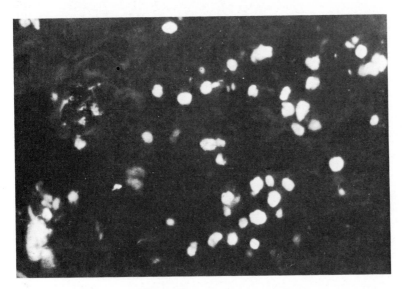

Fig. 7.16 Colloid bodies shown by immunofluorescence technique staining with labelled antibody to human IgM.

follicular in lupus erythematosus this distinction is not absolute. Wedge-shaped focal increase in the stratum granulosum favours a diagnosis of lichen planus but again this is not absolute. Both conditions show liquefaction degeneration of the basal layer but while in lichen planus this is usually continuous and in lupus erythematosis it tends to be patchy. This feature cannot therefore be relied upon to separate the conditions. The presence of hyaline degeneration of epidermal cells and of numerous colloid bodies in the upper dermis favours a diagnosis of lichen planus rather than lupus erythematosus, but again this is not a feature on which to base a definitive diagnosis. Thus, in some cases, differentiation by routine histological methods between the two is impossible. Fortunately, they can be separated by immunofluorescent staining, as a coarse band of immunoglobulin is deposited in the basement membrane zone in lupus erythematosus (Chapter 11). This is not usually seen in lichen planus, but numerous colloid bodies are a frequent finding (Fig. 7.16). These colloid bodies are best seen with antibody to IgM, when they appear as striking clumps or clusters, resembling a bunch of grapes.

Lichen nitidus

This condition may coexist with lichen planus and give rise to both clinical and pathological confusion. In fact, however, the conditions can be easily distinguished. Clinically the lesions are small, glistening, almost translucent papules and are usually non-itchy. Histological examination of one of these reveals a normal epidermis overlying discrete small granulomata set high in the papillary dermis with only a thin normal Grenz zone under the epidermis. A

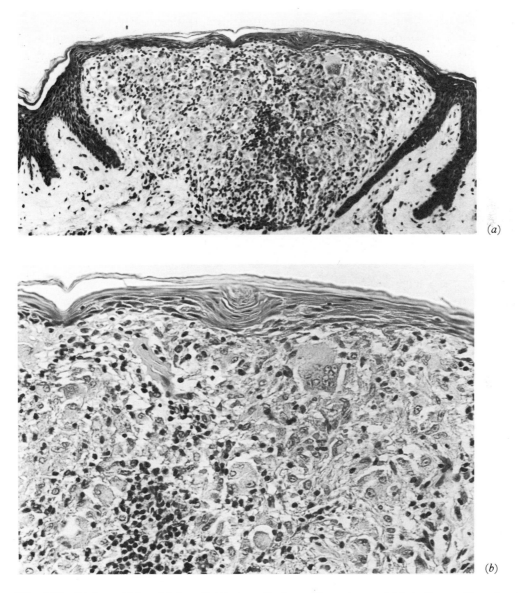

(a)

(b)

Fig. 7.17 Lichen nitidus. (*a*) A well-circumscribed granuloma is seen high in the papillary dermis with a claw-like invagination of epidermis at either side. (*b*) Higher magnification view. The Langhans-type giant cells are clearly seen in the infiltrate. Although somewhat thinned, the overlying epidermis is otherwise normal.

few Langhans-type giant cells may be present. On occasion these lesions appear to stretch the epidermis, giving it an attenuated appearance (Fig 7.17). The overlying epidermis is relatively normal with no evidence of basal cell degeneration or colloid body formation.

Graft versus host disease

Both acute and chronic cutaneous manifestations of this rare but important condition are currently recognised. They are arbitrarily subdivided into lesions occurring before 100 days post marrow transplant, and those developing after this time. Frequently, however, the two conditions merge. In the acute phase a lichen-planus-like eruption is seen clinically with striking involvement of the mucous membranes and the palms and soles (Fig. 7.18). The

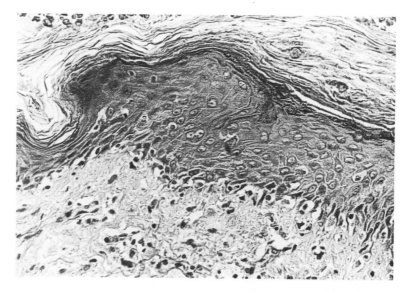

Fig. 7.18   Early lichenoid reaction in acute graft versus host disease. Note gross overlying hyper-keratosis, loss of normal polarity of cells of the epidermis and liquefaction degeneration of cells in the basal layer.

histological picture is that of a lichenoid tissue reaction with liquefaction degeneration of the basal layer.[12] The phenomenon of *satellite cell necrosis* has frequently been observed in the epidermis (Fig. 7.19). This term describes a lymphocyte in close apposition to a necrotic keratinocyte, and is strong supportive evidence of graft versus host disease. It is not, however, pathognomonic of the condition.

The late chronic form of graft versus host disease presents with a picture similar to generalised morphoea (scleroderma). Histologically there may be a persisting lichenoid pattern, but in addition there is evidence of destruction of adnexal structures and damage and shrinkage of dermal collagen.[13] At this stage satellite cell necrosis is not a common feature.

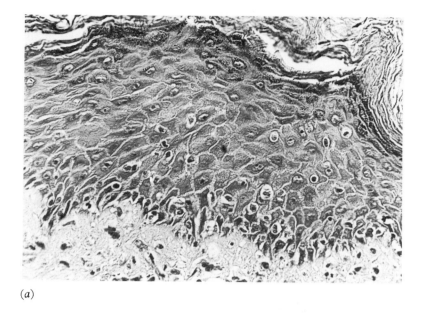

(a)

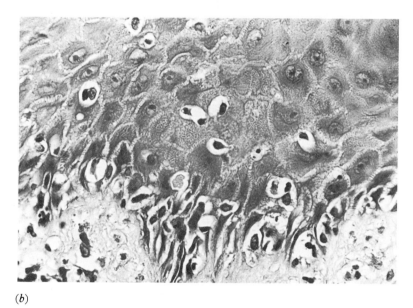

(b)

Fig. 7.19   Graft versus host disease. A more advanced case than that seen in Fig. 7.18 is shown. (a) Note the infiltration of lymphocytic cells into the epidermis and once again the underlying liquefaction of the basal layer. (b) Higher magnification view, showing clearly the 'satellite cell necrosis' which has been described in graft versus host diseases. A lymphocyte is seen in close apposition to a necrotic cell, presumably an epidermal keratinocyte. Two good examples of this are seen here.

References

1. Weinstein GD, Frost P. Abnormal cell proliferation in psoriasis. *J Invest Dermatol* 1968; **50:** 254-9.
2. Duffill M, Wright N, Shuster S. The cell proliferation kinetics of psoriasis examined by three *in vivo* techniques. *Br J Dermatol* 1976; **94:** 355-62.
3. Pinkus H, Mehregan AH. The primary histologic lesion of seborrhoeic dermatitis and psoriasis. *J Invest Dermatol* 1966; **46:** 109-16.
4. Baker H, Ryan TJ. Generalised pustular psoriasis. A clinical and epidermological study of 104 cases. *Br J Dermatol* 1968; **80:** 771-93.
5. Perry HO, Mayne JG. Psoriases and Reiter's syndrome. *Arch Dermatol* 1965; **92:** 129-36.
6. Burry JN, Kirk J. Lichenoid drug reaction from methyldopa. *Br J Dermatol* 1974; **91:** 475-6.
7. Skoven I, Thormann J. Lithium compound treatment in psoriasis. *Arch Dermatol* 1979; **115:** 1185-7.
8. Skegg DCG, Doll R. Frequency of eye complaints and rashes among patients receiving practolol and propranolol. *Lancet* 1977; **2:** 475-8.
9. DiGiovanna JJ, Aoyagi T, Taylor JR, Halprin KM. Inhibition of epidermal adenyl cyclase by lithium carbonate. *J Invest Dermatol* 1981; **76:** 259-63.
10. Ragaz A, Ackerman AB. Evolution, maturation and regression of lesions of lichen planus. *Am J Dermatopathol* 1981; **3:** 5-25.
11. Eady RAJ, Cowen T. Half and half cells in lichen planus. A possible clue to the origin and early formation of colloid bodies. *Br J Dermatol* 1978; **98:** 417-23.
12. Sale GE, Lerner KG, Barker EA, Shulman HM, Thomas ED. The skin biopsy in the diagnosis of acute graft versus host disease in man. *Am J Pathol* 1977; **89:** 621-33.
13. Shulman HM. Chronic cutaneous graft versus host disease in man. *Am J Pathol* 1978: **91:** 545-70.

8

Cutaneous Infection and Infestation

Although it is unusual to diagnose cutaneous infection—either bacterial or viral—by skin biopsy, this may be carried out on occasions when the diagnosis is in doubt, and while the appropriate bacteriological or serological tests are awaited. Two main areas of confusion arise. The first is in the differentiation between bacterial or viral infection giving rise to blisters and the immunobullous conditions discussed in Chapter 12. The second is between viral infections which cause benign hyperplasia and early epidermal malignancy. Chronic reactive changes due to persistence within the dermis of parts of biting insects or the scabies mite may also result in a histological picture mimicking early epidermal malignancy or cutaneous lymphoma. It is therefore important to be aware of these conditions. The wart virus, so long a rather tedious area of dermatology, has in the past decade been a subject of intensive and exciting research leading to the identification of several distinct types of papilloma virus with differing clinical expressions.[1] The current area of activity in this field is the accurate identification of subtypes of the human papilloma virus which have oncogenic potential. In the case of veneral warts, interaction between the human papilloma virus and herpes simplex is an area of particular interest.

Pyogenic infection of the skin

Impetigo contagiosa

This acute, superficial, bacterial infection of the skin is caused most often by the *Staphylococcus aureus*, although in a few instances by haemolytic streptococci. Histologically the lesion consists of a subcorneal pustule (Fig. 8.1) which is indistinguishable from subcorneal pustular dermatosis (Chapter 12).

Ecthyma

Ecthyma is another pyogenic infection of the skin which is usually seen in children with chronic skin disorders such as atopic dermatitis. The causal organism is usually a haemolytic streptococcus although a minority are staphylococcal in origin. The lesions are commonest on the lower limbs and buttocks, and while they bear a resemblance to impetigo they are obviously deeper-seated. When the superficial crusts are removed they leave shallow, punched-out ulcers. Sections show an acute pyogenic inflammatory process involving the epidermis and the upper dermis (Fig. 8.2). This heals by granulation tissue, leaving a small scar.

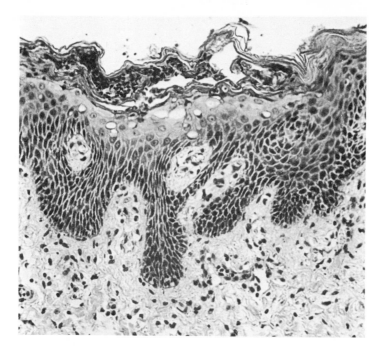

Fig. 8.1 Impetigo contagiosa. A small collection of neutrophil leucocytes, serous exudate, bacteria and cell debris is seen under the stratum corneum. There is an associated oedema of the dermis and a mild perivascular inflammatory infiltrate.

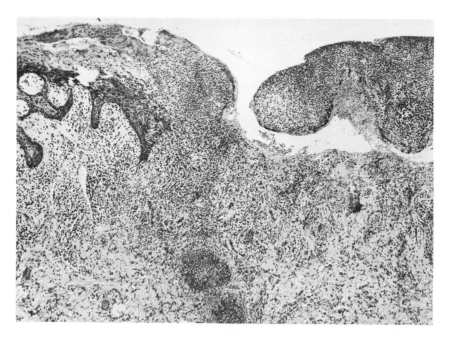

Fig. 8.2 Ecthyma. There is an ulcer in the centre of the field covered by the serous exudate containing many neutrophils. There is an acute pyogenic inflammation involving the upper and mid dermis. This lesion will heal by granulation tissue and, inevitably, leave a scar.

Staphylococcal pyogenic folliculitis

In this condition the pilosebaceous follicle is filled with pus (Fig. 8.3), and the surrounding dermis shows intense acute inflammation with vascular engorgement and dense polymorph infiltration. Should the inflamed follicle not discharge its contents rapidly through the duct opening, the wall disintegrates, allowing spread of infection into the surrounding dermis with the formation of a furuncle.

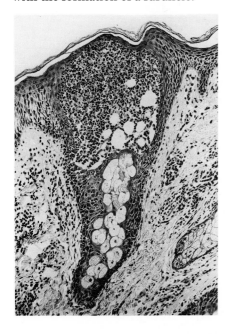

Fig. 8.3 Staphylococcal folliculitis. The upper portion of the pilosebaceous duct is dilated and filled with pus. There is some spongiosis of the surrounding epidermis and the related dermis shows acute inflammatory cell infiltrate.

Staphylococcal scalded skin syndrome[2]

This condition is characterised by superficial peeling of the skin associated with erythema and pain. It is most commonly seen in children and is now regarded as being identical with the condition named pemphigus neonatorum (Ritter's disease). It is associated with infection by *Staphylococcus aureus*, mainly of phage type 71.

Histological examination of the early lesion reveals a characteristic picture. At the level of the stratum granulosum a split appears in the epidermis and this is widened by an accumulation of serous fluid (Fig. 8.4). An occasional acantholytic-like cell may be seen in the floor of the lesion. Such cells tend to be elongated and lack the 'rounded off' appearance of the true acantholytic cell.

There is confusion in the literature regarding the histology of this condition. Much of it is due to the fact that biopsies are taken from old lesions at a time when secondary degenerative changes occur in the epidermal cells. A striking feature of the early lesion is the almost complete lack of cellular inflammatory response. In view of this it would appear that the lesions are not the result of actual staphylococcal invasion of the skin but are caused by a diffusible bacterial toxin.

In the past, reports of this condition have on occasion been confused with toxic epidermal necrolysis (TEN) (p. 217). This is easily distinguished on biopsy as the split in TEN is at the dermo-epidermal junction.

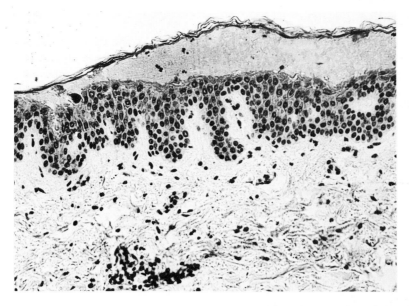

Fig. 8.4 Staphylococcal scalded skin syndrome. Note the elevation of the cornified layer above the surface of the rest of the epidermis and the collection of the serous fluid under this with a few neutrophils in the fluid. The rest of the dermis and epidermis shows remarkably little change other than dermal oedema. This picture illustrates well the site of action of the staphylococcal toxin. (Section by courtesy of Dr A. Lyell, Glasgow.)

Cutaneous viral infections causing epidermal necrosis

The viruses most commonly responsible for vesiculobullous changes in the epidermis and associated epidermal necrosis are herpes simplex, herpes zoster, varicella/variola and orf. The histological picture produced by these viruses is essentially similar, and differentiation must therefore be made on clinical, ultrastructural or serological grounds.

The earliest histological changes are an increase in size and chromatin content of individual keratinocyte nuclei in the basal and mid zone of the epidermis. The nuclei enlarge so as to almost fill the cytoplasm. After this has happened the cell itself enlarges, and some cells are seen to contain more than one nucleus (Fig. 8.5). Beyond this stage the cytoplasm becomes oedematous and the cell has a bloated appearance (balloon degeneration). Such cells eventually die but the cell walls often remain to form an irregular lattice-work stretching from the base to the roof of the vesicle (reticular degeneration). The fully formed lesion shows an intraepidermal bulla in which are floating altered epithelial cells (some showing balloon degeneration), leucocytes and cell debris. At the base or sides of the bulla may be seen the swollen hyperchromatic nuclei (Fig. 8.6). Secondary bacterial infection may soon mask the picture although it is usually still possible to distinguish the enlarged hyperchromatic nuclei (Fig. 8.7). Where there is no secondary infection, dermal inflammatory infiltrate is scanty.

Writers on the subject maintain that staining for viral inclusions will show them to be confined to the nucleus in herpes simplex, herpes zoster and varicella, whereas in variola inclusion bodies are said to be intracytoplasmic with only a few intranuclear ones. This is not always the case—in herpes zoster in particular both intracytoplasmic and intranuclear

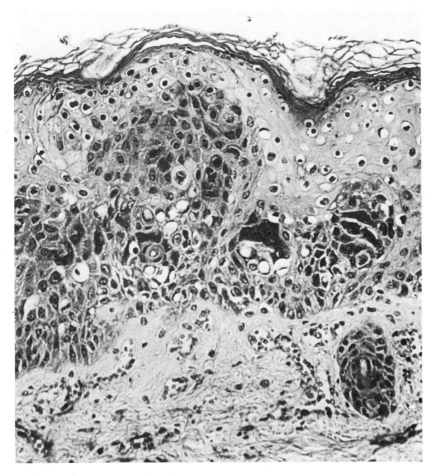

Fig. 8.5 Varicella (early lesion). Note the swelling of the keratinocytes and the enlargement and hyperchromatism of the nuclei in the lower and mid zones of the epidermis. Some keratinocytes contain two hyperchromatic nuclei. Many keratinocytes in the upper layers of the epidermis are vacuolated and contain pyknotic nuclei. (Section by courtesy of Dr A. Gibson, Glasgow.)

inclusions may be seen (Fig. 8.8). It may be that the location of the viral inclusions is related to age of the lesion rather than to specific affinities on the part of the virus.

Cutaneous viral infections causing epidermal hyperplasia

Molluscum contagiosum

This condition is caused by a pox virus closely related to the variola and paravaccinia group but gives rise to a quite distinct clinical picture. It is most commonly seen in young children and presents as clusters of raised pearly pink papules, each with a distinct central punctum. These are rarely biopsied as they are easily identified, and the more common histological

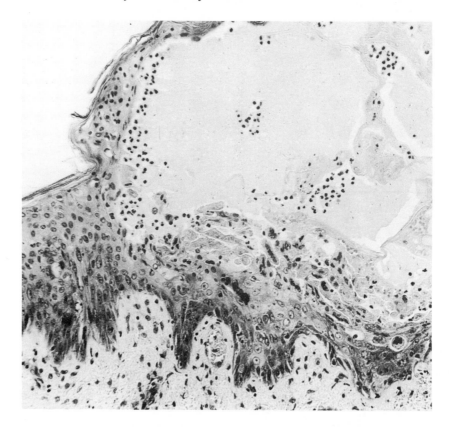

Fig. 8.6 Varicella (fully formed lesion). The bulla cavity is filled with serous exudate in which inflammatory cells and degenerate keratinocytes can be seen. Note the swollen keratinocytes with enlarged hyperchromatic nuclei in the base of the lesion and in the lower epidermis to the left of the actual blister.

specimen is an isolated lesion in an adult which may grow rapidly and be confused with a keratoacanthoma or basal cell carcinoma.

The central portion is formed by a lobulated mass of acanthotic epidermis with the normal epidermis at the periphery of the lesion running upwards and inwards, forming a shoulder. The invaginations of the acanthotic epidermis compress and seem to pull the dermal papillae upwards between them. In the centre of each pear-shaped lobule, as though extruded through the pore, are the elongated, deeply basophilic molluscum bodies. Sometimes in the basal layer but invariably just above it in the acanthotic epidermis there are inclusions. They are most easily seen half way up in the epidermis as well-defined acidophilic intracytoplasmic inclusions (Fig. 8.9) which eventually completely fill the cell, pushing the compressed nucleus to one side. As the cells ascend in the epidermis the inclusions alter their staining affinities to become more basophilic, at the level of the stratum granulosum or just beneath it. This basophilia increases until the inclusions are cast off as molluscum bodies.

No diagnostic difficulties should be encountered with this condition if the biopsy is orientated properly; otherwise, an oblique cut through the acanthotic epidermis may produce strands of what appears to be an epithelial tumour invading the dermis (Fig. 8.10). This

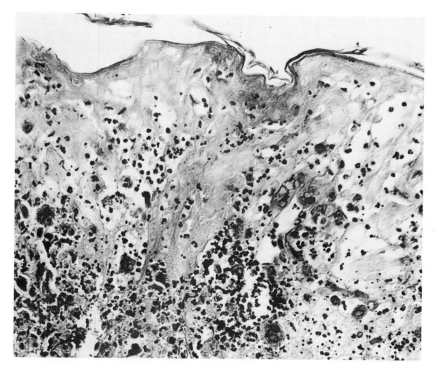

Fig. 8.7 Herpes zoster (old lesion). Although the epidermis is necrotic and infiltrated by inflammatory cells the enlarged hyperchromatic nuclei can still be seen.

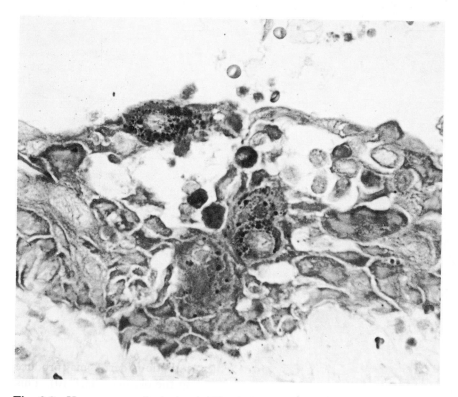

Fig. 8.8 Herpes zoster (inclusions). The darkly staining viral inclusions are predominantly cytoplasmic but an occasional intranuclear inclusion can be seen. Dilute Giemsa.

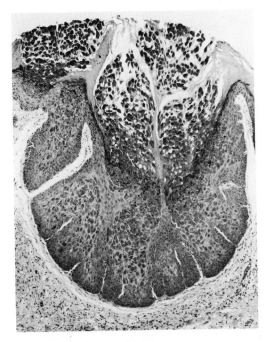

(a)

Fig. 8.9 Molluscum contagiosum. (*a*) The lobulated acanthosis of the epidermis and the slit-like compression of the dermal papillae are evident. Eosinophilic inclusions can be seen in the cytoplasm of the keratinocytes above the stratum basale. On the surface the basophilic molluscum bodies are being extruded through the pore. (*b*) Higher magnification view of lower right quadrant. Small, eosinophilic intracytoplasmic inclusions can be seen in some of the keratinocytes just above the stratum basale. These inclusions increase in size and about half way up the epidermis they can be seen pushing the nucleus to one side of the cell (arrowed). The inclusions near the surface are more darkly stained (basophilic)

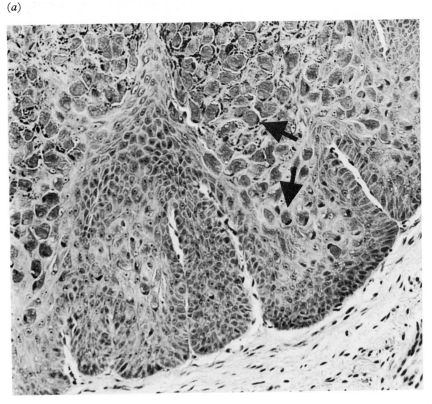

(b)

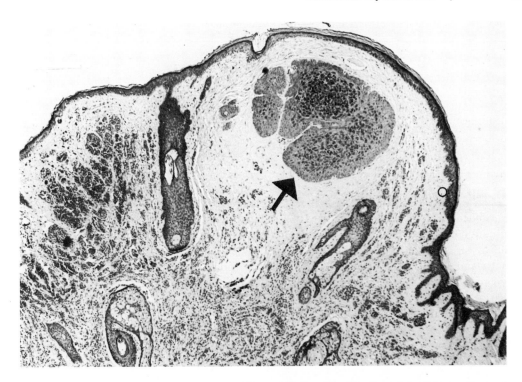

Fig. 8.10 Molluscum contagiosum. An oblique cut through the edge of the lobulated acanthotic epidermis produces an isolated strand of epithelium, containing darkly staining molluscum bodies, apparently invading the papillary dermis (arrowed). In this case the molluscum contagiosum was superimposed on a benign intradermal pigmented naevus, which can be seen to the left of the picture.

impression will at times be reinforced by the fact that no connection with the epidermis can be found.

In the solitary type encountered in the adult, secondary pyogenic bacterial infection may destroy so much of the lesion as to leave only fragments of epithelium or a few molluscum bodies, making a diagnosis difficult.

Viral warts

These common clinical problems are the result of infection with a group of DNA viruses, the human papilloma viruses (HPV). Extensive research in the past decade has demonstrated at least 16 distinct viruses, many of which give rise to distinct clinical pictures. Table 8.1 indicates the currently identified viruses. It has recently been suggested that these different viruses may give rise to histologically distinct patterns, but identification of these patterns certainly requires considerable experience of the study of HPV-infected epidermis.[3]

Verruca vulgaris This is the common wart of children and, while it can occur anywhere on the skin surface and on mucous membranes, it is most often seen on the fingers.

There is marked acanthosis and hyperkeratosis of the involved epidermis demarcated at each side by an elongated rete ridge which curves inwards almost enclosing the involved

Table 8.1 Clinical varieties of wart and type of HPV identified

Verruca vulgaris	HPV 1, 2 + 4	
'Butcher's wart'	HPV 7	
Verruca plana	HPV 3 + 10	
Epidermodysplasia verruciformis	{ HPV 5 + 8	Associated with carcinoma development
	HPV 3 +10	As yet no progression to carcinoma
Condyloma acuminatum	HPV 6	
Laryngeal papilloma	HPV 11	

area (Fig. 8.11). Within this area all the tips of the rete ridges tend to point towards the centre. The dermal papillae thus appear to radiate outwards from a central point. Closer examination of the spinous layer reveals columns of cells in its upper portion which, in the region of the stratum granulosum, have an empty vacuolated appearance with distorted, pyknotic and even fragmented nuclei. The cells in the stratum granulosum which are not vacuolated contain large irregular masses of keratohyalin. Overlying the streaks of vacuolated cells are columns of cornified cells containing spherical basophilic inclusions (Fig. 8.12), reminiscent of parakeratosis. The spherical nature of the inclusions, however, differentiates

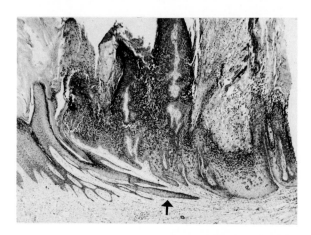

Fig. 8.11 Verruca vulgaris. This view shows the central acanthosis and hyper-keratosis, sharply demarcated from the normal epidermis by the elongated curved rete ridge (arrowed) pointing towards the centre of the lesion.

them from the flattened nuclei of parakeratotic cells. These pseudonucleated columns of stratum corneum alternate with columns of hyperkeratosis. In about half the cases of verruca vulgaris, in addition to the basophilic fragmentation of the nucleus (presumably due to viral invasion of the nucleus), many of the cells are packed with angular fragments of highly eosinophilic hyaline material (Fig. 8.13). While electron microscope and other studies have demonstrated the viral nature of the basophilic structures, the question as to whether the eosinophilic cytoplasmic 'inclusions' are aggregates of virus particles has not been fully settled.

Verruca plantaris   The histological appearances of verruca plantaris are essentially similar in detail to those of verruca vulgaris.

Verruca plana   In contrast to verruca vulgaris this lesion appears as a slightly elevated, smooth, flat-topped, angular, skin-coloured or brownish papule.

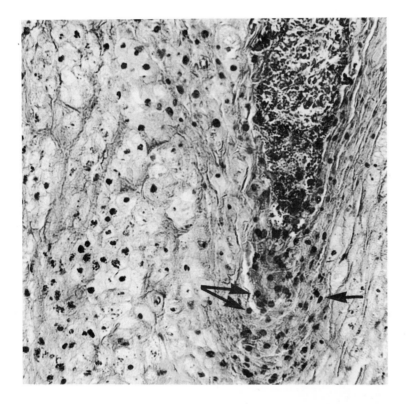

Fig. 8.12 Verruca vulgaris. This picture shows the vacuolated appearance of the cells in the region of the stratum granulosum and the distortion of their nuclei. To the right is a column of stratum corneum cells containing spherical basophilic nuclei inclusions (arrowed).

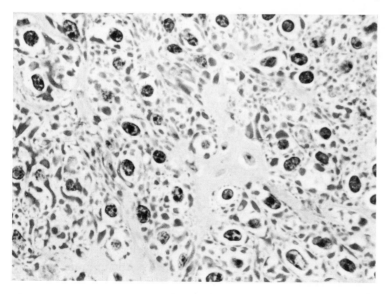

Fig. 8.13 Verruca vulgaris. The cytoplasm of the keratinocytes containing angular-shaped fragments of strongly eosinophilic material.

Sections show a moderate acanthosis with broadening of the rete ridges and some flattening of the dermal papillae. The acanthosis is most pronounced in the centre of the lesion and tapers off towards the periphery, to merge imperceptibly with the normal epithelium. In the upper epidermis and the stratum granulosum the most noticeable feature is the presence of vacuolated cells with small dense nuclei. Sometimes there are also small areas of thickened stratum granulosum and these contain the large angular basophilic masses seen in verruca vulgaris. In a fully developed lesion, irrespective of site, the stratum corneum shows an exaggerated basket-weave appearance (Fig. 8.14). No inclusions are seen in the cells of the stratum corneum.

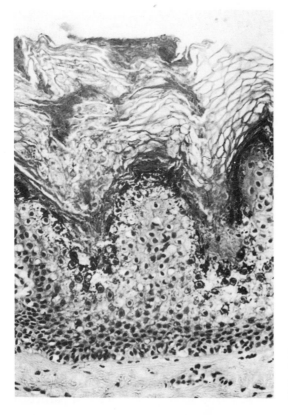

Fig. 8.14 Verruca plana. Vacuolated cells are seen in the upper layers of the acanthotic epidermis. Note the basket-weave appearance of the stratum corneum.

Genital warts (condylomata acuminata)[4]   These lesions do not generally show gross histological evidence of viral invasion. They are characterised by rapid growth and striking appearance. They are found in the perianal and vulvar regions and the glans penis. On histological examination they show marked acanthosis with elongation of the dermal papillae. Hyperkeratosis is variable but rarely marked. In the upper layers of the acanthotic epidermis there is a mild intercellular oedema. By contrast, intracellular oedema is usually marked, the cells of the stratum spinosum being enlarged to about twice their normal size and appearing much paler than normal (Fig. 8.15). There is considerable increase in mitotic activity, commensurate with their rapid growth.

The cauliflower-like configuration of these lesions means that an oblique cut through some of the acanthotic ridges is almost inevitable. The resulting areas of what seems

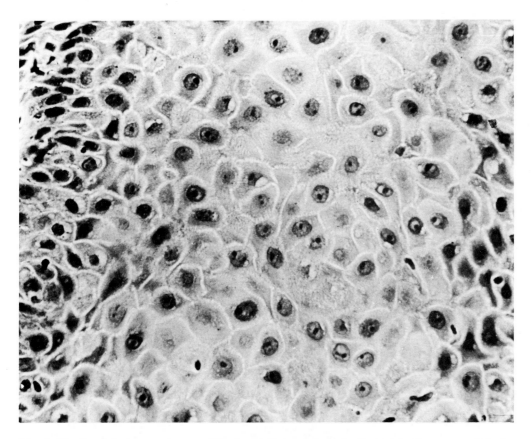

Fig. 8.15 Condyloma acuminatum. The intracellular oedema (pallor) and enlargement of the keratinocytes in the centre of this picture are clearly seen. There is also a mild intercellular oedema as evidenced by the prominent intercellular bridges running between adjacent keratinocytes.

proliferating epithelium, apparently unattached to the epidermis, seen in conjunction with the increased mitotic activity, may be mistaken for infiltrating squamous carcinoma.

Giant condylomata of Buschke and Loewenstein These lesions appear to be grossly enlarged genital warts and are presumed to have a viral aetiology. They are of particular interest in that malignant transformation has been reported in a small percentage of cases and the possibility of virus acting as a co-factor in carcinogenesis has therefore been postulated. The majority do not undergo true malignant change but tend to be relentlessly locally recurrent after excision or other forms of therapy. This is particularly true of lesions occurring in patients who are immunosuppressed.

Epidermodysplasia verruciformis[5] This rare, genetically determined condition is characterised by multiple warts on all body surfaces. HPV 3, 5, 8 and 10 have been located within these lesions and malignant transformation is associated at present only with HPV 5 and 8. Identification of the HPV type in these patients is thus of practical value in management.

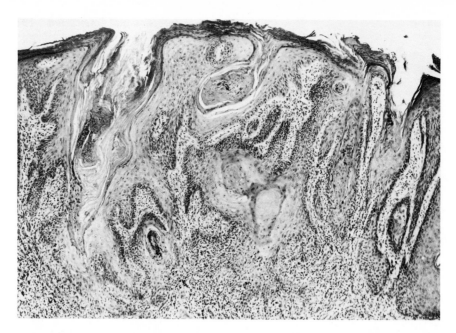

Fig. 8.16 Persistent insect bite. The surface is covered by a parakeratotic scale and there is a marked irregular acanthosis of the epidermis which appears to be 'invading' the upper dermis (pseudoepitheliomatous hyperplasia—Chapter 14). The details of the cellular dermal infiltrate are not apparent at this magnification.

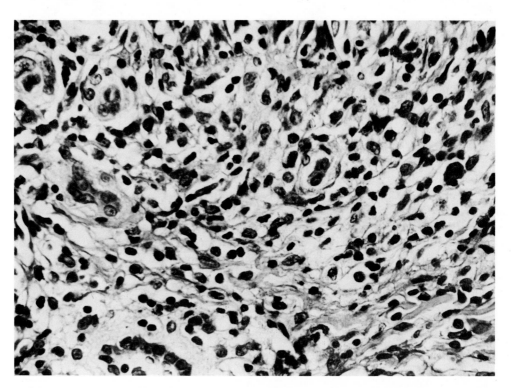

Fig. 8.17 Persistent insect bite. The dermal infiltrate is extensive and pleomorphic. It consists of lymphocytes, histiocytes, eosinophils and large, atypical mononuclear cells with hyperchromatic, often indented nuclei. These features may be easily mistaken for a malignant lymphoid neoplasm.

Persistent insect bite

Some individuals produce a peculiar and persistent reaction to the bites of certain insects which leave their biting parts in the host. The lesions are often solitary and continue to grow slowly over a period of months or years. Because of this they are often excised as possible neoplasms. Sections usually show a complex acanthosis. Because at first glance it seems to invade the upper dermis (Fig. 8.16), it is usually referred to as pseudoepitheliomatous hyperplasia. The dermis is occupied by a dense cellular infiltrate composed of lymphocytes, histiocytes, many eosinophils and atypical-looking mononuclear cells with hyperchromatic nuclei. This picture may be suggestive of an early cutaneous lymphoma (Fig. 8.17). Careful search, however, fails to reveal any abnormal mitosis. Material of this type should be sectioned at multiple levels, and if one is fortunate portions of the insect's biting apparatus may be found, putting the diagnosis beyond doubt. More often one has to rely on the presence of the pseudoepitheliomatous hyperplasia, the character of the infiltrate and the solitary nature of the lesion, which combined are highly suggestive of persistent insect bite.

Scabies and persistent nodular scabies

The female of the parasitic species *Sarcoptes scabiei* burrows into the stratum corneum where she deposits her eggs. It is rare for a biopsy to be performed in a case of scabies as the diagnosis is usually made on clinical grounds. Occasionally a massive infestation with the parasite is encountered (Norwegian scabies) which may present as an exfoliative dermatitis. Examination of one of the exfoliated scales from such a case, cleared in xylol, will reveal many parasites. If a biopsy is taken, tunnels in the stratum corneum will be seen containing either the eggs or the female acarus (Fig. 8.18).

A more common reason for biopsy is the presence of persistent nodules some time after apparently successful therapy. These would appear to develop as a response to retained parts of the mite and may present diagnostic problems if the clinical history is inadequate. The lesions frequently show evidence of pyknotic lymphocytic cells with a high nuclear/cyto-plasmic ratio and mitotic figures. The differential diagnosis from early lymphoma may thus cause problems. It is assumed that these lymphocytes are antigenically activated as no report of subsequent malignant change has ever been recorded.

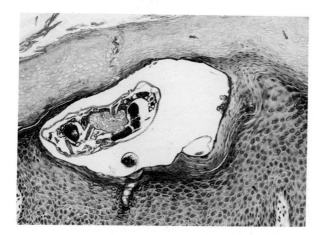

Fig. 8.18 Norwegian scabies. A tunnel is seen in the thick stratum corneum from this biopsy from the hand. Within the tunnel a cross-section of female aca-rus can be seen. (Section by courtesy of Dr F. Rickards, Lancaster.)

References

1. Orth G, Jablonska S, Breitburd F, Faure M, Croissant O. The human papilloma viruses. *Bull Cancer* 1978; **65**: 151–64.

2. Lowney ED, Baublis JV, Kreye GM, Harrell ER, McKenzie AR. The scalded skin syndrome in small children. *Arch Dermatol* 1967; **95**: 359–67.

3. Gross G, Pfister H, Hagedorn M, Gissmann L. Correlation between human papilloma virus type and histology of warts. *J Invest Dermatol* 1982; **78**: 160–4.

4. Dawson DF, Duckworth JK, Bernhardt H *et al.* Giant condylomata and verrucous carcinoma of the genital area. *Arch Pathol* 1965; **79**: 225–31.

5. Orth G, Jablonska S, Jasazabek-Chorzelska M, Obelez S, Rzese G, Faure M, Croissant O. Characteristics of the lesion and risk of malignant conversion associated with the type of human papilloma virus involved in epidermodysplasia verruciformis. *Cancer Res* 1979; **39**: 1074–82.

9

Granulomatous Inflammation of the Skin

Granulomatous inflammation of the skin includes a number of subacute or chronic inflammatory conditions in which the cellular infiltrate shows a tendency to form localised masses, often with a follicular arrangement. Essentially, a granulomatous process infers the presence of lymphocytes, plasma cells and epithelioid cells, frequently with the addition of varied types of multinucleated giant cells in varying numbers.

The causes of granulomatous infiltration are many, but fortunately the histological arrangement of the constituent elements is frequently such that in many cases a pattern is seen which permits conditional diagnosis of such conditions as tuberculosis, syphilis, leprosy and certain deep fungal infections, as well as sarcoidosis and the palisading granulomata.

Note on multinucleated giant cells

Three types of multinucleated giant cell are encountered in granulomatous infiltrates. The cells are large (60-100 μm), contain multiple nuclei (3-30) and have a pale, eosinophilic cytoplasm. The three types probably are all formed in a similar fashion by cell fusion rather than by repeated nuclear division of histiocytes.[1]

1. *Langhans type*. This is probably the commonest variety seen in the follicular granulomata, and consists of an oval or circular cell with a peripheral rim of nuclei arranged in a horseshoe configuration (Fig. 9.1).

2. *Foreign body type*. These are, as their name suggests, seen as a reaction to particulate foreign matter in the tissues, such as silica, keratin or suture material. The cells tend to be irregular in shape and the nuclei are scattered at random throughout the cell (Fig. 9.2). Foreign material may be seen within the cytoplasm or lying free in the tissue surrounded by the giant cells.

3. *Touton giant cell*. These are seen most frequently in granulomata formed as a reaction to lipids (xanthoma). The cells are circular and contain a perfect ring of nuclei situated mid way between the centre of the cell and the periphery (Fig. 9.3). The central portion of the cytoplasm within the ring of nuclei has a homogeneous 'ground glass' appearance, while the cytoplasm at the periphery of the cell is granular and often vacuolated.

It must be clearly understood that the identification of any one of these three types is of no specific diagnostic importance. All three may occur in the same section. This is hardly surprising, as it is likely that all three are essentially 'foreign body' in character, their differing structure probably being related to the physicochemical nature of the foreign material.

135

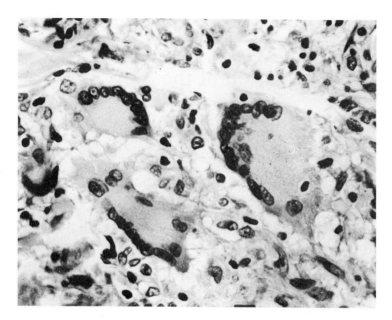

Fig. 9.1   Langhans-type giant cell. The peripheral rim of nuclei arranged in a horseshoe fashion can be clearly seen.

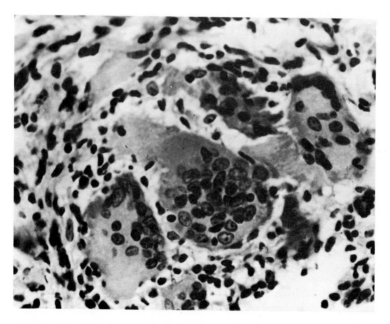

Fig. 9.2   Foreign-body-type giant cell. The nuclei in the central giant cell are arranged at random in the cytoplasm. To the right of centre there is a tendency in some cells to form the horseshoe arrangement seen in the Langhans type.

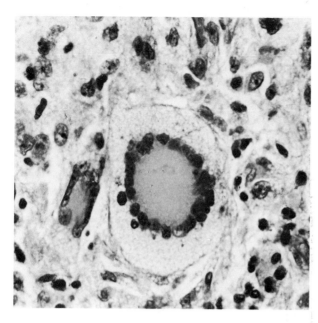

Fig. 9.3 Touton-type giant cell. This shows the characteristic 'ground glass' centre enclosed by a complete ring of nuclei, which in turn are surrounded by a zone of vacuolated, foamy cytoplasm.

The infective granulomata

This group is characterised by the formation of well-defined infiltrates composed of epithelioid cells, giant cells, lymphocytes and plasma cells in varying proportions. The central parts of these follicles may or may not show necrosis. The infecting agents are acid-fast bacilli, certain spirochaetes and some of the intermediate and deep fungi. It must be clearly stated at the outset, however, that all these agents can produce almost identical histological pictures. The final diagnosis must rest on the identification of the causative organism— preferably by culture—or indirectly by the appropriate serological investigations. A report which states that the histological appearances of a section are those of tuberculosis or one of the other infective granulomata must be questioned, unless it is supported by identification of the appropriate organism.

Cutaneous tuberculosis

Primary inoculation tuberculosis of the skin of children (equivalent to the Ghon focus) is rare in the UK. Inoculation tuberculosis in the immune or partially immune adult (tuberculosis verrucosa cutis) is still occasionally encountered. On histological examination such lesions show a varying degree of acanthosis of the epidermis, at times warty in character, and occasionally amounting to pseudoepitheliomatous hyperplasia. The dermal reaction varies from an acute inflammatory infiltrate composed mainly of polymorphonuclear leucocytes to a chronic lympho-histiocytic infiltrate which may contain follicular granulomatous lesions composed of epithelioid cells, giant cells and lymphocytes (Fig. 9.4). Small foci of caseation necrosis may be seen in the centres of some of the follicles. Prolonged search of sections (particularly where follicular granulomas are in evidence) stained by the Ziehl–Neelsen method may reveal an occasional acid/alcohol-fast bacillus. The finding of such organisms, however, cannot be regarded as diagnostic of tuberculosis and final proof must be obtained from culture or animal inoculation. Those lesions which show only an acute inflammatory

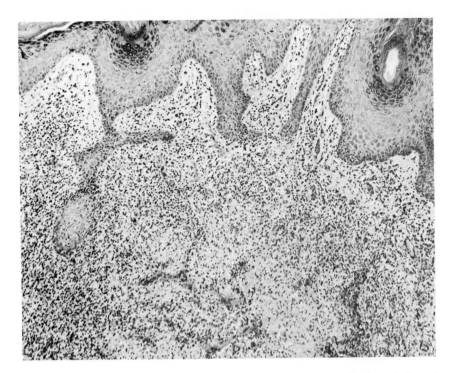

Fig. 9.4 Tuberculosis verrucosa cutis. The epidermis is acanthotic and there is a mild degree of pseudoepitheliomatous hyperplasia. The dermis contains a subacute inflammatory infiltrate in which are follicular aggregates of epithelioid cells. Early caseation necrosis can be seen in the follicles in the right lower portion of the photograph.

infiltrate can easily be misdiagnosed unless the histologist is alerted by the clinician to the possibility of a tuberculous infection.

Lupus vulgaris

While rare in incidence, this is probably the most common form of cutaneous tuberculosis now encountered and it occurs in susceptible individuals usually on the face and in infants on the lower limbs or buttocks. It consists of a soft yellow or reddish-brown nodule traditionally regarded as having an 'apple jelly' colour on diascopy. If untreated it tends to spread slowly by peripheral extension, while healing in the centre. The disease, if unchecked, may cause extensive scarring and tissue destruction.

Histological examination of an early lesion shows a well-defined follicular granuloma in the dermis composed of epithelioid cells, giant cells and a peripheral rim of lymphocytes (Fig. 9.5). This granulomatous inflammation often extends right up to the epidermis, gradually thinning it and eventually causing ulceration. This encroachment of the epidermis by the granulomatous infiltrate is suggestive of lupus vulgaris and when present can be helpful in its differentiation from sarcoidosis and leprosy. Unfortunately, involvement of the epidermis with ulceration may also occur in tertiary syphilis and some of the fungal infections so that it cannot be regarded as diagnostic of lupus vulgaris. The centres of some of the follicular collections of epithelioid cells may show small foci of necrosis (Fig. 9.6) or

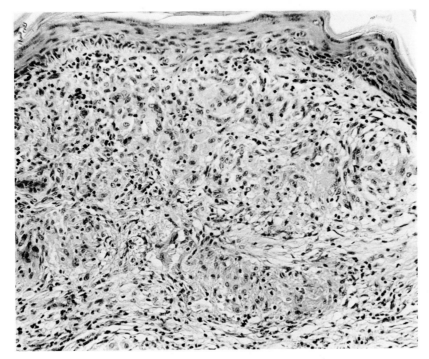

Fig. 9.5 Lupus vulgaris. Follicular aggregates in the dermis, composed of epithelioid cells, giant cells of Langhans type and, in this section, scanty peripheral lymphocytes, can be seen. Note that the granuloma extends to the underside of the epidermis.

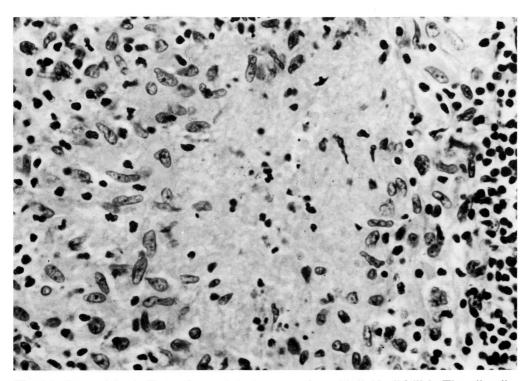

Fig. 9.6 Lupus vulgaris. Focus of necrosis in the centre of an epithelioid cell follicle. The cell outlines are lost and the nuclei pyknotic.

larger areas of caseation necrosis (Fig. 9.7). As such foci may occur in infective granulomata other than tuberculosis and even in sarcoidosis, they are not therefore diagnostic. Acid/alcohol-fast bacilli may, rarely, be found in appropriately stained sections and in this connection the use of the auramine O method plus fluorescent microscopy[2] allows rapid scanning of the section. Culture and animal inoculation permit definitive diagnosis but both are fraught with difficulties. The organism grows extremely slowly on artificial media and inoculated animals appear to thrive. If, however, the animal is sacrificed after 12–16 weeks, multiple follicular granulomata containing acid/alcohol-fast bacilli will usually be found in the viscera. In the absence of positive bacteriological proof the clinical picture, in conjunction with the histology and satisfactory response to specific chemotherapy, can be considered diagnostic.

Lupus vulgaris heals by fibrous scarring and may cause severe mutilation. Occasionally, after a period of 15–20 years, squamous carcinoma develops on the scarred areas. Whether this is a direct consequence of the scarring or is related to the methods of therapy (high-intensity ultraviolet lamp, destruction of tissue with acid nitrate of mercury) which were used before chemotherapy was available is not known.

Scrofuloderma

This term is used to describe direct infection of the skin from an underlying tuberculous infection of a lymph node, bursa or bone. It usually presents as an ulcer or sinus lined by pale, oedematous granulations. Sections show the lesion to be lined by chronically inflamed granulation tissue, often with numerous plasma cells. Follicular collections of epithelioid cells, giant cells and lymphocytes (Fig. 9.8) are seen. Caseation necrosis is often a prominent feature. Once again bacteriological proof or therapeutic response is necessary to confirm the diagnosis.

The tuberculides

In the past, a number of different eruptions have been grouped under this term on the assumption that either they were caused by haematogenous spread of tubercle bacilli in individuals with a high degree of immunity or they resulted from an allergic response to tuberculin. Such names as lichen scrofulosorum and lupus miliaris disseminatus faciei (the so-called rosacea-like tuberculid) can still be found in dermatological textbooks. These lesions were considered to be tuberculous because an epithelioid follicular granuloma was seen on histological examination and, as has been emphasised, this *per se* does not justify a diagnosis of tuberculosis. The so-called rosacea-like tuberculid, for example, is now considered to be related to papular rosacea.

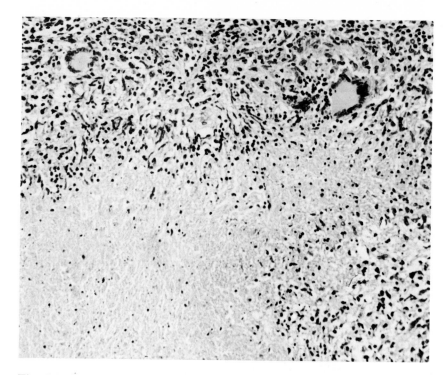

Fig. 9.7 Lupus vulgaris. An area of caseation necrosis containing numerous pyknotic nuclei is surrounded by a follicular granuloma with Langhans-type giant cells.

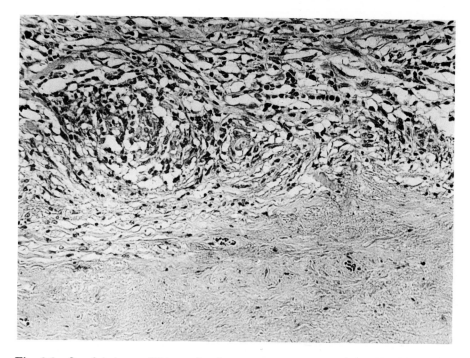

Fig. 9.8 Scrofuloderma. This section from a sinus track in the skin overlying tuberculous cervical glands shows an area of caseation necrosis surrounded by granulation tissue, in which can be seen rather poorly defined follicular granulomata composed mainly of epithelioid cells and lymphocytes.

Lupus miliaris disseminatus faciei, however, has a very distinctive histology. The dermis contains a confluent tuberculoid granuloma with central caseation, and when appropriately stained, a circle of elastic fibres is seen, probably representing the remains of a follicle.

Erythema induratum (Bazin's disease)

This now uncommon condition affects the backs of the calves of young and middle-aged persons, with a predominance in women. It consists of chronic persistent nodules which from time to time break down to form chronic, indurated discharging ulcers. Formerly thought to be a tuberculid, its aetiology remains unknown.

Sections from a lesion show an extensive area of inflammation in the dermis extending down to and involving the subcutaneous fat (Fig. 9.9). Depending on the age of the lesion, the fat shows changes varying from a subacute inflammatory infiltration to frank necrosis. Once fat necrosis has occurred the released lipid induces a foreign body granuloma which may include well-formed follicular aggregates of epithelioid cells and giant cells. Vascular involvement in the form of vasculitis or thrombosis is sometimes seen but, as the vessels affected are usually in the necrotic fat or running at the margin of it, it is not possible to assess whether the vascular lesion is cause or effect.

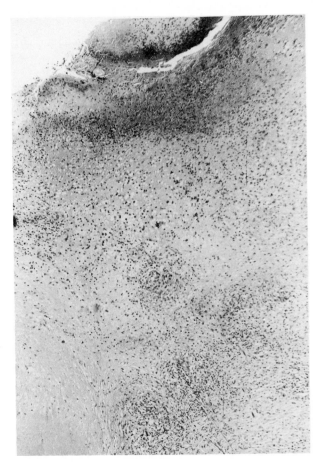

Fig. 9.9 Bazin's disease. There is ulceration of the epidermis. The dermis is occupied by a mass of caseous debris which is discharging on to the surface. At the bottom right of the picture is an area of granulation tissue containing a few poorly formed follicular aggregates of epithelioid cells and lymphocytes.

Papulonecrotic tuberculide

These lesions begin as small papules which break down, are slow to heal and, when they eventually do heal, leave a white atrophic scar.

If a section from an ulcerated lesion is examined, the histological findings are very reminiscent of those seen in pityriasis lichenoides acuta (Chapter 10). There is a wedge-shaped infarct of the dermis with ulceration of the overlying epidermis but without any free

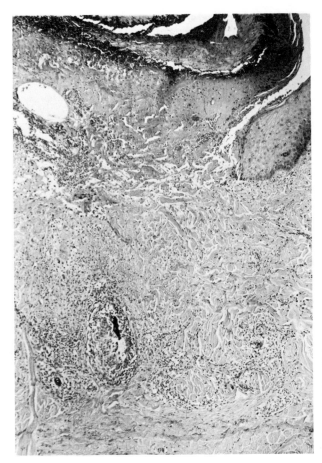

Fig. 9.10 Papulonecrotic tuberculide. The epidermis is ulcerated and the surface is covered by a serous crust. A wedge-shaped area of necrosis of the upper dermis can be seen and, at the apex of this, a well-defined follicle composed of epithelioid cells and lymphocytes.

haemorrhage (Fig. 9.10). Around the margins of the necrotic dermis, small, well-defined follicular collections of epithelioid cells and giant cells surrounded by a few lymphocytes are seen. Only the presence of the follicular granuloma separates this condition from pityriasis lichenoides acuta, as does the absence of free haemorrhage. It is, however, considered possible that the two conditions are related.

Swimming pool granuloma

Infection with some species of Mycobacterium (e.g. *M. balnei*, *M. kansasii*, *M. fortuitum*, *M. ulcerans*) which grow at low temperature may produce a clinical and histological picture suggestive of cutaneous tuberculosis. Infection is usually contracted following a minor abrasion while bathing in a swimming pool (hence the name). Lesions are commonest on the hands, elbows, knees and nose. They present either as slowly growing papules or nodules

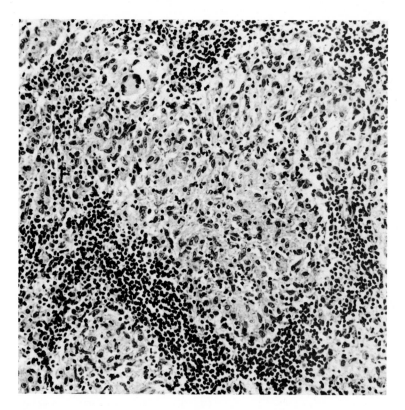

Fig. 9.11   Swimming pool granuloma. Follicles of epithelioid cells with an occasional giant cell of Langhans type can be seen surrounded by a heavy peripheral lymphocytic infiltrate. There is no necrosis. *Mycobacterium kansasii* was cultured from the lesion.

which soon become indolent ulcers. Secondary infections with pyogenic organisms is common.

Sections show in the dermis a rather poorly defined follicular granuloma, composed mainly of epithelioid cells with an occasional giant cell and a heavy peripheral lymphocytic infiltrate (Fig. 9.11). Necrosis is not a feature and acid/alcohol-fast bacilli are not usually seen. The diagnosis rests on the isolation of one of the atypical mycobacteria by the appropriate culture technique.

Syphilis

The histopathology of the primary syphilitic chancre is dealt with in detail in textbooks of

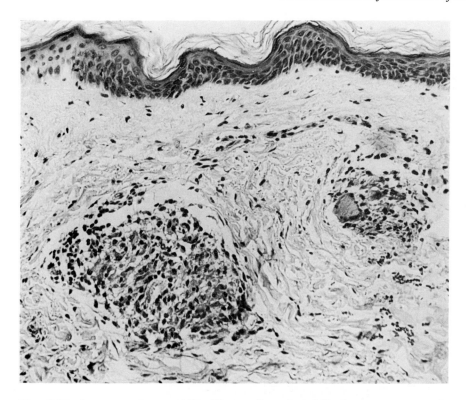

Fig. 9.12 Late secondary syphilis. Two well-marked follicular aggregations of epithelioid cells, lymphocytes and a giant cell of Langhans type can be seen in the mid dermis. No endarteritis is seen. The Wassermann reaction was strongly positive in this patient's serum.

general pathology and will not be discussed here. The histopathology of the various eruptions which constitute secondary syphilis is so variable and so often lacking in specific diagnostic features that histological diagnosis is unreliable. It is generally held that the plasma cell is the hallmark of the syphilitic tissue reaction. To a certain extent this is true, and if plasma cells are prominent syphilis must be considered in the differential diagnosis. It does not follow, however, that plasma cell infiltration is diagnostic of syphilis, as these cells may be seen in large numbers in conditions such as chronic sinus tracks. Conversely, it must be appreciated that absence or paucity of plasma cells does not exclude syphilis, as in the secondary or tertiary stages they may be hard to find. Figure 9.12 is a section from what was diagnosed as an 'atypical pityriasis rosea' of 4 months' duration. It shows well-marked follicular aggregates of epithelioid cells with an occasional giant cell and some peripheral lymphocytes. Neither plasma cells nor obliterative endarteritis are present. No organisms were seen in appropriately stained sections. Serology to exclude syphilis and a Kveim test were suggested. The Wassermann reaction was strongly positive and the lesions rapidly resolved with appropriate antibiotic therapy. Figure 9.13 is from a lesion of early tertiary syphilis and shows a follicular epithelioid granuloma with giant cells arranged around a pilosebaceous follicle. In this instance plasma cells were abundant but obliterative endarteritis absent. Because plasma cells were numerus, serology to exclude syphilis was again advised and found to be positive.

In the gumma of tertiary syphilis there is usually a large central area of caseation necrosis

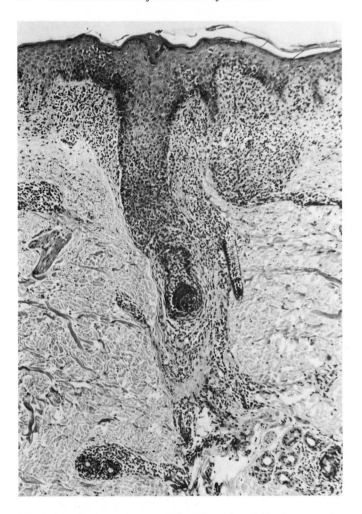

Fig. 9.13   Early tertiary syphilis. There is a follicular granulomatous infiltrate in the upper dermis which extends downwards as a sheath around the pilosebaceous follicle. The granuloma is composed of epithelioid cells, a few giant cells of the Langhans type, lymphocytes and plasma cells. The elongated body to the right of the hair bulb is an artefact.

(Fig. 9.14) surrounded by follicular granulomata composed of epithelioid cells, giant cells and, at the periphery, lymphocytes (Fig. 9.15). Eventually the granuloma involves the epidermis and ulceration follows. The epidermis at the margins of the gummatous ulcer often shows extreme hyperplasia (pseudoepitheliomatous hyperplasia: Chapter 14). Plasma cells may or may not be prominent. Obliterative endarteritis may be conspicuous but too much reliance should not be placed on this as most gummas occur in the middle and old age groups, when some degree of obliterative vascular disease is common. Plasma cells and obliterative endarteritis are also seen in some of the subcutaneous fungus infections.

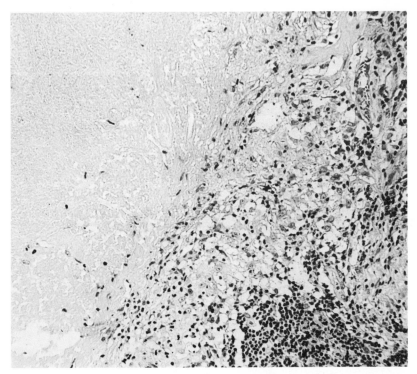

Fig. 9.14 Tertiary syphilis—gumma. A large area of caseation necrosis is surrounded by follicles of epithelioid cells and lymphocytes.

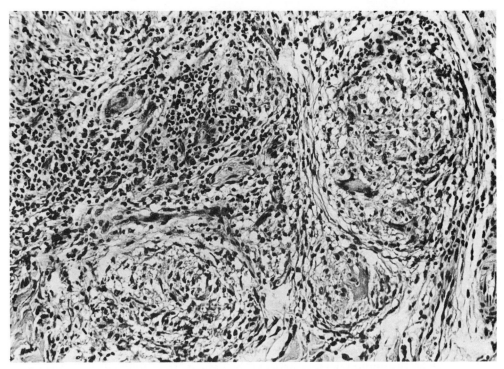

Fig. 9.15 Tertiary syphilis—gumma. This microphotograph from the inflammatory infiltrate at the margin of an area of caseation necrosis shows the follicles composed of epithelioid cells, Langhans-type giant cells and lymphocytes. Plasma cells were present in considerable numbers in this case but not obliterative endarteritis.

Fungus infections

Many of the fungus infections of the skin and subcutaneous tissues induce a follicular granulomatous reaction composed of epithelioid cells and giant cells. There is also a heavy infiltrate of lymphocytes, histiocytes and plasma cells. As in the syphilitic gumma of the skin, most of these granulomata are associated with pseudoepitheliomatous hyperplasia (Chapter 14). In lesions caused by some of the fungi (e.g. chromomycosis: Fig. 9.16) the organism can be seen in routine haematoxylin and eosin stained sections, but in those caused by *Sporotrichum* and *Cryptococcus*, among others, the periodic acid–Schiff (PAS) stain or other specific stain is needed to show the organisms. For details of the finer points of differentiation of these organisms the reader is referred to one of the numerous excellent textbooks of medical mycology.

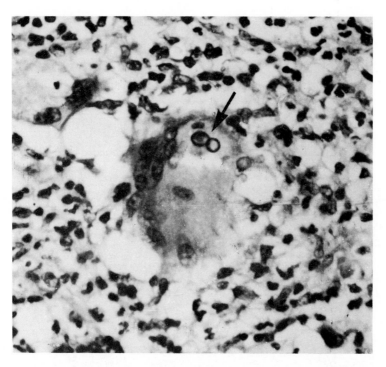

Fig. 9.16 Subcutaneous fungus infection—chromomycosis. The giant cell containing the thick-walled fungal cells (chlamydospores) (arrowed) is surrounded by an inflammatory infiltrate of lymphocytes, histiocytes and plasma cells. (Section by courtesy of Dr A.D. Bremner, Glasgow.)

Leprosy (Hansen's disease)

Leprosy is an infection of the Schwann cells of the peripheral nervous system by *Mycobacterium leprae*. Whether the organism gains direct access to the nerves through an abrasion in the overlying skin or whether it is carried there by the bloodstream from a distant site is still uncertain. The subsequent clinical picture and type of tissue response produced thereafter depend entirely on the immunological status of the patient. In individuals with low resistance, florid nodular lesions are produced (lepromatous leprosy) in skin, bone, mucous membranes and viscera, whereas in those with high resistance less dramatic lesions are confined to the skin and cutaneous nerves (tuberculoid leprosy). In persons whose immunological status fluctuates features of both lepromatous and tuberculoid types may be seen (dimorphous or borderline leprosy). An indeterminate type of leprosy is also described occurring in individuals whose immunological status is not defined. This type, although it may last for several years, is a phase in the development of one of the other three types.

Intradermal injections of lepromin, an antigen prepared from lepromatous leprosy (which is rich in *M. leprae*) is useful in estimating the degree of resistance of patients with leprosy. It is not a diagnostic test; a positive lepromin reaction indicates a high degree of resistance (tuberculoid leprosy) while a negative reaction indicates a low resistance (lepromatous leprosy). In dimorphous leprosy the lepromin reaction is negative as a rule, while in indeterminate leprosy both positive and negative reactions are seen.

Lepromatous leprosy   The lesions of lepromatous leprosy are composed of nodular aggregates of large vacuolated histiocytes (lepra cells or foam cells of Virchow) situated in the upper and middle parts of the dermis. These cells are usually separated from the epidermis by a narrow band of compressed collagen (Fig. 9.17). While the dermal infiltrate

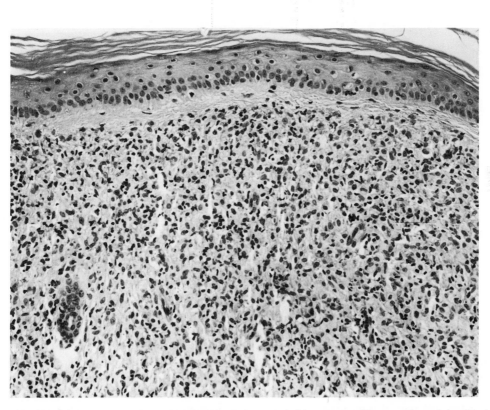

Fig. 9.17   Lepromatous leprosy. The dermis is occupied by a mass of large, pale-staining histiocytes with an admixture of small, darker-staining histiocytes and lymphocytes. Note that this infiltrate is separated from the epidermis by a narrow band of compressed dermal collagen.

is composed mainly of large macrophages with vacuolated foamy cytoplasm (Fig. 9.18), other cells (non-foamy small histiocytes, lymphocytes and occasional plasma cells) are also seen. Staining with modified Ziehl–Neelsen stain (Triff stain) reveals numerous acid-fast bacilli within the cytoplasm of the lepra cells (Fig. 9.19). The bacilli may be discrete or aggregated in globular clumps (globi). The cutaneous nerves are not involved by the inflammatory response although bacilli may be demonstrated in their Schwann cell sheaths.

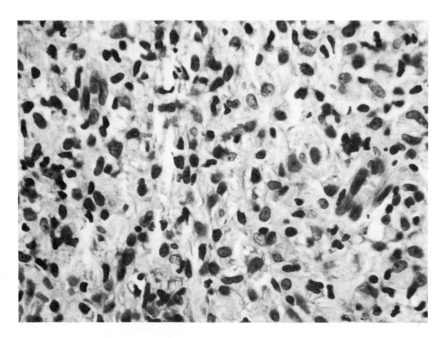

Fig. 9.18 Lepromatous leprosy. The vacuolated foamy appearance of the cytoplasm of the large histiocytes (foam cells of Virchow) can be seen at this magnification. Small histiocytes with darkly staining, indented nuclei and lymphocytes are scattered in between the foam cells.

Tuberculoid leprosy The histological features of this variety of leprosy consist of well-defined follicular granulomata composed largely of epithelioid cells and giant cells with a variable number of lymphocytes around the periphery (Fig. 9.20). Caseation necrosis in the centres of the follicles is not seen. The granulomata are scattered throughout the dermis, mainly in the vicinity of neurovascular bundles, and may be seen in dermal papillae adjacent to the epidermis. Acid-fast bacilli are not found in appropriately stained sections. The small nerve bundles in the subcutaneous fat and dermis should be examined for involvement of follicular granulomata; if necessary, multiple sections should be cut. The finding of nerve involvement makes a diagnosis of tuberculoid leprosy highly probable.

Dimorphous (borderline) leprosy The histology of dimorphous leprosy is intermediate between tuberculoid and lepromatous and shows features of both types. In the tuberculoid areas the follicle is composed mainly of epithelioid cells with many peripheral lymphocytes and few, if any, giant cells. In the lepromatous areas lepra bacilli may be demonstrated with the appropriate stain. The cutaneous nerves are involved by a granulomatous infiltrate and scanty acid-fast bacilli may be found.

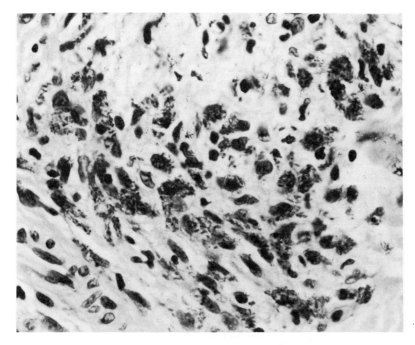

Fig. 9.19 Lepromatous leprosy. Abundant rod-shaped bacilli are seen both in clumps and discretely within the cytoplasm of the foamy histiocytes. Triff stain.

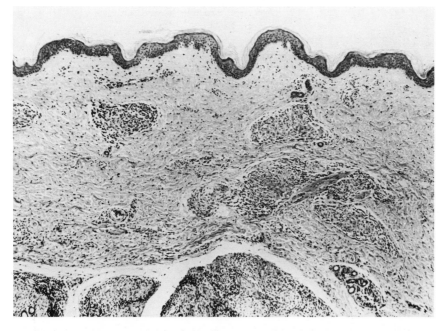

Fig. 9.20 Tuberculoid leprosy. Follicular granulomata composed of epithelioid cells, giant cells of Langhans type and a peripheral rim of lymphocytes are seen scattered throughout the dermis. No necrosis is seen in the follicular aggregates. Note the tendency for the granulomata to arrange themselves along the neurovascular bundles of the dermis.

Indeterminate leprosy The histological findings in this type in most instances are not diagnostic. There is a patchy lympho-histiocytic infiltrate in the dermis, mainly in relation to the skin appendages. The nerve bundles are devoid of inflammatory changes but in some cases scanty acid-fast bacilli are found after prolonged search. When searching for lepra bacilli in tissue great care must be taken with the staining as lepra bacilli are not so resistant to acid decolorisation as are tubercle bacilli. It is always advisable to stain at the same time a section known to contain abundant lepra bacilli which acts as a control.

Sarcoidosis

The view that sarcoidosis is a generalised disease, although still held by many, has been challenged, and the possibility that a form of the disease confined to the skin can occur, as well as a systematised form, has been raised.[3] The aetiology remains unknown, but it is accepted that a sarcoid-like tissue reaction can occur as a result of various stimuli (e.g. neoplasia, infections and foreign bodies, etc.) closely simulating the histology of true sarcoidosis.

The histology of the skin lesion, which may be a presenting feature of the generalised disease, has been aptly described as the 'naked granuloma'. Well-defined follicular arrangements of epithelioid cells with or without multinucleated giant cells and, unlike tuberculosis, devoid of any but a thin rim of lymphocytes at the periphery of the follicles (thus the term 'naked granuloma') are scattered through the dermis (Fig. 9.21). Caseation necrosis is not a feature of the sarcoid granuloma, and while the follicles tend to be scattered through the dermis without the same tendency to approach the undersurface of the epidermis as in lupus vulgaris, this is not an absolute finding. Some cases may be indistinguishable histologically,

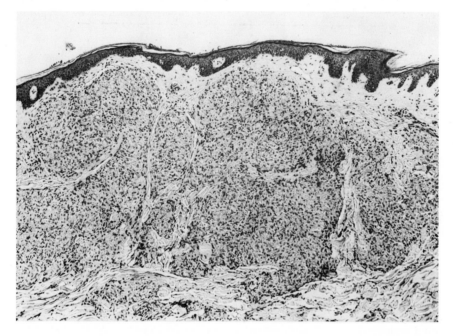

Fig. 9.21 Sarcoidosis. Follicular aggregates composed mainly of epithelioid cells with a scant peripheral rim of lymphocytes can be seen scattered haphazardly throughout the dermis.

and tuberculoid leprosy as well as foreign body granuloma must also be considered in the differential diagnosis. It is wise to report suspected cases of sarcoidosis in which a naked granuloma is found as showing a sarcoid-like granuloma and await the result of the Kveim test, one of the most important diagnostic tests.[4]

The Kveim test[5]   The Kveim antigen or reagent consists of a sterilised saline suspension of sarcoid tissue (preferably spleen) with an added preservative (usually phenol). The test is performed by the intradermal injection of 0.1 ml of this material, usually on the flexor aspect of the forearm, using a glass (not plastic) tuberculin syringe, kept solely for this purpose. The site of injection is fixed by a series of measurements from the bony points of the wrist, and carefully recorded. Some authors have suggested making a small tattoo mark at the site of the injection: this is to be avoided as the pigment may by itself induce the formation of a follicular granuloma (foreign body type).

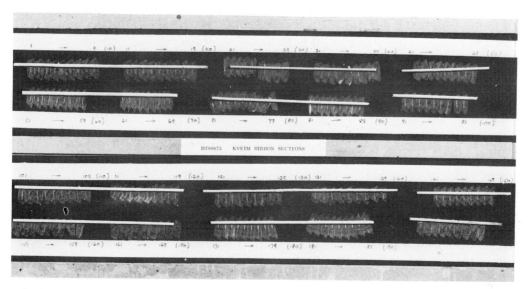

Fig. 9.22   Method of storing Kveim ribbons until the material has been sampled.

After a period of 6–12 weeks (earlier if a nodule has developed) the site of inoculation is excised and the specimen submitted in fixative to the laboratory.

Depending on size, the biopsy specimen is split in two after fixation. The tissue is embedded in wax and each block is then serially sectioned. The ribbons of paraffin sections are stored in order of cutting on slide trays and are held in place by orange sticks (Fig. 9.22). This normally produces two ribbons of approximately 300 sections each. Every tenth section is mounted and stained with haematoxylin and eosin for examination. If an indeterminate lesion is found, the neighbouring sections are stained and examined. Before reporting a negative Kveim test the sections from the entire excised area must be examined.

Care is necessary in the interpretation of a granulomatous reaction found at the site of a Kveim injection.

A true positive Kveim test consists of a well-formed follicular granuloma composed predominantly of epithelioid cells, with a few multinucleated giant cells of Langhans type and a scanty peripheral rim of lymphocytes (Fig. 9.23). This histological pattern may be seen in the absence of any obvious clinical lesion at the site of injection.

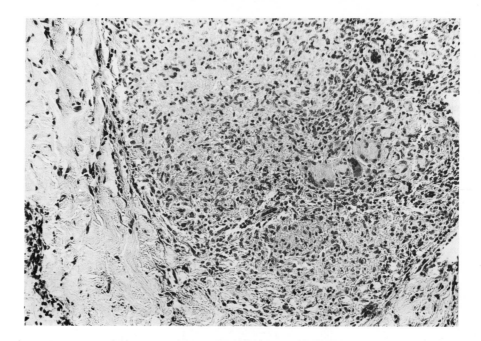

Fig. 9.23 Positive Kveim test. A well-defined follicular granuloma composed of epithelioid cells. Langhans-type giant cells and a scanty peripheral rim of lymphocytes is located in the mid dermis.

If the original injection has been made into the subcutaneous fat or the fat lobule supporting the secreting coils of the sweat glands, it may cause fat necrosis and the resulting follicular granuloma cannot be differentiated with certainty from that of a true positive Kveim. Such lesions in the fat should be regarded as false positive Kveim tests (Fig. 9.24). Should the original injection have been performed with a plastic syringe lubricated with silicone grease, a small follicular granuloma poor in epithelioid cells but with numerous foreign-body-type giant cells containing small oil droplets may be found (Fig. 9.25). Similar small granulomata in which the giant cells contain crystals of silica, doubly refractile when examined by polarised light, are sometimes seen even when glass tuberculin syringes have

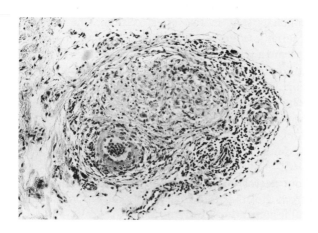

Fig. 9.24 False positive Kveim test. A small follicle composed of epithelioid cells and a foreign-body-type giant cell is seen in the upper part of the subcutaneous fat.

been used. Such foreign-body-type granulomata are interpreted as negative Kveim tests. If the Kveim antigen is injected while the patient is being treated with corticosteroids, the reaction may be suppressed. Treatment with corticosteroids may be started, if necessary, 2 weeks after the injection of the Kveim antigen without interfering with the development of the characteristic tissue changes.

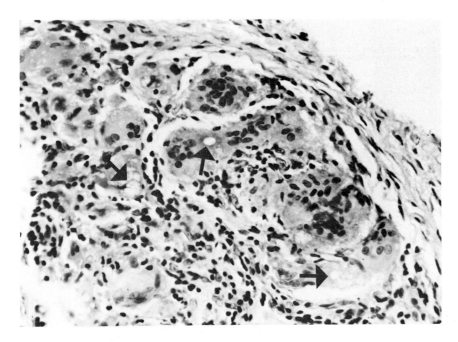

Fig. 9.25 Negative Kveim test (foreign body granuloma). A collection of foreign-body-type giant cells with vacuoles which contained droplets of oil (arrowed) can be seen. This lesion, which developed at the site of injection of Kveim antigen, was caused by using a plastic syringe lubricated with silicone grease.

Foreign body granulomata

A number of substances such as silica, mineral oils, starch, beryllium (fluorescent light tubes) and zirconium (deodorant sticks) can induce a follicular granuloma composed of epithelioid cells, giant cells and lymphocytes. In the case of silica, examination of the section in polarised light will reveal numerous doubly refractile crystals (Fig. 9.26). Beryllium produces large follicular granulomatous masses with central areas of caseation necrosis while zirconium produces small follicles without necrosis. Granulomas due to beryllium or zirconium cannot positively be separated from the other follicular granulomata except by the history of exposure.

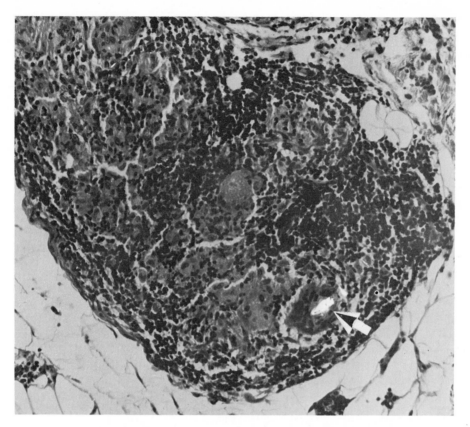

Fig. 9.26   Silica granuloma. A small bright crystal can be seen in the cytoplasm of a giant cell in this follicular granuloma. Partially polarised light.

More commonly, foreign body granulomata are seen in relation to keratin from a ruptured retention or inclusion cyst (Fig. 9.27) to suture material from previous surgical intervention, or to portions of hair shaft (Fig. 9.28) from ruptured pilosebaceous follicles. Small, isolated, multinucleated giant cells may be seen in relation to some of the altered elastic tissue fibres in solar elastosis.

It will be clear from the foregoing account that the recognition of a follicular granuloma with or without caseation necrosis is not diagnostic of any one condition, but merely a prelude to a series of investigations designed to elucidate the agent responsible.

The laboratory investigations which must be undertaken are:

1. Examination of section in polarised light.
2. Staining for acid-fast bacilli by Ziehl–Neelsen and Triff stains (control sections should be stained simultaneously).
3. Staining for fungi by PAS or methenamine silver.
4. Bacteriological and mycological culture and/or animal inoculation of fresh tissue.
5. Serology (Wassermann reaction, TPI).
6. Kveim test.

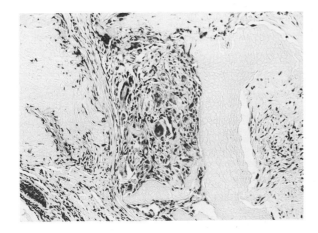

Fig. 9.27 Foreign body granuloma (keratin). A foreign body granuloma can be seen in the centre of the microphotograph in relation to the masses of keratin released as the result of rupture of an inclusion cyst.

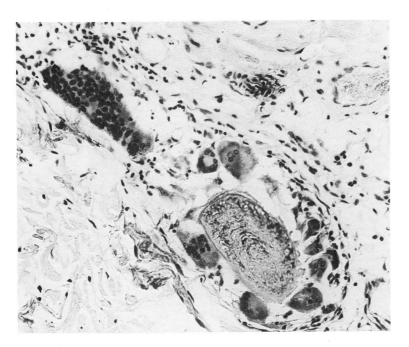

Fig. 9.28 Foreign body granuloma (hair shaft). A portion of hair shaft is seen surrounded by multiple foreign-body-type giant cells.

The aetiology of any follicular granuloma can be established only by selective use of these investigations. Table 9.1 summarises the diagnostic features of the main follicular granulomata.

Table 9.1 Differential diagnosis of follicular granulomata

Disease	Histological features	Diagnostic tests
Lupus vulgaris	Sharply delineated follicles. Caseation necrosis present or absent.	Identification of acid/alcohol-fast bacilli in sections (presumptive). Culture and animal inoculation.
Tuberculosis verrucosa cutis	Infiltrate may be acute inflammatory with a few follicular granulomata. Pseudoepitheliomatous hyperplasia of epidermis.	Identification of acid/alcohol-fast bacilli in sections (presumptive). Culture and animal inoculation.
Tuberculosis cutis colloquativa	Sinus track lined by granulation tissue containing follicular granulomata. Caseation + +.	Identification of acid/alcohol-fast bacilli in sections (presumptive). Culture and animal inoculation.
Swimming pool granuloma	Poorly defined follicular granuloma combined with heavy chronic inflammatory infiltrate. No caseation.	Culture at various temperatures (room). Identification of an atypical mycobacterium.
Syphilis, tertiary	Well-defined follicles. Caseation −ve to + + +. May or may not be associated with plasma cell infiltrate and obliterative endarteritis.	Wasserman reaction, TPI, etc.
Fungi	Well- to poorly defined follicles. Pseodoepitheliomatous hyperplasia of epidermis. Caseation −ve to + +. Plasma cell infiltration and obliterative endarteritis may be prominent.	Demonstration of fungus or spores in sections stained with periodic acid–Schiff or methenamine silver. Direct examination of fresh tissue for fungal elements. Culture and animal inoculation.
Leprosy	*Tuberculoid type*: well-formed follicles. No caseation. *Lepromatous type*: mass of foamy macrophages. Small band of fibrous tissue between infiltrate and epidermis.	*Tuberculoid*; careful search for neural involvement. Lepromin test. *Lepromatous*: acid/alcohol-fast bacilli (Triff stain) in foamy cells.
Sarcoidosis	Well-formed follicles. Central necrosis of follicles present or absent. No caseation.	Kveim test.
Beryllium, zirconium	*Beryllium*: large follicular aggregates. Caseation + + + *Zirconium*: small discrete follicles. No caseation.	No confirmatory laboratory tests available.
Silica and other particulate matter	Poorly to well-formed follicular granuloma. Foreign-body-type giant cells predominate. No necrosis. Often mixed chronic inflammatory infiltrate including plasma cells.	Birefringence in polarised light or recognition of foreign material (e.g.) keratin, starch grains, suture material) in sections.

Palisading granulomata

There is a type of granulomatous reaction where a central area of collagen degeneration or necrosis is surrounded by an epithelioid cell infiltrate in such a way that the long axes of these cells are perpendicular to the degenerate or necrotic centre. While this is the general arrangement, frequently small follicular granulomata are seen arranged around the periphery.

Granuloma annulare

This benign condition is seen predominantly in children and young adults and consists of annular groups of asymptomatic skin-coloured papules, often over the backs of the hands or

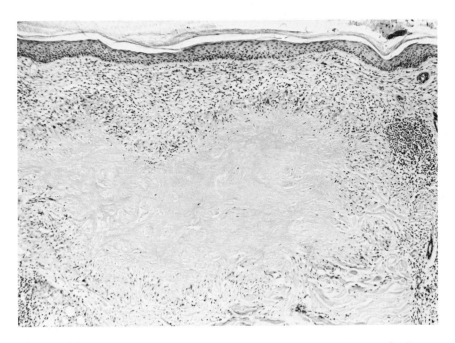

Fig. 9.29 Granuloma annulare. In the mid dermis an oval-shaped area of collagen necrosis is seen surrounded by radially arranged epithelioid cells and histiocytes.

fingers. A possible relationship with diabetes in some cases has been postulated.[6] In established cases at low magnification there is an oval area in the upper or mid dermis in which the collagen appears to have lost its nuclei and its normal staining properties (Fig. 9.29). Not all of the collagen fibres are always involved. This is seen on closer examination in early lesions when in addition some nuclear dust may be seen in the central part of the lesion and

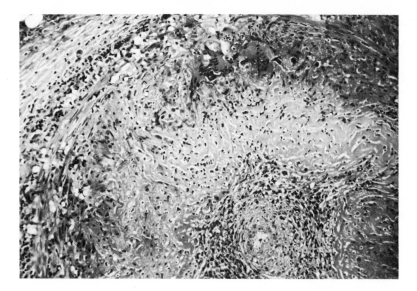

Fig. 9.30   Granuloma annulare. There is a central area of necrosis of collagen with nuclear dust and a damaged blood vessel.

is part of a leucocytoclastic vasculitis with necrosis of the vessel wall (Fig. 9.30). Usually there are also small foci of amorphous material which is metachromatic with toluidine blue. Elastic tissue stain may show that, while there are some fragmented fibres, most are preserved intact. There is a loose infiltrate of radially arranged epithelioid cells and histiocytes surrounding the central damaged area, and scattered among them are multinucleated Langhans giant cells (Fig. 9.31). Occasionally, small, well-defined follicular aggregates of epithelioid cells and giant cells may be detected scattered throughout the looser arrangement of epithelioid cells and histiocytes. Usually the epidermis is normal, but on occasion cases of perforating granuloma annulare occur where there is focal necrosis of the epidermis (Fig. 9. 32), seen especially on the fingers. A useful point of differentiation from necrobiosis lipoidica is the presence of greater quantities of Alcian blue positive mucin in granuloma annulare.

In most instances the lesions of granuloma annulare, unlike those of necrobiosis lipoidica (see below), occur in the upper and mid dermis, but occasionally a solitary lesion of granuloma annulare involving the subcutaneous fat occurs. Such lesions must be differentiated from the rheumatoid nodule (Chapter 9). More recently, widespread follicular and palisading granulomata have been called disseminated granuloma annulare.[7] In these reports the differentiation from other follicular granulomata has not been fully clarified and must await further study.

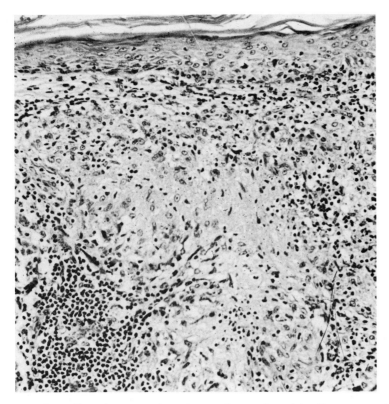

Fig. 9.31 Granuloma annulare. A central area of partial collagen necrosis containing some pyknotic nuclei is seen in the upper dermis. This is surrounded by a loose palisade of epithelioid cells, histiocytes, lymphocytes and an occasional multinucleated giant cell.

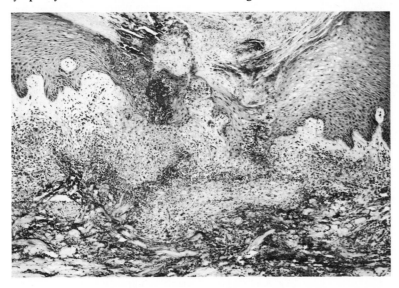

Fig. 9.32 Perforating granuloma annulare. Focal loss of epidermis with extrusion of debris from dermis. Abundant nuclear dust is present and several foci of collagen necrosis.

Necrobiosis lipoidica (necrobiosis lipoidica diabeticorum)

This condition is customarily called necrobiosis lipoidica diabeticorum. In view of the fact that in some 40 per cent of cases encountered there is no evidence of diabetes, overt or latent, it would seem logical to abandon the qualifying 'diabeticorum'. The condition appears most frequently in the lower limbs, as slow-spreading, usually symmetrical, reddish-coloured patches with a mottled yellowish centre. As the lesion spreads, the centre tends to heal by atrophic scarring. Sections show a picture very like that of granuloma annulare except that the areas of collagenous change are much more numerous, are scattered throughout the entire thickness of the dermis in a rather haphazard fashion and are usually much more conspicuous (Fig. 9.33).

Closer examination reveals areas of severely damaged, swollen collagen which fails to stain well with eosin. The elastic tissue in this area is either fragmented or absent. Small deposits of amorphous material, metachromatic when stained with toluidine blue, and similar to those seen in granuloma annulare may be seen. The granulomatous infiltrate around these areas is much more pronounced than in granuloma annulare (Fig. 9.35). Although it still shows a palisading arrangement, many more foci with a follicular architecture are seen. Perhaps the most striking differential feature is the heavy deposit of lipid in the central area. This is seen in frozen sections of fresh tissue stained with Sudan red (Fig. 9.34). If necrobiosis is suspected, the skin biopsy should be submitted unfixed to the laboratory. Many authors have commented on obliterative vascular changes as a differentiating feature from granuloma annulare. However, necrobiosis tends to occur more frequently after middle age and obliterative vascular changes in the vessels of the lower limbs are common at this time; vascular

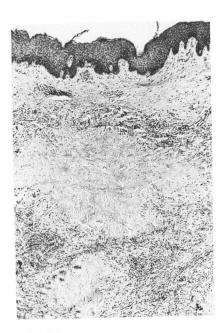

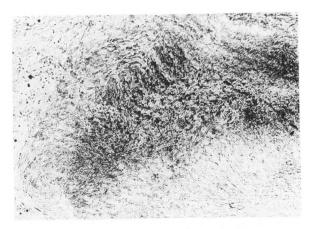

Fig. 9.33 (left)   Necrobiosis lipoidica. Numerous areas of collagen necrosis can be seen scattered throughout the entire depth of the dermis.

Fig. 9.34 (right)   Necrobiosis lipoidica. Note the heavy deposit of lipid droplets in the central necrotic area. Frozen section, Sudan IV.

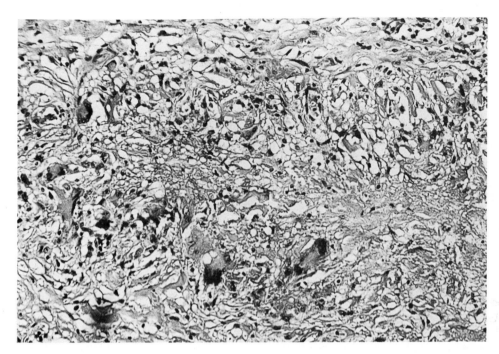

Fig. 9.35 Necrobiosis lipoidica. A focus of necrotic collagen in the lower dermis is surrounded by both a palisade and follicular aggregates of epithelioid cells. Many of the follicular aggregates contain Langhans-type giant cells.

changes in cases of necrobiosis lipoidica in the younger age groups are not usually seen. Nothing is really known concerning the aetiology of either granuloma annulare or necrobiosis lipoidica.

Rheumatic and rheumatoid nodules

Nodules occurring during the course of acute rheumatic fever or rheumatoid arthritis are more common in the subcutaneous tissue, but they can occur also in the skin. Although they

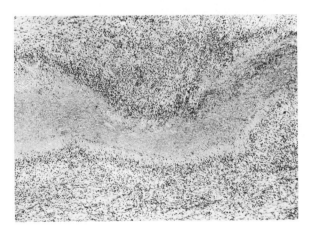

Fig. 9.36 Rheumatic nodule. An elongated area of fibrinoid necrosis of collagen in the centre of the microphotograph is surrounded by an epithelioid cell granuloma in which palisading is very pronounced.

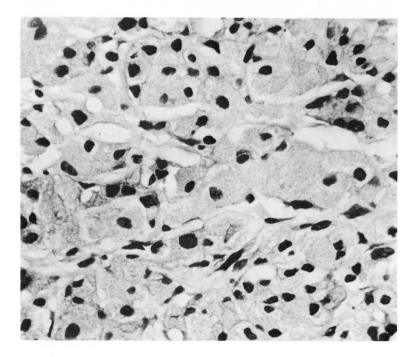

Fig. 9.37 Xanthoma. The large histiocytes with granular, vacuolated cytoplasm, and relatively small, darkly staining nuclei, which are characteristic of all types of xanthoma, are seen in this microphotograph.

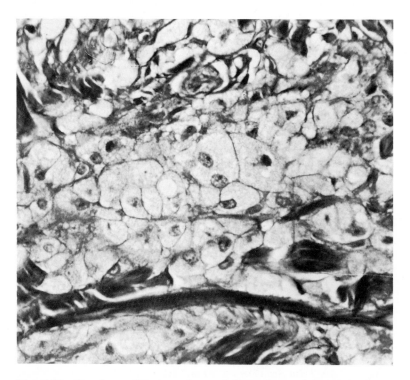

Fig. 9.38 Xanthoma. The use of one of the variants of the trichrome stain accentuates the foamy nature of the cytoplasm of the xanthoma cells. Mallory's trichrome.

can be confused with either granuloma annulare or necrobiosis lipoidica, with rheumatic or rheumatoid nodules the necrosis is more complete, occupies a relatively larger central area, stains heavily with eosin (fibrinoid necrosis) and the palisading granulomatous reaction surrounding it is more pronounced (Fig. 9.36).

At times, however, histological differentiation is impossible and the diagnosis can be reached only by careful screening of the patient for evidence of active rheumatism.

Xanthoma

Extracellular deposits of lipid become phagocytosed by macrophages which aggregate into nodules in the dermis and constitute the essential lesion of a xanthoma. There are numerous clinical types of xanthoma, from the yellowish plaques on the eyelids (xanthelasma) to the larger nodular masses which occur on extensor surfaces (xanthoma tuberosum), to the widespread eruption of small, acuminate, yellow papules (eruptive xanthoma). They are classified according to the basic defect by extensive analysis of serum lipids and lipoproteins. The essential histological lesion in all types is similar, and while minor histological criteria may suggest one type or the other, the differences are not sufficient for accurate separation. In haematoxylin and eosin stained paraffin sections collections of large foamy cells with small, deeply staining nuclei are seen (Fig. 9.37). These cells lie in the dermis and are usually separated from the epidermis by a narrow band of collagen. The foamy appearance, caused by the dissolving of the lipid droplets during processing, is more obvious in sections stained by one of the many modifications of Mallory's trichrome stain (Fig. 9.38). This is particularly useful in early lesions when the cells may be scanty. Staining of frozen sections of unfixed tissue by a fat stain such as Sudan IV shows abundant orange-stained droplets within the cells. If the clinician suspects xanthoma, the biopsy specimen should be submitted to the laboratory unfixed. Scattered among the foamy macrophages are scanty multinucleated giant cells. These are predominantly of the Touton type, but giant cells of either Langhans or foreign body type may be encountered.

After a time the foamy cells are gradually replaced by progressive fibrosis. Examination at this stage shows strands of collagen breaking up the mass of foamy cells. Some of these cells are destroyed and their lipid is released into the tissue where it may induce a foreign body granuloma. In paraffin sections of late lesions foreign body giant cells surround cholesterol clefts.

References

1. Black MM, Epstein WL. Formation of multinucleate giant cells in organized epithelioid cell granuloma. *Am J Pathol* 1974; **74:** 263–74.
2. Bancroft JD, Stevens A. *Theory and Practice of Histological Techniques.* 2nd ed. Edinburgh: Churchill Livingstone, 1982: pp. 284–316.
3. Hanno R, Needelman A, Eiferman RA, Callens JP. Cutaneous sarcoidal granulomas and the development of systemic sarcoidosis. *Arch Dermatol* 1981; **117:** 203–7.
4. Poole GW. The diagnosis of sarcoidosis. *Br Med J* 1982; **285:** 321–2.
5. Veien NK, Stahl D, Genner J, Hou-Jensen K. Kveim test in sarcoidosis. A report of a Danish Kveim material. *Dan Med Bull* 1979; **26:** 6–9.
6. Anderson BL, Verdich J. Granuloma annulare and diabetes mellitus. *Clin Exp Dermatol* 1979; **4:** 31–7.
7. Muhlbauer JE. Granuloma annulare. *J Am Acad Dermatol* 1980; **3:** 217–30.

10
Disorders of the Vasculature and Subcutaneous Fat

The term 'vasculopathy' refers to any pathological process affecting blood vessels, and may or may not include inflammatory damage to the vessel walls.

Vasculitis[1] (angiitis) is an inflammatory process affecting blood vessels in which there is damage to the vessel wall which may be accompanied by the traversing of the damaged area by inflammatory cells, and on occasion by the appearance of thrombus in the lumen. Strict adherence to those definitive criteria will ensure that the pathologist does not interpret perivascular accumulations of inflammatory cells as vasculitis. The changes in the vessel wall in vasculitis may vary from slight blurring of its outline, fibrinoid change in the wall or swelling of endothelial cells, to actual necrosis affecting any of the constituent parts of the vessel. All sizes of vessels may be affected, and all types of inflammatory cells may be seen. Thus acute neutrophilic vasculitis represents one end of this spectrum, and granulomatous vasculitis the other. Like any inflammatory process, the degree of damage seen and the preponderance of one cell type over others may well be a reflection of the stage of the disorder at which biopsy is performed, rather than of diagnostic significance.

Urticaria and capillaritis

In acute urticaria from whatever cause the earliest histological sign is that of oedema affecting the papillary and, later, the upper reticular dermis. It is difficult when examining haematoxylin and eosin sections to be certain that oedema is present, and a useful hint is to close the substage diaphragm of the microscope by about 25 per cent. This permits easier recognition of the accumulation of fluid between collagen bundles, pushing them slightly apart.

If the urticaria fails to resolve, the picture develops into one of oedema in the dermis together with superficial perivascular accumulations of acute inflammatory cells among which eosinophils may sometimes be seen (Fig. 10.1). The capillaries may also show evidence of inflammatory change by swelling of their endothelial cell nuclei and loss of clarity of outline of their walls.[2] In some cases more acute changes occur in the vessel walls and the picture gradually merges with that of leucocytoclastic vasculitis.

Leucocytoclastic vasculitis

This is characterised by the presence of fragments of disintegrating neutrophil nuclei around damaged small vessels forming the so-called 'nuclear dust' (Fig. 10.2). There is, of course, a varying degree of free haemorrhage, and while polymorphonuclear cells predominate, eosinophils and lymphocytes may also be present in varying numbers. Damage to vessel walls includes marked endothelial swelling and, later, fibrin seepage, going on to focal or

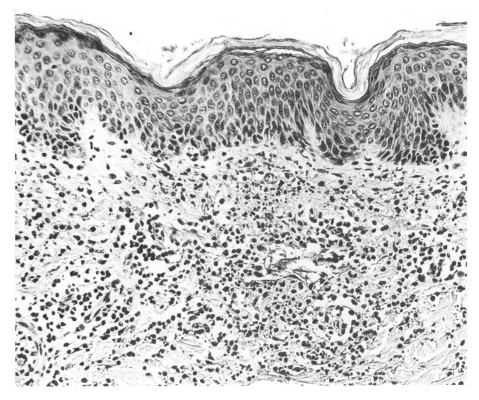

Fig. 10.1 Acute capillaritis (leucoclastic vasculitis). The epidermis shows mild intercellular oedema. There is haemorrhage into the papillary dermis and a marked acute inflammatory infiltrate in and around the dermal capillaries. Many of the inflammatory cell nuclei are pyknotic and fragmented. This biopsy was taken from an adolescent with classic anaphylactoid purpura (Henoch–Schönlein).

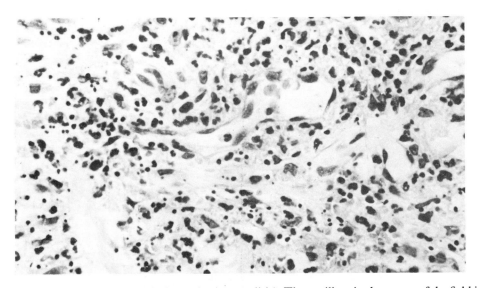

Fig. 10.2 Acute capillaritis (leucoclastic vasculitis). The capillary in the centre of the field is lined by swollen endothelium, and neutrophils can be seen migrating through the wall, forming a cuff around it. Many of the nuclei of the neutrophils are pyknotic and fragmented (nuclear dust, leucoclasia). This biopsy was taken from a child with anaphylactoid purpura (Henoch–Schönlein).

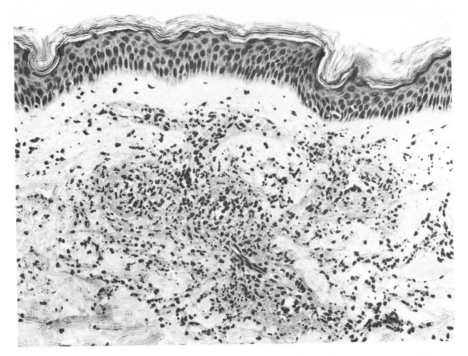

Fig. 10.3 Acute necrotising vasculitis (allergic vasculitis). All the vessels in this microphotograph show acute fibrinoid necrosis of their walls and are surrounded by fibrin seepage. There is a moderate perivascular infiltrate composed mainly of neutrophils, the nuclei of which are pyknotic and fragmented.

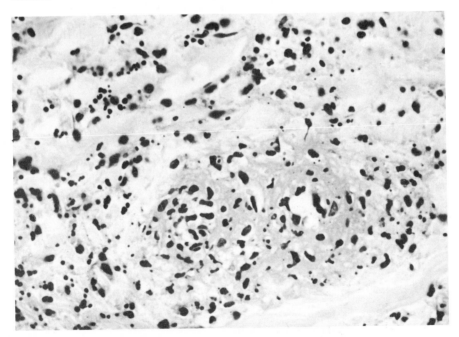

Fig. 10.4 Acute necrotising vasculitis (allergic vasculitis). The walls of the two vessels in the centre of the field show fibrinoid necrosis and are surrounded by fibrin seepage. There is a perivascular inflammatory cell infiltrate consisting of neutrophils, histiocytes and lymphocytes. The nuclei of many of the neutrophils are pyknotic and fragmented.

total necrosis of the walls, may be seen (Fig. 10.3). The papillary vessels are affected but in some cases there is extension of the process to include small vessels in the reticular dermis.

It must be emphasised that these appearances are not specific to one designated disease[3] but occur in such widely differing clinical conditions as allergic vasculitis (Fig. 10.4) including the capillaritis of Henoch–Schönlein purpura, nodular vasculitis, some adverse drug reactions, acute systemic lupus erythematosus (rarely),[4] erythema multiforme, some types of urticaria,[5] erythema elevatum diutinum and granuloma faciale.

Polyarteritis nodosa (periarteritis nodosa)[6, 7]

Polyarteritis nodosa may occur at any age but is most commonly seen between 20 and 40 years of age. Males are affected more frequently than females. Two types of the disease have been described: one in which only the skin is involved; the other being a multisystem disease affecting the kidneys, gastrointestinal tract, liver, pancreas, and both the peripheral and the central nervous systems. The histological findings in the skin are identical in each type and classically show segmental necrosis of the walls of small and medium-sized vessels in the mid and deep dermis (Fig. 10.5). Sometimes a panvasculitis occurs when the whole vessel

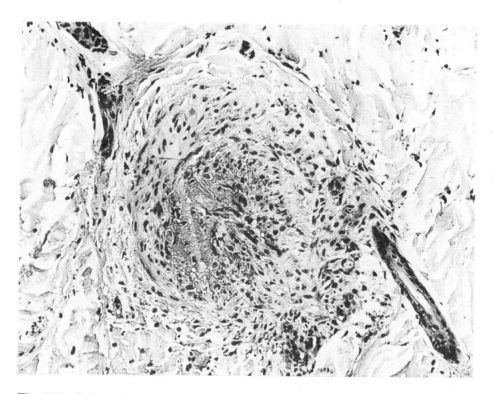

Fig. 10.5 Polyarteritis nodosa (periarteritis nodosa). In the wall of this dermal arteriole there is an area of fibrinoid necrosis which is infiltrated with and surrounded by an inflammatory infiltrate composed of neutrophils, eosinophils and a few lymphocytes and histiocytes. This is an old lesion and the inflammatory infiltrate is not so prominent as in the early stages.

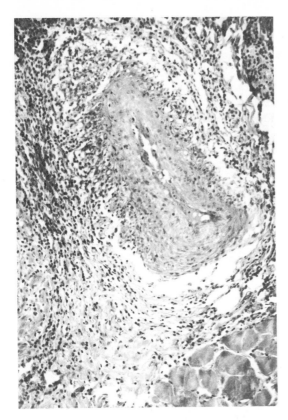

Fig. 10.6 Polyarteritis nodosa (muscle biopsy). There is a damaged vessel with surrounding inflammatory cell infiltrate and muscle fibre necrosis.

wall is affected, and in early cases bulging of part of the vessel wall is seen, giving an appearance of small vessel aneurysm formation. There is an accompanying inflammatory infiltrate of neutrophils, eosinophils, with some lymphocytes and histiocytes. The use of an elastic tissue stain will reveal defects in the integrity of the vessel elastica, and there may be a leucocytoclastic phase in the natural history of the disease. Diagnosis of the systemic form of the disease may be confirmed by muscle biopsy in some of the cases (Fig. 10.6), and positive results are more likely to be obtained if the biopsy is taken from a muscle which is tender. Subcutaneous lesions also occur which may be palpable, especially after thrombosis and infarction.

Pernio (chilblain)

In pernio, which on occasion may be biopsied because it is not clinically typical, there is a most striking oedema of the papillary dermis, sometimes to the extent of forming a subepidermal bulla (Fig. 10.7). The small dermal blood vessels stand out clearly through marked prominence of the endothelial cells, and there is a perivascular lympho-histiocytic infiltrate. Both the deep dermis and the subcutis may be involved with vessels there showing similar appearances to the superficial vessels, and may also show thrombus formation. The subcutaneous fat as a result may undergo necrosis with reactive changes.

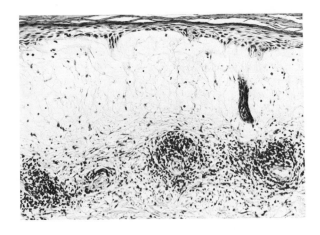

Fig. 10.7 Pernio (chilblain). The epidermis is thinned and shows mild spongiosis. There is intense oedema of the papillary dermis, which has resulted in virtual separation of the epidermis from the dermis. The small dermal vessels appear prominent due to endothelial proliferation and thickening of their walls. There is a dense perivascular lymphocytic inflammatory infiltrate.

Granulomatous vasculitis

A number of conditions have in common a granulomatous reaction seen in association with blood vessels. Their aetiology is not known and their early development is obscure in terms of histology.

Allergic granulomatosis[8]

Allergic granulomatosis is a multisystem disease which in many respects is similar to polyarteritis nodosa. In addition to damage to medium-sized vessels, there is a copious infiltrate of eosinophil leucocytes and polymorphonuclear cells both through and around the vessel walls. Fibrin and eosinophilic 'mush' are also seen, and, depending on the stage, a greater or less component of the infiltrate is granulomatous,[9] including small multinucleated giant cells. Differentiation from polyarteritis is possible because of the eosinophilia present, the granulomatous element in the vasculitis and the pulmonary involvement in allergic granulomatosis.

Wegener's granulomatosis

In this, a necrotising vasculitis with leucocytoclasia and thrombosis leads to necrosis of surrounding tissue, especially affecting the upper respiratory tract. The skin is involved in about half the cases and histologically the lesions may closely resemble those seen in allergic granulomatosis.[10] In that variety known as lethal midline granuloma, necrosis of the skin over the nose and mouth may be seen and the appearances histologically may, in addition to the granulomatous aspect, be indistinguishable from a non-Hodgkin's lymphoma.

Giant cell arteritis (temporal arteritis)

In addition to the temporal artery, arteries in the kidney, heart and retina may be affected with resultant consequences of potentially severe damage to those organs. Blindness is a particularly possible result, but early diagnosis with treatment by corticosteroids can usually prevent this. Clinically, headache on one side may be the presenting symptom, but skin manifestations such as ulceration over the temporal artery distribution are rare. It has become standard practice to biopsy the temporal artery when the diagnosis is considered,[11] and, because of the difficulties in sampling, it is imperative that the entire biopsy specimen be examined and, if necessary, ribboned. In a well-developed case tight stenosis of the vessel

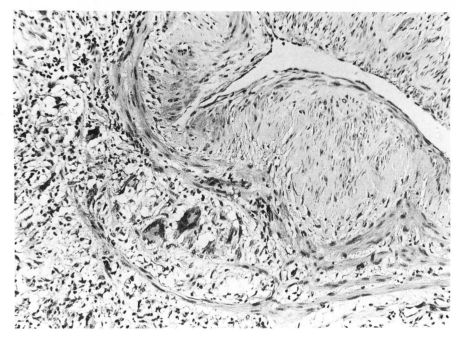

Fig. 10.8 Giant cell arteritis (temporal arteritis). This branch of the temporal artery shows a marked subendothelial fibrous thickening with consequent narrowing of its lumen. In the media between the internal and external elastica lamina there are follicular granulomata composed of rather poorly formed epithelioid cells, multinucleated giant cells of Langhans type and some lymphocytes.

due to intimal proliferation and fibrosis of the vessel wall is seen histologically (Fig. 10.8). There is swelling and fragmentation of the elastica, and between the elastic laminae are granuloma composed of epithelioid cells, lymphocytes, some eosinophils and occasional multinucleated giant cells. No bacteria or fungi can be demonstrated, nor is there any fibrin deposition within the vessel wall.

Lymphomatoid granulomatosis

This is a rare disorder seen mostly in middle-aged to elderly males, and primarily affects the lungs as a necrotising and granulomatous vasculitis.[12] Other systems, including the central nervous system, may be affected, and skin lesions[13] are seen in about one-third of the cases. The dermis contains a lymphoid infiltrate with small multinucleated giant cells seen particularly in association with small and medium-sized blood vessels, and there is hyperplasia of the eccrine sweat glands. Some cases resolve spontaneously, while a few have been reported as progressing to malignant lymphoma, and the precise pathogenesis of the condition remains to be settled.

Diabetic microangiopathy

In diabetic microangiopathy, the small vessels of the papillary and reticular dermis are affected. Their outlines are less clear on examination of a haematoxylin and eosin section, and staining by the periodic acid–Schiff method shows the deposition of minute red threads and beads within those vessel walls. This is a not infrequent finding on routine examination of a vulval biopsy on account of pruritus, and invariably satisfies the pathologist while surprising the clinician!

Erythema elevatum diutinum

Erythema elevatum diutinum presents clinically as reddish-purple to reddish-brown nodules and plaques on the extensor surfaces of the limbs, usually symmetrical in distribution, and with a predilection for the extensor aspects of small joints. Sometimes small bullae[14] may be seen on some of the lesions, and growth is very slow indeed. In the early stage histological examination reveals an acute leucocytoclastic vasculitis throughout the dermis with large numbers of inflammatory cells extending to the undersurface of the epidermis (Fig. 10.9). Eosinophilic fibrinoid material is seen in and around affected vessels, forming the 'toxic hyaline' described in the older literature. In the later stages a somewhat laminated fibrosis occurs, but still present focally is the abundant neutrophil response, thus producing the paradox of an acute histological picture in a chronic clinical condition.

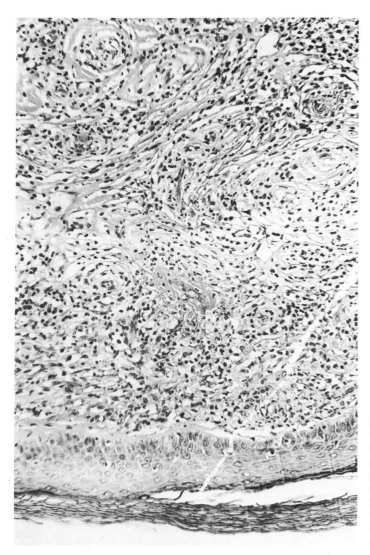

Fig. 10.9 Erythema elevatum diutinum. There is an acute vasculitis associated with an intense acute inflammatory infiltrate. All the vessels in the section are involved and the inflammatory infiltrate extends up to the under surface of the epidermis (cf. granuloma faciale, Fig. 10.10).

Granuloma faciale

Granuloma faciale is another chronic disorder seen almost always on the face and ears as slowly growing reddish-purple asymptomatic patches. Histologically, a dense inflammatory infiltrate is seen in the dermis in which, in the early stages, eosinophils predominate. In this disorder the epidermis shows no abnormality, and is separated from the inflammatory infiltrate in the dermis by a narrow band of collagen known as the Grenz zone (Fig. 10.10). Both eosinophil and polymorphonuclear cells disintegrate, forming nuclear dust, and a vasculitis can be detected (Fig. 10.11), thus giving the picture of leucocytoclastic vasculitis. Within the cellular infiltrate are also seen histiocytes, lymphocytes and plasma cells in varying numbers depending on the timing of the biopsy. In well-established cases the connective tissue assumes a fibrinoid appearance in the vicinity of affected capillaries, and,

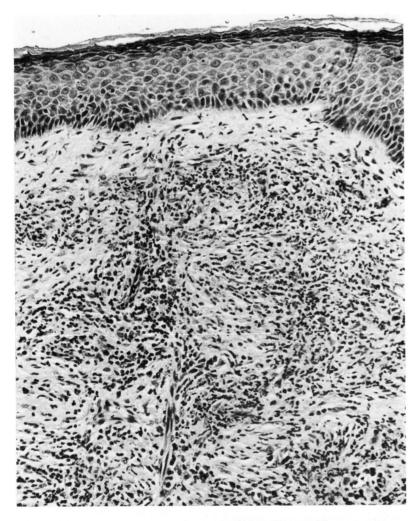

Fig. 10.10   Granuloma faciale. Patches of dense inflammatory infiltrate are centred around the dermal blood vessels. Many of the inflammatory cells are polymorphonuclear leucocytes. Note the band of normal dermis between the undersurface of the epidermis and the infiltrate.

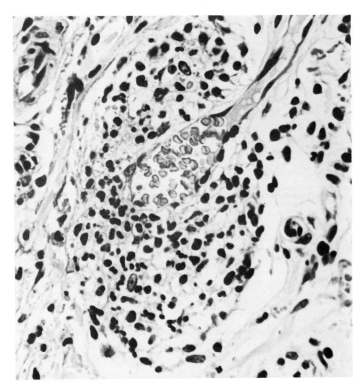

Fig. 10.11 Granuloma faciale. A dilated dermal capillary with a prominent endothelial lining is surrounded by inflammatory cells. Many of these are polymorphonuclear leucocytes, the nuclei of which are fragmented and pyknotic.

still later, fibrosis occurs. At this stage the acute inflammatory cells are not in evidence, having been replaced by lymphocytes, histiocytes and plasma cells together with varying amounts of haemosiderin deposition. Eventually only scar tissue with a few scattered foci of chronic inflammation is seen.

Progressive pigmented purpuric dermatoses

Majocchi–Schamberg disease

In the past this disorder was known as Majocchi's disease or Schamberg's disease depending on the clinical appearances, but it is now generally accepted that they have the same pathological basis and are merely different stages of the same disease.[15] It occurs usually on the lower limbs, but can present elsewhere, either as an annular purpuric eruption, or as small patches of purpura which eventually develop into hyperpigmented plaques. At first the epidermis is normal and there appears to be an increased number of papillary blood vessels present with endothelial swelling. Slight papillary oedema is present and there may be a few free red blood cells in the fine collagen adjacent to the vessels together with a very sparse lympho-histiocytic infiltrate (Fig. 10.12). No haemosiderin is detectable, and the findings at this stage are thus non-specific. Later the epidermis may show focal flecks of

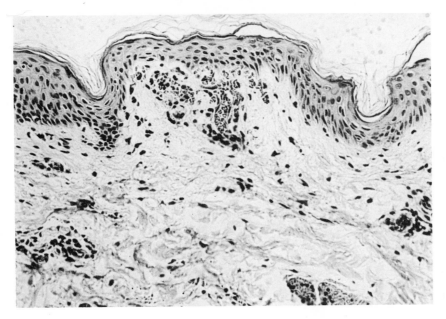

Fig. 10.12 Pigmented purpuric eruption (Majocchi–Schamberg disease). In the dermal papilla in the centre of the field the capillaries show endothelial swelling and proliferation. The vessels are engorged with blood and a small focus of extravasated erythrocytes can be seen between the capillaries and the undersurface of the epidermis.

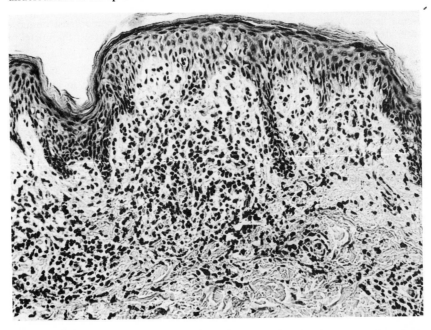

Fig. 10.13 Pigmented purpuric eruption (Majocchi–Schamberg disease). There is a patchy oedema of the epidermis. Foci of extravasated erythrocytes can be seen in the dermal papillae. The moderately dense lymphocytic infiltrate in the upper dermis invades the dermo-epidermal junction at one point. The density of this infiltrate masks the new capillary formation.

parakeratosis, and the infiltrate described above becomes much more evident and scattered between the small blood vessels which are also considerably increased in number (Fig. 10.13). Free pigment and pigment-laden macrophages can now be seen in varying amount, most easily by closing the iris diaphragm of the microscope a little. Staining with Prussian blue shows that this pigment is haemosiderin, and that there is much more of it than is evident on examination of a haematoxylin and eosin section (Fig. 10.14).

Diagnosis of this condition should be made only when there is good clinical correlation because the lower legs suffer frequent minor injuries in everyday life which may produce similar microscopic appearances. Another differentiation is from stasis dermatitis resulting from chronic venous insufficiency. The changes in Majocchi–Schamberg disease are confined to the upper dermis, while those of stasis dermatitis are more extensive and may involve the deeper dermis with subcutaneous fibrosis and vascular thickening. Moreover, stasis dermatitis shows a varying degree of the dermatitis reaction, and scarring of the dermis is usually a prominent feature.

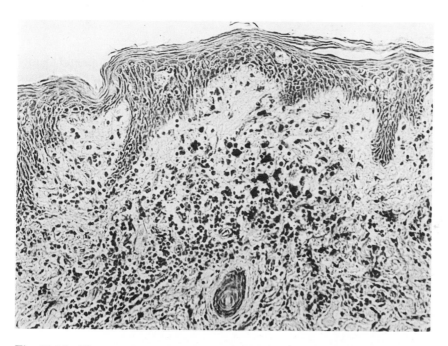

Fig. 10.14 Pigmented purpuric eruption (Majocchi–Schamberg disease). In haematoxylin and eosin stained sections the density of the lympho-histiocytic infiltrate masks the pigment-laden macrophages as well as the new capillary formation. This section, from the same block of tissue from which Fig. 10.13 was taken, shows the numerous darkly stained haemosiderin-containing macrophages. Perl's Prussian blue-neutral red.

Lichenoid purpura

This is also known as the lichenoid dermatitis of Gougerot and Blum. It starts as purpuric papules on the skin which tend to spread radially, and which have a predilection for the lower limbs. Histologically, there is a marked increase in the number of capillaries noticeable in the papillary and upper reticular dermis, with a mixture of lymphocytes, histiocytes and extravasated red blood cells deposited in those areas. Haemosiderin deposition is considerable, and the Prussian blue reaction shows this to be lying freely and within macrophages in the superficial dermis. The epidermis shows slight focal acanthosis with some elongation of rete ridges, and in general the appearance is somewhat lichenoid. Close clinical correlation is essential because of the liability of repeated minor trauma producing a similar picture histologically.

Lichen aureus[16]

Lichen aureus is the name applied to a condition where groups of rust- to golden-coloured papules are seen on the skin in any area of the body. These purpuric lesions are symptom free and are not associated with trauma. Histologically very similar changes to those found in lichenoid purpura are seen but are much more circumscribed and thus less extensive. A distinguishing feature is that the epidermis in lichen aureus shows no significant abnormality.

Pityriasis lichenoides

This is a condition of unknown aetiology which occurs in the younger age groups and mainly affects males. An acute form is described and a chronic form also occurs, but intermediate

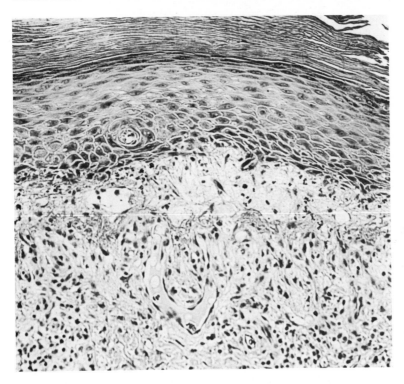

Fig. 10.15 Pityriasis lichenoides et varioliformis acuta (early lesion). There is intense oedema of the papillary dermis (almost amounting to a subepidermal bulla) associated with some free haemorrhage and a lympho-histiocytic infiltrate. Towards the centre of the field there is a Y-shaped dilated capillary. The epidermis shows only mild oedema of its lower portion.

forms of the disorder which are arbitrarily called 'subacute' are also seen. Pityriasis lichenoides in all its forms is not a common disease of skin and the acute form, known as pityriasis lichenoides et varioliformis acuta (Mucha–Habermann disease), is rare. The eruption consists of a scattered maculopapular rash which develops into varicelliform and papulonecrotic lesions. Histologically, in an early lesion there is marked oedema of the papillary dermis with the impression of a developing subepidermal bulla (Fig. 10.15). The papillary dermis shows a considerable extravasation of red blood cells together with a mixture of lymphocytes and histiocytes. The epidermis at this stage may be normal or show both intra- and intercellular oedema. Later a wedge-shaped infarct of the epidermis and the papillary dermis is seen with

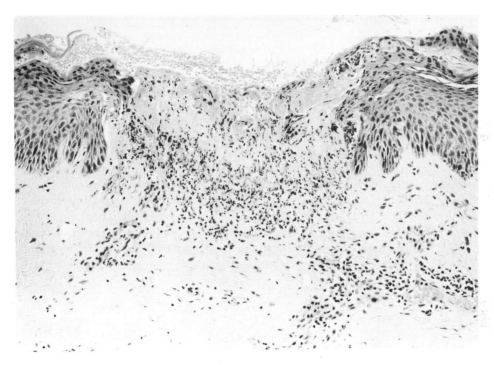

Fig. 10.16 Pityriasis lichenoides et varioliformis acuta (fully formed lesion). There is a wedge-shaped area of necrosis (infarct) involving the upper dermis and epidermis. Numerous erythrocytes can be seen within this area and it is surrounded by a lympho-histiocytic infiltrate. No vasculitis is seen in this section.

sharply circumscribed necrosis of those areas (Fig. 10.16). At the base of the infarct, vessels showing swollen endothelial cells and lymphocytes in association with vessel walls may be seen, but not as a constant feature. When present, therefore, the picture is one of a lymphocytic vasculitis. In the subacute and chronic forms of pityriasis lichenoides the epidermis shows perhaps only slight thickening and is surmounted focally by a disc-like scale of orthokeratin and parakeratin. Only a sparse upper dermal perivascular lymphoid cellular infiltrate may be present, which in the subacute form becomes more noticeable. Some of these cells are seen in the epidermis, and again depending on the stage of the disease, papillary oedema and an occasional free red blood cell in the papillary dermis are present.

Pyoderma gangrenosum

This condition is included in this chapter because the early lesions show evidence of inflammation affecting small blood vessels in the dermis and subcutis, with breakdown of their walls and the extrusion of red blood cells and neutrophils into the adjacent tissue. As time goes on, non-specific ulceration of the epidermis occurs, and the picture becomes obliterated by the accumulation of necrotic debris and a massive inflammatory cell infiltrate which extends through the dermis and subcutis. Later still, foreign body giant cells appear randomly situated among what is now inflamed granulation tissue, and eventually healing occurs with the formation of dense scar tissue causing retraction of the epidermis.

It must be emphasised that the overall histological picture is not diagnostic, and interpretation of a section from such a case can only be reported as consistent with the clinical diagnosis.

Nodular lesions of the lower limbs

A varied collection of clinical entities may present as palpable, sometimes tender, swellings on the lower legs. Among such are erythema nodosum, nodular vasculitis and erythema induratum. Thrombophlebitis may also manifest itself in this fashion, and should not present any clinical doubt, but nodular migratory panniculitis of the legs which has as its basis thrombophlebitis may on occasion provide difficulty in diagnosis. It is essential, when the decision to proceed to biopsy has been made, to ensure that the sample taken is deep enough to include the whole thickness of the subcutaneous fat. Tissue samples which include only the deep dermis must be regarded as failed biopsies in this respect, as no opinion can be offered on the state of the fat. If an early representative lesion is selected, it is useful to try to assess the site of origin of the disease process. Inflammatory change in a large vessel, either a vein or an artery in the deep dermis or subcutaneous fat, seen before reactive changes have obscured the picture, suggests nodular vasculitis (Fig. 10.17). Origin of an inflammatory

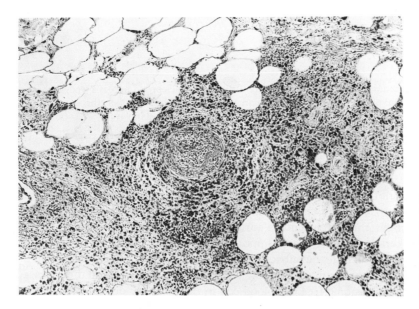

Fig. 10.17 Nodular vasculitis. There is an acute necrotising inflammatory process affecting the vessel wall with a surrounding area of fat necrosis.

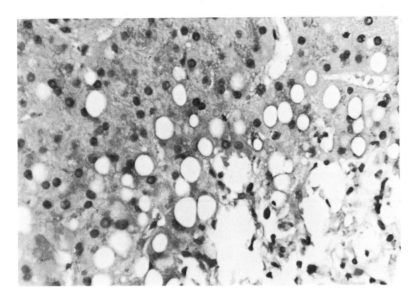

Fig. 10.18 Lobular panniculitis. This shows early fat necrosis before any granulomatous reaction has occurred.

process in the interlobular septae of the subcutaneous fat with the presence of a few multinucleated giant cells in the mixed infiltrate there suggests erythema nodosum (Fig. 10.18). Primary involvement of the fat lobule in the subcutis with fat necrosis and a spreading granulomatous reaction with giant cells, polymorphonuclear cells, lymphocytes and histiocytes may be seen in nodular vasculitis, the Weber–Christian syndrome and subcutaneous sarcoid among others. Eventually, however, as the inflammatory process becomes more established, both the septae and the lobules become involved, and any diagnostic criteria are lost (Fig. 10.19). In this situation all that can be reported is a panniculitis with an opinion on its stage of evolution (e.g. whether still active or at the stage of sclerosis).

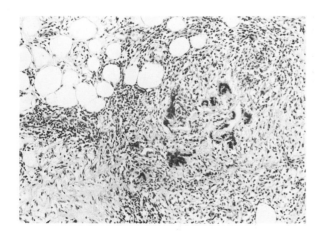

Fig. 10.19 Nodular vasculitis. An early lesion before fat necrosis has extended through the lobule.

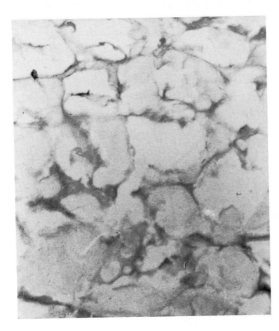

Fig. 10.20   Panniculitis of pancreatic disease, showing the ghost-like appearance of cells which have undergone necrosis. Their indistinct appearance is typical of the condition.

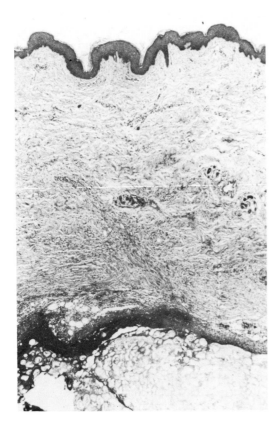

Fig. 10.21   Panniculitis of pancreatic disease. This is a later stage than in Fig. 10.21, showing the ghost-like appearance of fat cells with a dense chronically inflamed shelf of fibrous tissue at the interface with the dermis.

Pancreatic panniculitis

The panniculitis associated with pancreatic disease,[17] either inflammatory or neoplastic in origin, begins as a scattered focal lobular panniculitis. Necrosis of groups of fat cells occurs, characterised first by granular degeneration and later by a ghost-like appearance of the cells (Fig. 10.20). Eventually varying degrees of spotty calcification occur, and a granulomatous reaction develops, with a characteristic condensed inflamed zone of fibrous tissue at the interface with the dermis (Fig. 10.21).

References

1. Wolff K, Winkelmann RK. *Vasculitis*. Oxford: Blackwell Scientific 1980.
2. Monroe EW, Schulz CL, Maize SC, Jordon RE. Vasculitis in chronic urticaria: an immunopathologic study. *J Invest Dermatol* 1981; **76**: 103-7.
3. Mackel SE, Jordon RE. Leucocytoclastic vasculitis. *Arch Dermatol* 1982; **118**: 296-301.
4. O'Loughlin S, Schroester AL, Jordon RE. Chronic urticaria-like lesions in systemic lupus erythematosus. *Arch Dermatol* 1978; **114**: 879-83.
5. Gammon WR, Wheeler CE Jr. Urticarial vasculitis. *Arch Dermatol* 1979; **115**: 76-80.
6. Borrie P. Cutaneous polyarteritis nodosa. *Br J Dermatol* 1972; **87**: 87-95.
7. Diaz-Perez JL, Winkelmann RK. Cutaneous periarteritis nodosa. *Arch Dermatol* 1974; **110**: 407-14.
8. Churg J, Strauss L. Allergic granulomatosus. *Am J Pathol* 1951; **27**: 277.
9. Dicken CH, Winkelmann RK. The Churg-Strauss granuloma. Cutaneous necrotizing, palisading granuloma in vasculitis syndromes. *Arch Pathol Lab Med* 1978; **102**: 576-80.
10. Le T, Pierard GE, Lapière ChM. Granulomatous vasculitis of Wegener. *J Cutaneous Pathol* 1981; **8**: 34.
11. Allsop CJ, Gallagher PJ. Temporal artery biopsy in giant cell arteritis a reappraisal. *Am J Surg Pathol* 1981; **5**: 317.
12. McDonald DM, Sarkany I. Lymphomatoid granulomatosis. *Clin Exp Dermatol* 1976; **1**: 163-73.
13. James WD, Odom RB, Katzenstein A-LA. Cutaneous manifestations of lymphomatoid granulomatosis. *Arch Dermatol* 1981; **117**: 196-202.
14. Vollum DI. Erythema elevatum diutinum—vesicular lesions and sulphone response. *Br J Dermatol* 1968; **80**: 178-83.
15. Randall SJ, Kierland RR, Montgomery H. Pigmented purpuric eruptions. *Arch Dermatol Syph* 1951; **64**: 177-91.
16. Waisman M, Waisman M. Lichen aureus. *Arch Dermatol* 1976; **112**: 696-7.
17. Hughes PSH, Apisarnthanarax P, Mullins JF. Subcutaneous fat necrosis associated with pancreatic disease. *Arch Dermatol* 1975; **11**: 506-10.

11
The Connective Tissue Disorders (Collagen Diseases)

It has become customary to group under this heading a number of disorders in which collagen, if not primarily affected, is at least secondarily affected in the disease process. Although these disorders are classified[1] under separate headings their identity is not always easy to define; thus, in this group intermediate and transitional forms are frequently found and even the term 'mixed connective tissue disease'[2] is used to describe certain clinical and pathological features which do not fit concisely into one of the more defined disorders.

Lupus erythematosus

In practice two main forms are recognised: (1) chronic discoid lupus erythematosus and (2) systemic lupus erythematosus.

Chronic discoid lupus erythematosus (CDLE)

In this type the lesions are confined to the skin with occasional mucous membrane involvement. Two variants are recognised, one being the localised form where lesions are seen in, for example, the face or hands, and the other a disseminated form where skin lesions are widespread. The course of CDLE on the whole is benign but an occasional sequel in the development of squamous carcinoma in a long-standing lesion of CDLE.

In CDLE erythematous, slightly raised, scaly patches are seen on the skin together with follicular plugs. Later a varying degree of atrophy may be seen.

Histologically (Figs. 11.1–11.5), in a typical case the findings include:

1. Hyperkeratosis.
2. Follicular plugging, usually conical in shape.
3. A varying degree of epidermal atrophy with, occasionally, areas of epidermal thickening.
4. Liquefaction degeneration of the basal layer of the epidermis.
5. A thickened and focally broken basement membrane best seen with the PAS stain.
6. A scattered chronic inflammatory infiltrate throughout the dermis, sometimes encroaching the epidermis, containing lymphocytes, histiocytes with a few plasma cells, and often seen concentrated around appendages.
7. Depending on the stage of the lesion, some degree of papillary oedema may be seen with dilated capillaries and a few free red blood cells.
8. Melanin pigment incontinence beneath the epidermis in long-standing cases.

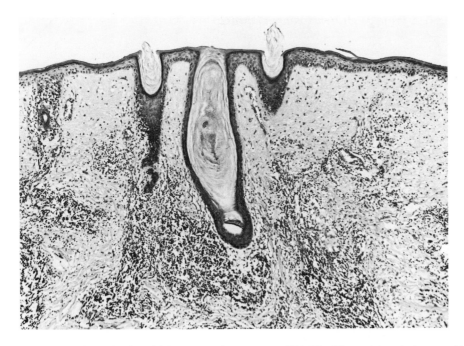

Fig. 11.1 Chronic discoid lupus erythematosus (CDLE). The epidermis is atrophic and shows follicular plugging. Liquefaction degeneration of the basal layer of the epidermis is seen affecting the two follicles to the left of the picture. Dilated blood vessels and a lympho-histiocytic infiltrate occupy the dermis.

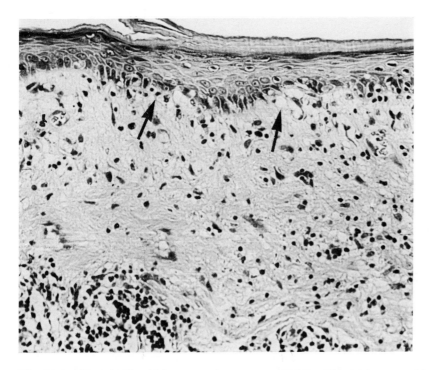

Fig. 11.2 Chronic discoid lupus erythematosus (CDLE). This higher magnification shows hyper-keratosis, basal cell liquefaction degeneration (arrowed) and a patchy lympho-histiocytic infiltrate in the dermis.

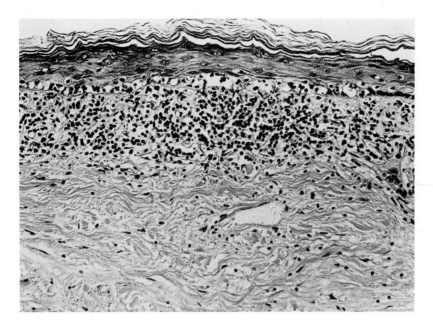

Fig. 11.3   Here liquefaction degeneration is more widespread than in Fig. 11.2, and the lympho-histiocytic infiltrate in the subjacent dermis is more dense.

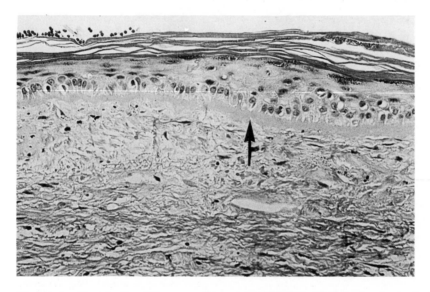

Fig. 11.4   Chronic discoid lupus erythematosus (CDLE). This section from a lesion on the forehead shows a diffuse thickening of the basal lamina (arrowed).

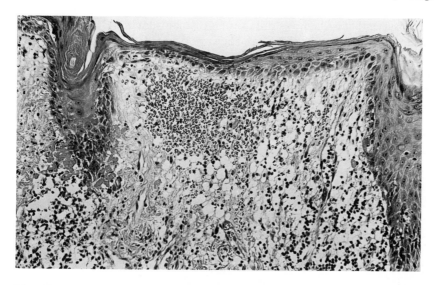

Fig. 11.5 Subacute lupus erythematosus. Epidermal atrophy and liquefaction degeneration of the basal layer, hyperkeratosis and follicular plugging are obvious. In addition, dermal oedema is prominent and free haemorrhage is present just beneath the epidermis; an area of fibrinoid necrosis is seen in relation to the follicle at the left of the picture. The term 'subacute' is used here in the pathological sense, as most cases showing these features are clinically CDLE.

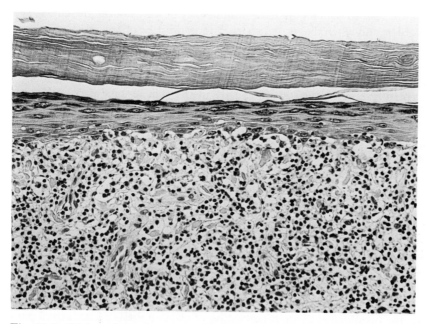

Fig. 11.6 Lichen planus (compare with Fig. 11.3). There is hyperkeratosis with epidermal atrophy, liquefaction degeneration of the basal layer, and a dense lympho-histiocytic infiltrate in the dermis. This picture emphasises the need for a good clinical history when attempting to interpret such a histological appearance.

It is a useful rule to observe that a diagnosis of lupus erythematosus should *not* be made in the absence of liquefaction degeneration of the basal layer of the epidermis, whether focal or more widespread. In doubtful cases multiple sections should be examined from the block of tissue to ensure that this finding is not missed. Useful but not diagnostic is the presence of tiny accumulations of Alcian blue positive material in the dermis, usually as fine threads or stippling. Such appearances may also be seen in other conditions, notably dermatomyositis (p. 190).

Varying degrees of the picture of CDLE are encountered in practice, and, as is customary in histopathology, some attempt is usually made to assess the severity and activity by arbitrarily ascribing the terms 'subacute' or 'chronic' depending on the presence of oedema, haemorrhage, fibrinoid necrosis etc.[3]

Many of the histological features described above may also be seen in lichen planus, especially during the involuting period (Fig. 11.6). Colloid bodies, seen typically in lichen planus, may also be seen occasionally, but to a lesser extent, in lupus erythematosus. In lichen planus, however, the increase in the granular layer is often more focal in nature and is likely to be wedge shaped. It has to be stated, however, that on occasion the two conditions may be indistinguishable histologically and it is thus imperative to have good clinical information. It is fortunate, moreover, that the use of direct immunofluorescence tests can distinguish between the two conditions.

Systemic lupus erythematosis (SLE)

This is multisystem disorder in which cutaneous lesions may or may not be present. It is a potentially fatal disorder, and when diagnosed strict criteria must be observed. Transitions between CDLE and SLE have been reported but are rare and it is sometimes difficult to decide whether such transition has actually occurred. It should also be noted that an SLE-like syndrome may be induced by certain drugs.[4]

While a variable picture may be seen histologically in the skin lesions associated with SLE, essentially the appearances are the same as those seen in CDLE. Occasionally the only recognisable histological abnormality is of the type described in the acute capillaritis of Henoch–Schönlein. If this is seen in adults the differential diagnosis should include SLE high on the list. Sometimes fibrinoid deposits in the dermis may be the only abnormality seen, but are not diagnostic. When there is papillary oedema and marked liquefaction degeneration of the basal layer of the epidermis, seen in conjunction with vascular changes including fibrin seepage and focal haemorrhage (Fig. 11.7), the diagnosis of SLE may be suspected. The view held in this laboratory is that in general a firm diagnosis of SLE should not be made on the grounds of skin histology alone.

Lupus erythematosus profundus   This is a rare finding in lupus erythematosus where the deep dermis and subcutaneous fat are affected. While seen more often in the course of SLE, its occurrence during the course of CDLE has also been reported on very rare occasions. It would be preferable to use the term *lupus panniculitis* because this more accurately describes the histological picture, consisting of either a non-specific septal panniculitis or, later, a more lobular panniculitis. In each case collections of lymphocytes, plasma cells and histiocytes are seen which later assume a more granulomatous appearance, including the presence of multinucleated giant cells.

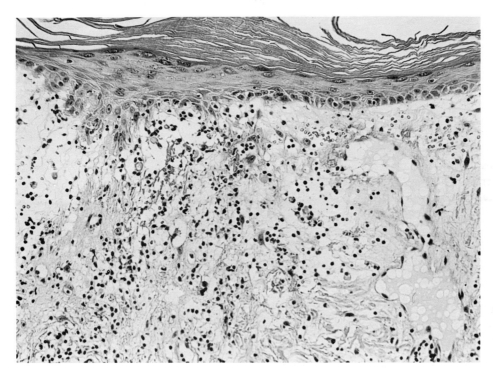

Fig. 11.7 (Acute) systemic lupus erythematosus (SLE). In this example there is hyperkeratosis of the epidermis associated with extensive focal liquefaction of the basal layer. There is gross oedema of the dermis with an area of haemorrhage and an inflammatory infiltrate consisting of lymphocytes, histiocytes and neutrophil leucocytes. Such changes are compatible with, but not diagnostic of, SLE.

Diagnostic immunopathology of lupus erythematosus Direct immunofluorescence tests using the patient's skin as substrate have been found to be most useful in both the diagnosis and the differentiation of CDLE and SLE.[5] The skin specimen is snap-frozen, cryostat sections are cut, and inclubation of these with fluorescein-labelled antibody against human IgG, IgM and complement (C3) is performed. When examined microscopically using a fluorescent light source, positive results consist of the appearance at the basement membrane zone (BMZ) of a characteristic immunofluorescing band, continuous and either coarsely or finely microgranular in nature (Fig. 11.8). Either IgG or IgM produces the band, and sometimes both are found; C3 is found in a similar fashion in active lesions. When CDLE is suspected, an active lesion, at least 1 month old and which has not been treated with topical corticosteroid preparations for at least 2 weeks, is selected for biopsy. Positive results are obtained in over 90 per cent of cases of CDLE, and only active lesions show the 'lupus band'. In SLE, skin lesions show similar results to CDLE, but in addition about 80 per cent of active cases exhibit a lupus band in clinically unaffected light-exposed skin. In both forms of the disease, lesions may show positive immunofluorescence of colloid bodies in the dermis, but this is a non-specific finding which has no diagnostic significance.

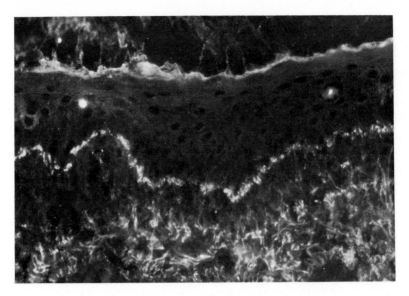

Fig. 11.8 Lupus erythematosus. Direct immunofluorescence test using IgM. The granular fluorescence along the basement membrane zone is typical of the lupus band seen in lesions of SLE and CDLE and in the clinically normal exposed skin in SLE.

Dermatomyositis

Polymyositis is an acquired inflammatory myopathy which may show clinically and histologically as an acute, subacute or chronic condition. When there are associated skin lesions the term 'dermatomyositis' is used. Both children and adults may be affected. In children the disease may remain undetected until the chronic stage is reached, when complications such as calcinosis and contractures have occurred. The adult form of the disease may in some cases be associated with visceral malignancy[6, 7] and occasionally patients in younger adult age groups may die of such complications as the Hamman–Rich syndrome. It should be remembered that apart from the specific entity known as dermatomyositis, polymyositis may be seen as part of a symptom complex associated with such conditions as polyarteritis nodosa, systemic lupus erythematosus, rheumatoid disease, rheumatic fever, progressive systemic sclerosis and Sjögren's syndrome. Sarcoidosis may also involve skeletal muscle and on occasion mimic polymyositis or even limb girdle muscular dystrophy. When polymyositis is associated with malignant disease the patients are usually over 40 years of age and the neoplasm is likely to be epithelial, but cases have been reported during the course of the lymphomas.

Clinically the classic appearance is a heliotrope swelling affecting the face and most obvious on the eyelids. Linear erythematous streaks may also be seen on the backs of the fingers, and bluish-red knuckle pads may be present. Scaling, redness and focal hyperpigmentation may occur anywhere on the skin and occasionally the appearance is that of poikiloderma.

In suspected cases the creatine phosphokinase (CPK) level in the serum is often raised, sometimes considerably, but on occasion is normal. Urinary creatine excretion is often greatly increased. Electromyographical studies may be helpful, but are not specific and may not in any case be readily available.

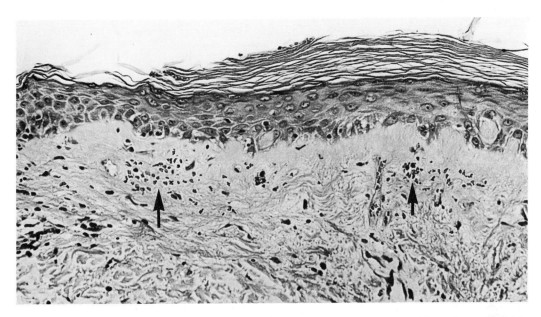

Fig. 11.9 Erythematous lesion in dermatomyositis. Hyperkeratosis, some epidermal atrophy with loss of rete ridges and tiny foci of liquefaction degeneration of the basal layer are seen. There is mild oedema in the papillary dermis with tiny aggregates of free red blood cells (arrowed). Only a very sparse inflammatory infiltrate is seen.

Pathology of the skin lesions   The histological changes in the erythematous lesions of the skin are non-specific and consist of minute foci of liquefaction change of the basal layer of the epidermis, variable dermal oedema, and scanty perivascular accumulations of lymphocytes with a few plasma cells occasionally (Fig. 11.9). In children but not usually in adults a microangiopathy may be demonstrated in the dermis, and deposition of immunoglobulins (IgG and IgM) and the C3 fraction of complement may be demonstrated in and around the vessel walls by immunofluorescent microscopy in some cases. Patients of all ages may show the presence of Alcian blue positive material in the dermis as gossamer threads and focal stippling. In sections which are otherwise non-informative the presence of prominent 'vascular clusters' of small dilated blood vessels high in the dermis should at least suggest consideration of the possibility of dermatomyositis.

In the poikilodermatous lesions seen in dermatomyositis the histological appearances may be very similar to those seen in LE, but as a rule liquefaction degeneration is not nearly so marked and the dermal infiltrate tends to be just beneath the epidermis, consisting of lymphocytes, histiocytes and a few plasma cells (Fig. 11.10). Focal haemorrhage with haemosiderin deposition may be seen and sometimes there is melanin incontinence.

Histopathology of muscle   It is essential to obtain a well-orientated, atraumatic core of muscle in order to prevent the many artefacts associated with faulty biopsy technique. Cryostat sections provide the best preparations, obviating the shrinkage artefact seen in paraffin sections which has led to misdiagnosis in the past. It must also be clearly stated that even in the presence of an elevated CPK, random muscle biopsy may show no signs of a

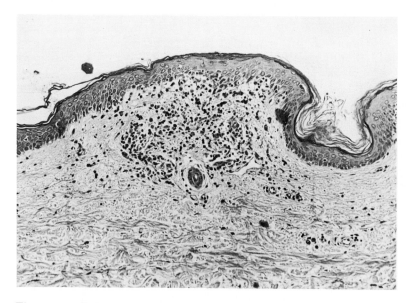

Fig. 11.10 Poikiloderma in dermatomyositis. There is moderate hyperkeratosis, some epidermal thinning with loss of rete ridges and focal liquefaction degeneration of the basal layer. Some papillary oedema is present with vascular dilatation, and a lympho-histiocytic infiltrate which includes some free red blood cells is seen beneath the epidermis.

necrotising myopathy. In doubtful or apparently negative biopsies, recourse should be made to one of the expert opinions on muscle pathology available in certain centres.

Transverse sections should always be studied, with the addition of longitudinal sections if enough material is available. An early sign is dilatation of the capillaries associated with individual muscle fibres (Fig. 11.11). Fibre rounding, variation in fibre diameter, with the

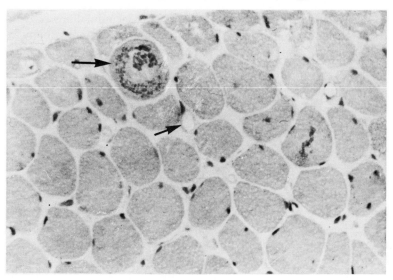

Fig. 11.11 Early polymyositis. Fibre rounding, variation in fibre size, some internal nuclei, dilatation of capillaries (lower arrow) and haemorrhage into one fibre are seen (upper arrow).

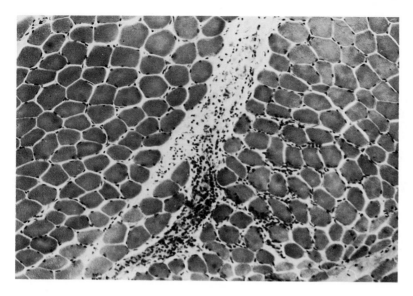

Fig. 11.12 Oedema separates the fibres and there is a chronic inflammatory infiltrate both in the interstitium and between muscle fibres.

presence of increasing numbers of internal sarcolemmal nuclei and a variable degree of myoedema may all occur, but, significantly, hypertrophic fibres are not seen (Fig. 11.12). Necrosis of fibres with loss of sarcoplasm through phagocytosis by histiocytes entering the damaged fibre (myophagia) (Fig. 11.13) and the appearance of small basophilic fibres with large 'potato eye' nuclei (regenerating fibres) point to the coexistence of processes of damage and repair. Many or few muscle fascicles may be involved, and the degree of damage also

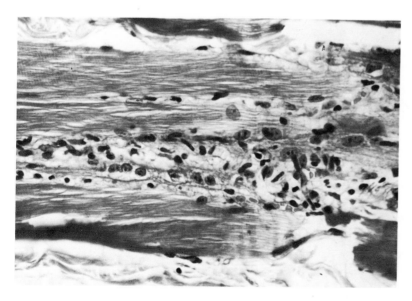

Fig. 11.13 Myophagia. Damaged fibre is being digested by macrophages (longitudinal section).

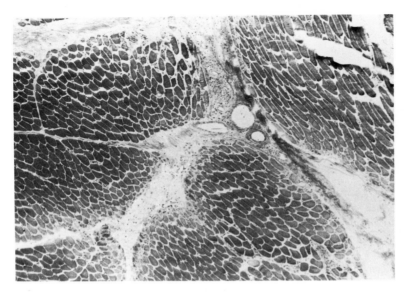

Fig. 11.14   Perisfascicular atrophy. Fibres at the periphery of the muscle fascicles are much smaller than those in the centres.

varies. There may be a heavy inflammatory component, or it may be seen only as a few lymphocytes and plasma cells cuffing medium-sized blood vessels after examination of multiple sections. A very useful sign which strongly supports a diagnosis of polymyositis, especially in children, is the appearance of perifascicular fibre atrophy (Fig. 11.14), particularly in less severely affected fascicles. Oedema of the muscle fascicles may also be seen, and, as the condition becomes more chronic, degeneration outstrips regeneration with

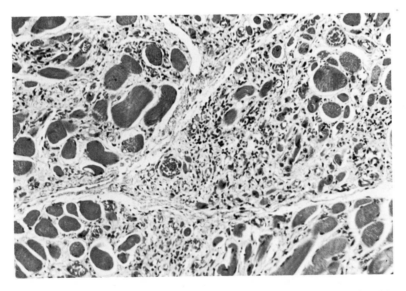

Fig. 11.15   Chronic continuing polymyositis. Extensive fibrosis with evidence of chronic inflammatory cell infiltrate is still present. There is much destruction of muscle tissue.

ensuing fibrosis which, in severe cases, extends from the interstitial tissue throughout the fascicles (Fig. 11.15). There have been reports variously of the finding of virus-like particles[8] on ultrastructural examination, but so far no clear evidence exists that activated viral infection is responsible for the aetiology of dermatomyositis.

In the polymyositis of SLE, polyarteritis nodosa, sarcoidosis[9] etc., a variety of changes may be seen in the muscle biopsy, and the reader is referred to the specialist literature[10] on the subject. In Sjögren's syndrome and progressive systemic sclerosis the findings may be similar to those seen in dermatomyositis, and are non-specific.

Scleroderma (systemic sclerosis and morphoea)

The term 'scleroderma' is used in the literature to describe two entirely different disease processes: one in which the skin is involved along with other viscera, and the other limited to the skin with no visceral involvement. Both conditions show clinical evidence of hardening of the skin but beyond that the similarities cease.

Systemic sclerosis (diffuse scleroderma)

This condition is most often seen in women. The onset is preceded for a period of several years by Raynaud's phenomenon. Gradually the patient notices stiffness of the hands or feet, and at this stage is often referred to a rheumatology clinic with a tentative diagnosis of early rheumatoid arthritis. The lesions, however, are not in the joints but in the skin, which is shrinking and prevents joint movement. At about the same time dysphagia may develop, or if the patient wears dentures these require frequent reshaping because the contours of the mouth are continuously altering. The progression of the disease is slow but relentless, and in the later stages the skin over the hands and feet is taut, shiny, devoid of creases and appears to be bound down to the underlying bone. Small ulcers which may discharge calcareous granules appear sometimes on the fingers or toes. The skin of the face shrinks so that there may be difficulty in opening the mouth; the features become sharpened and eventually all patients suffering from the disease have a similar facies. Dysphagia increases and various gastrointestinal symptoms appear. There is progressive pulmonary fibrosis, usually complicated by repeated attacks of respiratory infection. There is also myocardial fibrosis and often progressive renal involvement. All of these cause and may subsequently aggravate cardiac failure. Death occurs after many years, although in some cases the disease burns itself out leaving the patient more or less crippled.

On histological examination the entire gastrointestinal tract from mouth to anus shows an extensive fibrosis. The same findings in the lungs are associated with cyst formation, and the myocardium also reveals extensive fibrosis. The renal lesions resemble those seen in (acute) systemic lupus erythematosus ('wire loop' changes in the glomeruli) with added changes due to hypertension.

If the skin, even in the late stages, is examined it shows that its normal microarchitecture is maintained (Fig. 11.16) unless the calcification of the dermis results in ulceration and repair by scarring. The epidermis retains its rete ridges and there is a normal complement of vessels and sweat glands. It will be noticed, however, that the dermis has shrunk and the subcutaneous fat is much nearer the epidermis than normal. In other words, it is a normal skin in miniature. If silver impregnation for nerve endings is performed it will be seen that these appear to be increased in number because dermal shrinkage brings them closer together.

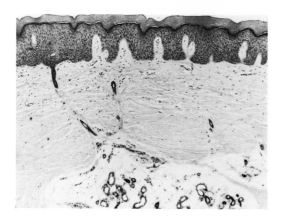

Fig. 11.16 Systemic sclerosis. This photograph is from the skin of the finger. The normal microarchitecture of the skin is maintained and the dermal appendages are present in normal numbers. The dermis is reduced in thickness, which results in the subcutaneous fat being nearer to the epidermis than normal (cf. Fig. 11.17).

Morphoea (localised scleroderma)

This condition may affect any part of the skin surface, and varies from a small, circular plaque to entensive involvement of a large area. There is no association with Raynaud's phenomenon and viscera are not involved.

The initial lesion is a localised thickening of the skin surrounded by a violaceous inflammatory border. It spreads for a while, then ceases, eventually undergoing partial involution and leaving a hardened disc in the skin covered by hyperpigmented atrophic epidermis. In the initial stages the collagen in the mid portion of the dermis becomes thick, swollen and somewhat hyalinised-looking. The elastic fibres become stretched, and in the reticular dermis appear thereby to lie straighter and more parallel with the surface. In addition, some longitudinal splitting of the fibres may be observed. As they approach the margin of the lesion these changes merge gradually with the normal dermis. A perivascular lymphocytic infiltrate may be seen at this site. While the changes in the collagen may stay in the mid zone of the dermis, as the condition progresses they tend to spread upwards to involve the papillary dermis, obliterating and replacing its fine structure by dense hyaline girders of collagen. In the late stage the epidermis is atrophic with flattening of the rete ridges. The entire dermis is replaced by thick strands of acellular collagen, lying parallel with the epidermis. In haematoxylin and eosin preparations this collagen looks hyalinised, and the distinction between the papillary and reticular dermis becomes obliterated (Fig. 11.17).

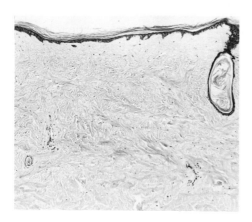

Fig. 11.17 Morphoea (localised scleroderma). The epidermis is atrophic. The entire dermis has been replaced by strands of acellular hyaline collagen obliterating the distinction between the papillary and reticular layers. The dermal appendages are destroyed (cf. Fig. 11.16).

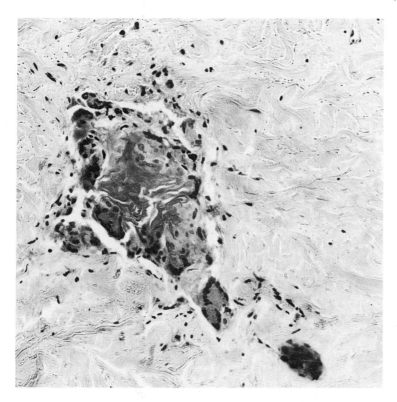

Fig. 11.18   Morphoea (localised scleroderma). A portion of hair shaft in the mid dermis is surrounded by multinucleated giant cells.

Similarly, elastic tissue stains show that the fibres in both the papillary and reticular dermis, though preserved, are all now lying parallel with the surface. Sweat glands and pilosebaceous follicles are completely destroyed although here and there an odd fragment of sweat gland (Fig. 11.18) or hair may be seen surrounded by a multinucleated foreign-body-type giant cell. If morphoea involves a limb or the scalp during childhood, the growth of the underlying bone structure may be affected, resulting in shortening of the limb or asymmetry of the skull.

Eosinophilic fasciitis

This condition, first described by Shulman[11] in 1974, is being reported more frequently as clinical awareness develops. It is characterised by localised hardening of the skin, with muscle fatigue and stiffening following exertion. At some stage in its evolution, transient eosinophilia may be found in the peripheral blood, together with elevation of the ESR, and there is usually hypergammaglobulinaemia. The histopathology of Shulman's syndrome is found in the deep fascia,[12] and to make a histological diagnosis, an unusually deep biopsy is required. This means an incision down to and including the fascia of the skeletal muscle in the area involved, with atraumatic removal of the tissue as described in Chapter 2. Within the fascia an inflammatory cell infiltrate is seen scattered throughout, and this infiltrate may or may not contain numbers of eosinophils. As the condition progresses, there is involvement of the subcutaneous fat by the inflammatory process, and eventually a shelf of sclerosis is seen in the fat with only a few remaining inflammatory cells.

Undoubtedly many such cases in the past have been diagnosed as variants of progressive systemic sclerosis,[13] and because the prognosis in Shulman's syndrome is so very much better, it is of importance to make the distinction.

Pretibial myxoedema

Paradoxically this condition is usually seen in association with thyrotoxicosis, in which there is concomitant exophthalmos. Coarse nodular yellow-white plaques develop on the shins and the dorsa of the feet. Histologically, on routine haematoxylin and eosin sections all that can be seen is an appearance of oedema affecting the dermis, most intense in the deep dermis, and separation of collagen bundles (Fig. 11.19). The collagen fibres appear to be stretched

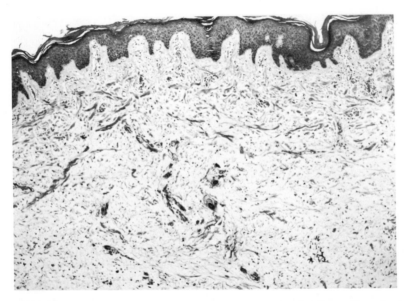

Fig. 11.19   Pretibial myxoedema. There is separation of collagen fibres in the mid dermis by mucin deposits.

and form a lattice-like arrangement, best seen by reducing the iris diaphragm of the microscope. Using an appropriate stain for tissue mucin, such as Alcian blue, shows that what appears to be oedema is in fact deposition of mucin. The mucin is present in large amounts as threads and small pools which separate the collagen fibres and is PAS-negative.

Papular mucinosis

In papular mucinosis, an asymptomatic condition, deposits of mucin are seen in the dermis, but in a more discrete fashion than in pretibial myxoedema. Fibroblast activity is seen virtually surrounding the foci of mucin deposits. A variant of papular mucinosis, scleromyxoedema,[14] also shows deposits of mucin in the dermis. In addition, fibroblast activity is considerable, with the formation of coarse collagen bundles distributed irregularly in the deep dermis.

Lichen sclerosus et atrophicus

This condition occurs most frequently as an itching vulvar dermatosis, but is also seen on the glans penis and on the skin, notably the perianal area, the neck and the upper trunk. It presents clinically as flat-topped white papules which unite to form irregular plaques, and, in the vulva, if they show slight induration, may be regarded as 'leucoplakia' (Chapter 4).

In fully developed lesions the histology shows considerable thinning of the epithelium, over which is dense lamellar hyperkeratosis. Follicular plugging may be seen, and there is liquefaction degeneration of the basal layer, with, in some cases, the development of a subepidermal cleft which in turn may progress to frank bulla formation.

While these appearances are regarded as those of the 'classic' case, it must be stated that on occasion the epidermis appears normal in thickness, or even shows focal acanthosis.

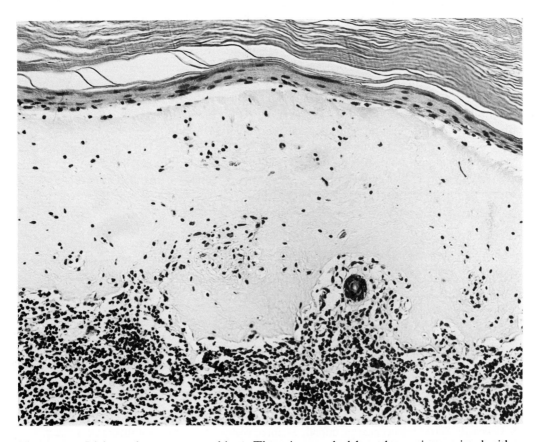

Fig. 11.20 Lichen sclerosus et atrophicus. There is a marked hyperkeratosis associated with an extreme degree of epidermal atrophy. The almost complete liquefaction degeneration of the stratum basale has resulted in separation of the dermo-epidermal junction. The papillary layer of the dermis has a pale homogeneous (ground glass) appearance. There is a dense linear band of lymphocytes with a few histiocytes at the junction of the papillary and reticular dermis.

Fortunately the changes seen in the dermal collagen are striking and diagnostic. In the papillary dermis there is an area of pale, homogeneous collagen remnant which has a very typical ground glass appearance (Fig. 11.20), and within this there is considerable oedema. Elastic tissue stains show that only a very few elastic fibre fragments remain in this area, while those in the reticular dermis remain intact. An inflammatory cell infiltrate of histiocytes and lymphocytes is present at the base of the homogeneous zone, and in early cases may be quite dense. In long-standing cases, however, the infiltrate becomes less dense and may eventually disappear.

Cutaneous amyloid[15]

Various clinical forms of primary cutaneous amyloid have been defined, including a generalised form, a macular and a papular, with overlaps occurring in the latter two.

Histologically the finding of melanin pigment incontinence in the papillary dermis should alert the pathologist to consideration of the diagnosis. Closer inspection of the area will reveal the presence of what may be only minute deposits of the pink, globular amorphous amyloid in a haematoxylin and eosin section. In the primary systemic or generalised form the deposits of amyloid are much easier to detect, and as the condition progresses, not only the papillary dermis is affected but also the reticular dermis around blood vessels and sweat glands, and even the subcutaneous fat. Seldom is there any accompanying inflammatory response in any of those forms of the disorder.

Over the years a number of staining methods have been developed for the identification of amyloid, but none is specific. The most useful method remains that of the Congo red stain with confirmatory apple-green birefringence on polaroscopy. The thioflavine T method is a very simple procedure giving spectacular positive results, but has the disadvantage of producing false positive results on occasion. Clearly the definitive method for the identification of amyloid is by the use of the electron microscope, when the characteristic short non-branching filaments are readily recognised.

References

1. Sharp GC, Anderson PC. Current concepts in the classification of connective tissue diseases. *J Am Acad Dermatol* 1980; **2**: 269–79.
2. Black C. Mixed connective tissue disease. *Br J Dermatol* 1981; **104**: 713–19.
3. Harper JI. Subacute cutaneous lupus erythematosus (SCDLE): a distinct subset of lupus erythematosus. *Clin Exp Dermatol* 1982; **7**: 209–12.
4. McQueen A. Skin disease. In D'Arcy PF, Griffin JP, eds. *Iatrogenic Diseases*. Oxford: Oxford University Press, 1979: p. 83.
5. Harrist TJ, Mihm MC Jr. Direct and indirect immunofluorescence techniques in dermatologic disease. *Hum Pathol* 1979; **10**: 625–53.
6. Barnes BE. Dermatomyositis and malignancy. *Ann Intern Med* 1976; **84**: 68–76.
7. Talbott JH. Acute dermatomyositis-polymyositis and malignancy. *Semin Arthritis Rheum* 1977; **6**: 305–60.
8. Pearson CM. Myopathy with viral-like structures. *N Engl J Med* 1975; **292**: 641–2.
9. Callen JP. Sarcoidosis appearing initially as polymyositis. *Arch Dermatol* 1979; **115**: 1336–7.
10. Currie S. In: Walton SRJ, ed. *Inflammatory Myopathies in Disorders of Voluntary Muscle*. 4th ed. Edinburgh: Churchill Livingstone, 1981: p. 525.
11. Shulman L. Diffuse fasciitis with hypergammaglobulinemia and eosinophilia: a new syndrome? *J Rheumatol* 1974; **1**: 46.
12. Torres VM, George WM. Diffuse eosinophilic fasciitis. *Arch Dermatol* 1977; **113**: 1591–3.

13. Fleischmajer R, Jacotot AB, Shore S, Binnick SA. Scleroderma, eosinophilia and diffuse fasciitis. *Arch Dermatol* 1978; **114:** 1320-5.
14. Chanda JJ. Scleromyxedema. *Cutis* 1979; **24:** 549-52.
15. Westermark P. Amyloidosis of the skin: a comparison between localized and systemic amyloidosis. *Acta Derm Venereol (Stockh)* 1979; **59:** 341-5.

12
Bullous Diseases

The bullous skin diseases comprise a group of eruptions of widely differing aetiology and prognosis which share as a common characteristic the formation of blister cavities within or under the epidermis. By convention blisters over 3 mm in size have in the past been called bullae, and those up to 3 mm vesicles. As the actual size of the blister is often related to its age the distinction is not a practical one. In many instances vesicles and bullae are present in the same area of skin, or even in the same section. In this chapter the term 'blister' will be used for lesions of any size.

Blistering disorders can be divided broadly into three main groups. The first, the *mechano-bullous* group, arise as a result of a structural defect in normal epidermal–dermal adhesion. These mainly comprise the various types of epidermolysis bullosa and have already been described (Chapter 5). The second group are the *immunobullous* disorders which arise in association with autoantibody formation against components found in the epidermis, the basement membrane zone and the papillary dermis.[1] Conditions in this category include pemphigus, pemphigoid and dermatitis herpetiformis. Proof that the circulating antibody in pemphigus plays an aetiological role is reasonably well established. The third group of bullous disorders are the *metabolic/bullous* disorders, such as porphyria, in which blisters arise in association with abnormal deposits in the papillary dermis. In addition to these three main groups, cutaneous viral infections may cause blistering. They are discussed in Chapter 8.

This discussion will be limited to those conditions where blister formation is the main and constant feature. In the differential diagnosis of these blisters the dermatitis reaction (Chapter 6), benign familial pemphigus (Chapter 5) and Darier's disease (Chapter 5) must be considered. It should also be remembered that in early childhood the dermo-epidermal junction is less cohesive and many of the acute inflammatory skin disorders such as lichen planus and urticaria, which are not normally associated with blisters, may present with bullae. There are probably no other dermatological conditions, with the possible exception of tumours, in which such clear-cut diagnostic information can be obtained as in the bullous disorders—*provided the blister chosen for biopsy is not more than 12 hours old*. This cannot be overemphasised, as beyond this time degenerative changes in the epidermis or superimposed pyogenic infection may convert a primarily intraepidermal bulla into an apparent subepidermal bulla, while the regenerating epidermis spreading across the dermis may convert a subepidermal bulla into an intraepidermal one. If the '12-hour rule' is adhered to strictly, if necessary by admitting the patient to hospital to await the development of a fresh blister, most of the diagnostic pitfalls will be eliminated. It is a common practice to carry out immunofluorescence studies in blistering conditions to detect site-specific deposits of both antibody and complement in pemphigus vulgaris, pemphigoid and dermatitis herpetiformis.

A small piece of *perilesional* skin should therefore be biopsied and snap-frozen for immunopathological studies, and a serum sample taken for examination for circulating antibody.

Sites and mechanisms of bulla formation

Before considering the individual diseases which comprise this group, it is necessary to have a clear appreciation of the sites of bulla formation in the skin. The two basic locations are (1) within the epidermis—*intraepidermal* bullae—and (2) between the epidermis and dermis—*subepidermal* bullae.

Intraepidermal bullae

These arise as a consequence of focal areas of epidermal cell damage, which by altering the local osmotic pressure result in tissue fluid accumulating in the area. Such damage may be caused by invasion of the epithelial cells by virus particles whose subsequent multiplication within the cell leads to its eventual death, as is seen in herpes zoster. This is termed *balloon* or *reticular degeneration* (Chapter 4). It may result from immunological cell damage, as seen in allergic contact dermatitis (Chapter 6). Lymphokine release results in *spongiosis* or intercellular oedema (Chapter 4). Damage to the cell surface adhesive material may also be mediated by an immunological mechanism, as in the pemphigus group of disorders. This results in *acantholysis* and the classic acantholytic bulla. The various types of intraepidermal bullae are illustrated in Fig. 12.1 and a key to their histological differentiation is given in Table 12.1 Intraepidermal bullae tend to be flaccid and easily ruptured, as their roof is often only three or four cell layers thick. Care must therefore be taken during both biopsy and subsequent processing to retain them intact.

Subepidermal bullae

In this type the separation is at the dermo-epidermal junction so that the roof of the bulla is formed by the full thickness of the epidermis. Because of this, considerable fluid pressure can build up and clinically such lesions appear more tense than intraepidermal bullae, and are sometimes referred to as tension bullae. The subcellular changes in this type appear to affect either the attachment of the basal keratinocyte to the basal lamina or the basal lamina itself, followed by increased exudation from the blood vessels of the papillary dermis. The fine detail of these changes is detectable only with the electron microscope, and on light microscopic examination subepidermal bullae tend to look remarkably alike (Fig. 12.2).

A key to the differential diagnosis of subepidermal bullae is given in Table 12.2.

Pemphigus

This term, derived from the Greek word for a blister, has in the past been used to name widely differing conditions (pemphigus neonatorum, butcher's pemphigus etc.). It should be reserved to cover a group of serious chronic relapsing bullous mucocutaneous disorders which prove fatal if left untreated. On histological and immunological grounds these are divided into two main groups: (1) pemphigus vulgaris with its variant pemphigus vegetans, and (2) pemphigus foliaceus. There is a possible third group which combines the clinical, histological and immunological features of pemphigus and lupus erythematosus, to which

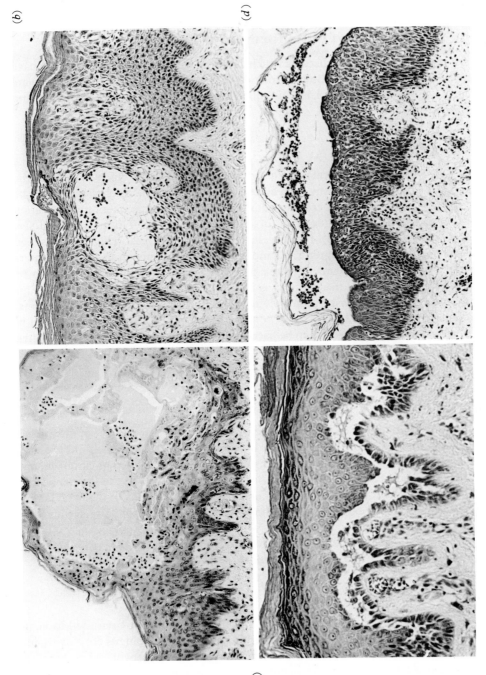

Fig. 12.1 (*a–d*) Different types of intraepidermal bullae. (*a*) Viral bulla (varicella). (*b*) Spongiotic vesicle (acute dermatitis). (*c*) Acantholytic bulla (pemphigus vulgaris). (*d*) Subcorneal bulla (subcorneal pustular dermatosis).

Table 12.1 Key to the differential diagnosis of intraepidermal bullae

Disease	Area of skin involved	Mucosal involvement	Site of lesion within epidermis	Basic pathological process	Differential microscopic features	Diagnostic immunopathology *in situ*	Circulating antibody
Herpes simplex Herpes zoster Vaccinia and variola	Localised to generalised	Yes. Sometimes	Intraepidermal. No specific location	Degeneration and swelling of epidermal cells. Balloon degeneration	Balloon degeneration of epidermal cells. Multinucleated cells. Intracytoplasmic or intranuclear inclusion bodies	No	No
Acute dermatitis	Localised to generalised	Seldom	Intraepidermal. No specific location	Spongiosis	Intra- and intercellular oedema. Microvesicles	No	No
Pemphigus vulgaris	Widespread	May precede skin lesions. Oral mucosa usually involved	Suprabasal initially	Acantholysis	Location and extent of bulla. 'Tombstone' appearance of basal layer	Intercellular IgG and C3	Yes
Pemphigus vegetans	Initially as pemphigus vulgaris. Later confined to moist areas: axillae, groins, perioral and perineal regions	Nearly always	Suprabasal initially	Acantholysis	Later stages characterised by acanthosis. Abscesses composed mainly of eosinophil leucocytes in rete ridges and dermal papillae	Intercellular IgG and C3	Yes
Pemphigus foliaceus	Widespread	No	Subcorneal	Acantholysis	Site of bulla. Bulla easily lost in processing	Intercellular IgG and C3	Yes
Subcorneal pustular dermatosis	Generally trunk and body folds	No	Subcorneal	Acantholysis, presumably by proteolytic enzymes from polymorphs	Cannot be differentiated on histological grounds from impetigo contagiosa	No	No
Chronic benign familial pemphigus	Localised. Sides of neck, axillae, groins	Yes	Suprabasal	Slow acantholysis	Dyskeratosis. Histological differentiation from Darier's disease or even pemphigus may be impossible	No	No
Darier's disease	Solitary to confluent on seborrhoeic areas. Bulla rare. If present may be produced by sunlight	Yes	Suprabasal	Slow acantholysis	Acantholytic splits small as a rule. Dyskeratosis. Differentiation from benign familial pemphigus may be difficult	No	No

Table 12.2 Key to the differential diagnosis of subepidermal bullae

Disease	Mucosal involvement	Differential microscopic features	Diagnostic immunopathology *in situ*	Circulating antibody
Bullous erythema multiforme	Yes	Associated with characteristic coagulative necrosis. There may be a vasculitis of the small dermal vessels. Dermal infiltrate mainly lymphocytes and histiocytes with occasional eosinophil	May be weak perivascular C3	No
Dermatitis herpetiformis	Occasionally	Presence of leucocyte microabscesses in dermal papillae adjacent to bullae	Granular IgA in dermal papillae. Rarely linear IgA at dermo-epidermal junction	No
Bullous pemphigoid	Yes	Fresh bulla contains serofibrinous exudate with few inflammatory cells. Eosinophil leucocytes vary in number. Mild dermal inflammatory infiltrate	Linear IgG and C3 at dermo-epidermal junction	Basement membrane zone Ab (usually IgG)
Benign mucous membrane pemphigoid	Yes, extensive later synechiae	Cannot be differentiated from bullous pemphigoid	As for bullous pemphigoid	No
Herpes gestationis	Rarely	Identical to bullous pemphigoid	Coarse linear granular C3 at dermo-epidermal junction	Rarely (HG factor)
Chronic benign bullous dermatosis of childhood (CBBDC)	Rarely	Similar to bullous pemphigoid	Linear IgA at dermo-epidermal junction	No
Porphyria, congenital erythrocytic and hepatic cutaneous	No	Slightly oedematous dermal papillae covered by basal lamina project upwards into cavity of bulla (seen only if biopsy is from area of skin with well-marked dermal papillae). Inflammatory infiltrate conspicuous by its absence	No	No
Protoporphyria, congenital erythropoietic	No	Bulla as in other porphyrias. Histochemistry: dermal capillaries surrounded by mantle of an acidic carbohydrate–protein–lipid complex (in light-exposed areas)	No	No
Epidermolysis bullosa (simple and dystrophic)	Yes (in dystrophic type)	Degenerative changes with vacuolation of stratum basale (in simple type)	No	No

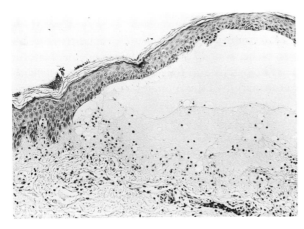

Fig. 12.2 Subepidermal bulla. The roof of the bulla is formed by the entire thickness of the epidermis. Bullous pemphigoid.

the name pemphigus erythematosus (Senear–Usher syndrome) is given. Many authors consider the last to be a variant of pemphigus foliaceus.

The basic mechanism in all forms of true pemphigus is acantholysis (Chapter 4; Fig. 4.4). The most recent observations with the electron microscope indicate that acantholysis begins in the cell surface adhesive material which is interspersed between adjacent cells. As this material disperses, spaces appear between the cells; these become filled with serous fluid. As the gap between the cells widens, cell processes bearing desmosomes elongate and are eventually disrupted.

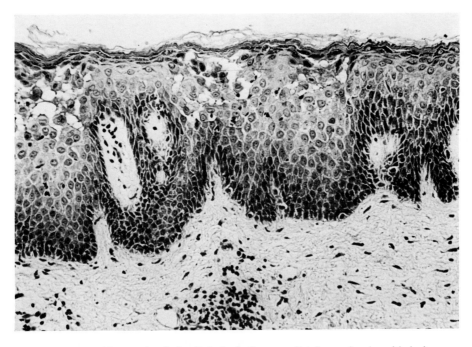

Fig. 12.3 Pemphigus vulgaris (early lesion). On superficial examination this lesion suggests patches of intercellular oedema. The partially separated keratinocytes are, however, assuming the characteristic 'rounded off' appearance of acantholytic cells. The lesion is commencing unusually high in the epidermis for pemphigus vulgaris, the usual location being suprabasilar.

Pemphigus vulgaris

The earliest lesion in pemphigus vulgaris is reminiscent of the acute dermatitis reaction (Chapter 6), the keratinocytes appearing to be separated by intercellular oedema. Careful examination, however, reveals this change to be patchy and to lack the elongated cells with their prominent 'prickles' which surround the margin of the spongiotic vesicle of dermatitis (Chapter 6). In pemphigus, even the partially separated keratinocytes assume the characteristic enlargement and 'rounding off' of the acantholytic cell (Fig. 12.3). In pemphigus vulgaris and pemphigus vegetans, acantholysis usually commences in the suprabasilar regions but it may begin higher in the epidermis. The fully developed lesion of pemphigus vulgaris is illustrated in Fig. 12.4.

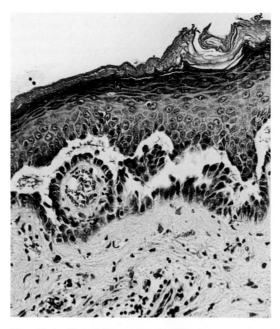

Fig. 12.4 Pemphigus vulgaris. The intact stratum basale projects into the blister cavity. Just above this, groups of acantholytic keratinocytes and a small amount of serous exudate can be seen.

The basal layer of the epidermis may appear intact. Often the acantholytic process has caused separation of the basal keratinocytes at their lateral points of contact. The cells are then referred to as 'tombstone' cells and they are seen to project upwards into the cavity of the bulla. The cavity itself contains some serous exudate, an occasional polymorphonuclear leucocyte and free-floating rounded-off acantholytic cells which are most often seen just below the roof of or at the lateral margins of the blister. Involvement of the epithelium of the sweat ducts and the pilosebaceous follicle is commonly seen (Fig. 12.5). Inflammatory infiltration of the dermis by lymphocytes and histiocytes is minimal and confined to the papillary dermis. Oral mucous membrane lesions may precede cutaneous lesions, but sometimes they appear simultaneously. Genital mucosa is frequently affected.

Histological confirmation of the nature of the mucosal lesions may be extremely difficult. Trauma from eating or, in the case of the genital mucosa, friction from clothing, usually

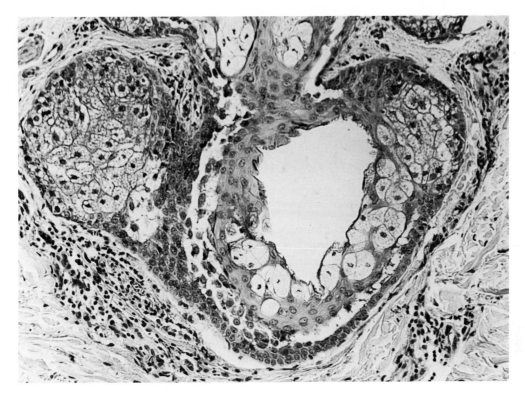

Fig. 12.5 Pemphigus vulgaris. Involvement of the epithelium of the duct of a pilosebaceous follicle by acantholysis.

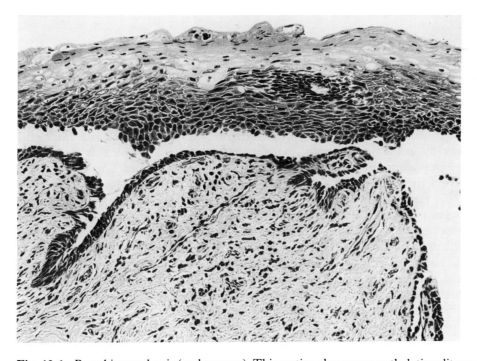

Fig. 12.6 Pemphigus vulgaris (oral mucosa). This section shows an acantholytic split occurring just above the stratum basale of the oral mucosa. A few acantholytic cells may be seen on the undersurface of the roof of the lesion. Note the involvement of the ducts of the mucus glands. (cf. Figs. 12.4 and 12.5).

quickly ruptures these fragile bullae. Figure 12.6 shows an early mucosal lesion which has the same histological characteristics as the skin lesion. Inflammatory infiltrate in the sub-epithelial tissues tends to be much more pronounced in the mucosa than in the skin.

If the roof of a mucous membrane blister is lost either during biopsy or in the subsequent processing, these lesions can very easily be missed and interpreted as chronic non-specific inflammation. One helpful feature is that, as in the skin, the process of acantholysis may involve duct epithelium. Acantholytic splits can therefore usually be seen extending down the ducts of the mucous glands or the minor salivary ducts (see Fig. 12.6).

Pemphigus vegetans

In the early stages of this variant the mucocutaneous lesions are clinically and histologically indistinguishable from pemphigus vulgaris. When, however, there is involvement of the groins, axillae, inframammary and perianal regions, the raw surfaces develop a heaped-up, granular appearance which progresses to warty excrescences or vegetations. Histological examination of the edge of such a lesion may show some acantholysis but often it is absent or it is masked by inflammatory changes. There is, however, a marked acanthosis of the epidermis and long, sometimes branched, rete ridges extend into an oedematous upper dermis. In the tips of some of these elongated ridges, and often also involving the adjacent dermal papillae, are circumscribed collections of inflammatory cells, composed mainly of eosinophil leucocytes with some lymphocytes and plasma cells (Fig. 12.7). This lesion can be regarded as almost specific for pemphigus vegetans. The only other condition in which it is encountered is the fungating granuloma seen in halogen-induced drug sensitivity. The dermis in pemphigus vegetans is oedematous and there is a dense inflammatory infiltrate composed mainly of eosinophil leucocytes, lymphocytes, histiocytes and plasma cells.

Pemphigus foliaceus

The early lesions of this condition consist of very transient flaccid bullae confined to the face and neck. After a few weeks, however, spread occurs to involve the entire skin, and at this stage the clinical picture may resemble an exfoliative dermatitis. Involvement of mucous membranes does occur, but is rare and often insignificant. The acantholysis affects the epidermis, usually in the upper part of the stratum granulosum adjacent to the stratum corneum. The changes are not pronounced and can easily be overlooked. Small areas of the stratum corneum are lifted up and below this are seen a few, rather elongated, acantholytic cells (Fig. 12.8). There is remarkably little reaction to this change, although at a later stage the cavity becomes filled with serous fluid and a patchy dermal infiltration with lymphocytes and histiocytes can be seen. Because of the evanescent nature of the blisters it may be extremely difficult to obtain a really fresh lesion. In older lesions there is some acanthosis of the epidermis associated with hyperkeratosis. Small fracture-like clefts may be seen in the region of the stratum granulosum. The cells in these are small, shrunken and contain dark-staining pyknotic nuclei resembling the grains of Darier's disease (Fig. 12.9). According to Lever[2] these occur in old acantholytic areas in the stratum granulosum and are diagnostic of pemphigus foliaceus. The histological appearances in the early lesions of pemphigus foliaceus are identical to those seen in the staphylococcal scalded skin syndrome (Chapter 8) and bullous impetigo (Chapter 8).

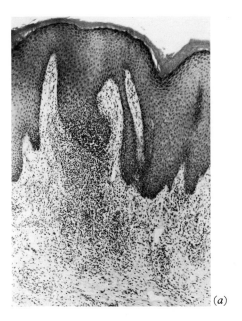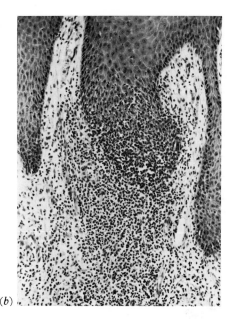

(a) (b)

Fig. 12.7 Pemphigus vegetans. (*a*) The epidermis is acanthotic and covered by hyperkeratosis. In the tip of one of the elongated ridges and involving the adjacent dermis is a collection of inflammatory cells. (*b*) Higher magnification view. The lesion in the tip of the elongated rete ridge and adjacent dermis is composed mainly of polymorphonuclear leucocytes (eosinophils).

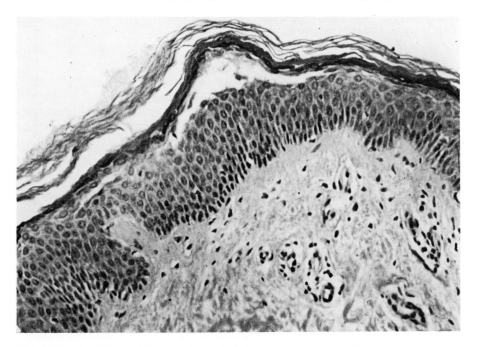

Fig. 12.8 Pemphigus foliaceus. A small cleft can be seen immediately under the stratum corneum containing a few rather elongated acantholytic keratinocytes. Note the absence of inflammatory reaction.

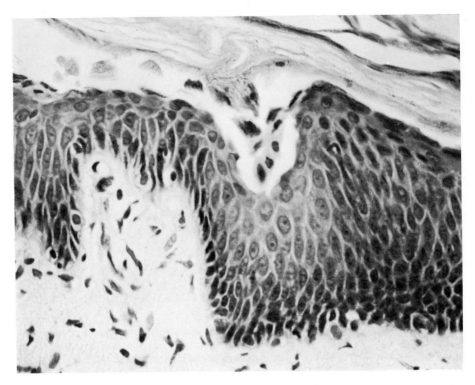

Fig. 12.9 Pemphigus foliaceus. The small cleft in the region of the stratum granulosum contains shrunken cells with pyknotic, rather elongated, nuclei.

Pemphigus erythematosus (Senear–Usher syndrome)[3]

This is a relatively benign condition where evanescent blisters form on the chest and back in association with a facial eruption which resembles lupus erythematosus. The histology of the bullous lesions is similar to that seen in pemphugus foliaceus and the two cannot be distinguished on histological grounds. In view of the original clinical description which suggested elements of pemphigus and lupus erythematosus, it is of interest that immuno-fluorescence studies have confirmed the presence of both intercellular and antinuclear antibody.

Immunopathological studies in pemphigus vulgaris

In the past 10 years the place of immunofluorescence or immunoperoxidase studies in the diagnosis of bullous disorders has become firmly established, and in many departments these are now routine diagnostic procedures. More experience has been gained with the immuno-fluorescence technique but comparable results can be obtained with the immunoperoxidase method and the choice of method will depend on local expertise and equipment.

Although it is theoretically possible to use paraffin-processed material for such studies[4] there is an unacceptable level of false negative results and the use of snap-frozen tissue is therefore recommended. At the time of biopsy of an area *adjacent* to a blister the tisse should be immediately frozen in a hexane cooling bath or by contact with carbon dioxide snow. It

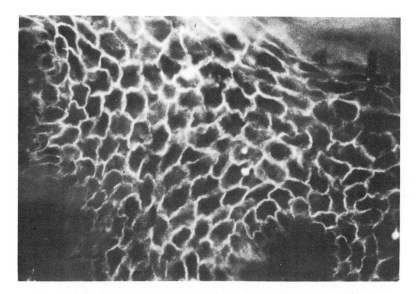

Fig. 12.10   Pemphigus vulgaris. Direct immunofluorescence (IgG) shows clearly the intercellular staining between epidermal keratinocytes.

then should be stored at -70°C until cut at 5–6 μm on a cryostat. Tissue sections are then overlaid with appropriate dilutions of fluorescence-conjugated antisera or taken through the peroxidase immunoenzyme bridge technique. Excellent technical results are available with either of these methods.[5,6]

In the case of pemphigus, an antibody (usually of the IgG class) will be found deposited in the intercellular areas of the epidermis, giving a striking and diagnostic picture (Fig. 12.10).[7,8] Complement deposits are generally seen in association with this antibody deposition. In pemphigus vulgaris and pemphigus vegetans the antibody deposition is maximal in the lower layers of the epidermis while in pemphigus foliaceus it is usually more striking in the upper layers, reflecting the site of damage in these variants. False negatives of this direct immunopathological test are rare in untreated patients, while false positive results may rarely be seen in association with the rash of secondary syphilis, severe burns and some drug eruptions.

In addition to the direct demonstration of antibody deposition at the site of pathological damage, a circulating antibody can also be demonstrated by the indirect test. This test requires use of a mucosal substrate such as monkey oesophagus, guinea-pig lip or human vaginal mucosa. The chosen tissue is cut on a cryostat at 5–6 μm, layered with the patient's serum and thereafter with fluorescein-labelled antiserum. A clear intercellular deposition of antibody is demonstrated. This test can be quantified by diluting out the patient's serum until the positive reaction is lost. Prior absorption of the patient's serum with blood group A and B red cells will guard against false positive results due to antibodies to blood group substances.

Subcorneal pustular dermatosis (Sneddon–Wilkinson disease)[9]

This chronic disorder, which usually affects middle-aged and elderly women, presents as flaccid bullae which rapidly become pustular. The lesions, which tend to arrange themselves in serpiginous groups, occur mainly on the lower abdomen, inner aspects of the thighs, the groins, the axillae and inframammary regions. The contents of the pustules are sterile.

Histological examination shows a collection of leucocytes just under the stratum corneum (Fig. 12.11). There is no true acantholysis, although an occasional isolated flattened keratinocyte may be seen in the floor of the pustule. This presumably is caused by the high concentration of proteolytic enzymes, released from disintegrating polymorphonuclear

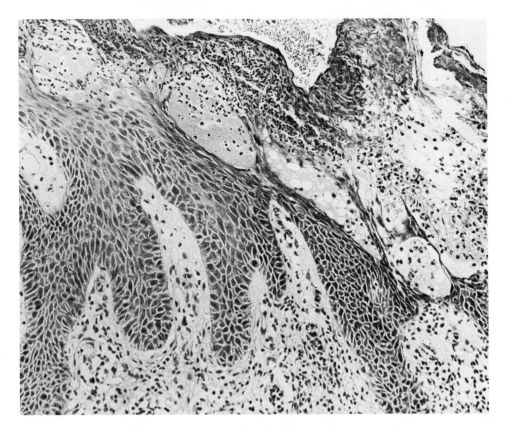

Fig. 12.11   Subcorneal pustular dermatosis (late stage). The epidermis to the right of the picture has disintegrated and has been replaced by polymorphonuclear leucocytes and serous exudate. The underlying papillary dermis is oedematous and infiltrated by polymorphonuclear leucocytes.

leucocytes, present in the pustule. There is some oedema of the dermis with an associated mild perivascular infiltrate in which polymorphonuclear leucocytes predominate. As the disease progresses the epidermis shows marked intra- and intercellular oedema, becomes infiltrated by polymorphs and finally disintegrates completely. The papillary dermis becomes increasingly oedematous and the inflammatory infiltrate more pronounced. Some workers believe this condition to be a variant of pustular psoriasis. The author does not subscribe to this belief but there are certainly resemblances between the later stages of subcorneal pustular dermatosis and the Munro microabscesses and spongiform pustules of pustular psoriasis. Cutaneous immunopathological studies are negative.

Diseases characterised by subepidermal bullae

Erythema multiforme

This term has come to mean separate entities on either side of the Atlantic. In the UK it is used to define a specific disorder characterised by the appearance of 'target lesions' on the skin surface. These are concentric rings of alternating oedema and inflammation which in time develop into necrotic blisters. In severe cases (the Stevens–Johnson syndrome) there may also be extensive involvement of the mucosa of the buccal cavity, genitalia and respiratory passages. In North America, however, the term is used much more widely to describe a rather mixed group of annular, macular and occasionally papular erythematous eruptions in addition to the specific target-lesion-associated condition. From a pathological viewpoint

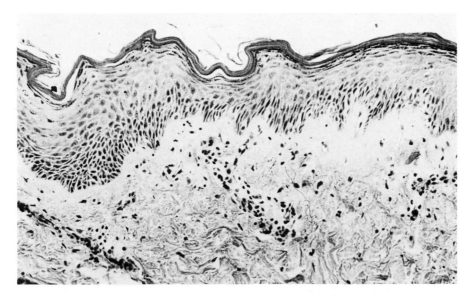

Fig. 12.12 Erythema multiforme (early lesion). The epidermis is normal. There is intense oedema of the papillary dermis which is most evident to the right of the picture as an area of pallor just under the epidermis. There is minimal perivascular lympho-histiocytic inflammatory infiltrate.

the disorder would appear to represent a reaction, perhaps allergic or toxic, to a variety of unrelated stimuli such as drugs and micro-organisms or their products.

The histological changes are numerous and may be related to the age of the lesion biopsied. As far as can be determined, the earliest changes consist of intense oedema of the papillary dermis without an associated cellular component (Fig. 12.12). This may be followed by separation of the epidermis from the dermis with the formation of a subepidermal bulla (Fig. 12.13) which, when complete, may be histologically indistinguishable from bullous pemphigoid (see below). In other cases an intense spongiosis of the epidermis with microvesicle formation similar to that of an acute dermatitis reaction (Chapter 6) may follow the early dermal oedema. The roof of the fully formed bulla in erythema multiforme shows coagulative necrosis (Fig. 12.14). This unique characteristic is an invaluable differential diagnostic feature. The underlying dermis shows a varying amount of oedema and perivascular

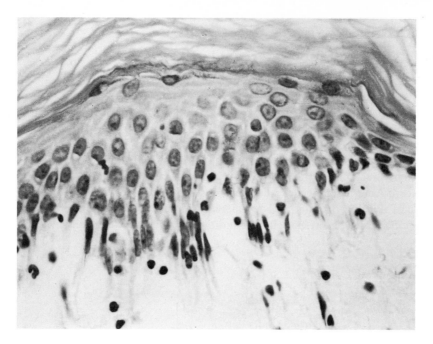

Fig. 12.13 Erythema multiforme (early bullous lesion). There is gross oedema of the papillary dermis, and the epidermis is on the point of separating from it at the level of the dermo-epidermal junction.

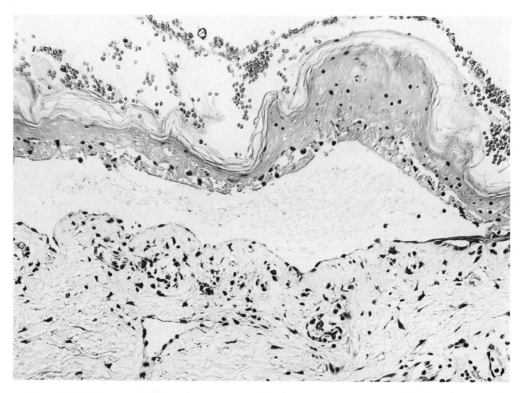

Fig. 12.14 Erythema multiforme (bullous lesion). There is a subepidermal bulla containing fibrin and an occasional inflammatory cell. The epidermal roof of the bulla shows coagulative necrosis. A small tongue of regenerating epithelium can be seen at the extreme right of the photograph. In the dermis there is vascular dilatation with sparse perivascular lymphocytic infiltration.

lympho-histiocytic infiltration. In some instances a capillaritis or frank necrotising vasculitis is seen in the vessels of the upper dermis. The cause of the coagulative necrosis of the epidermis is as yet unknown. It is often seen in the absence of a recognisable vasculitis, and conversely in acute allergic or necrotising vasculitis (Chapter 10) such epidermal changes are not encountered. Sometimes histology of the skin surrounding these blisters shows small foci of keratinocytes which have undergone coagulative necrosis (Fig. 12.15). This suggests, at least in some cases of erythema multiforme, a toxic or allergic effect on the keratinocytes themselves. In bullous erythema multiforme epithelial regeneration along the exposed der-

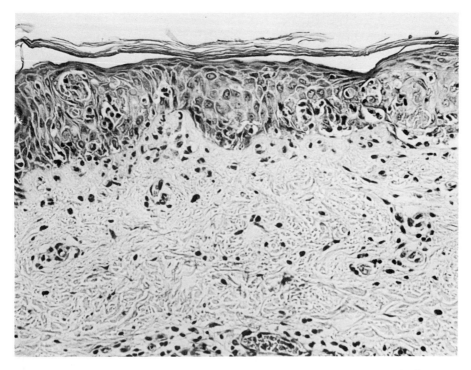

Fig. 12.15 Erythema multiforme. This section from skin adjacent to a bulla shows scattered foci of keratinocytes undergoing coagulative necrosis.

mis occurs with surprising rapidity, and reference to Fig. 12.14 will show a tongue of regenerating epithelium creeping over the dermis. This may rapidly convert the bulla into a pseudointraepidermal one. Whatever the nature of the disease process in erythema multi-forme, it appears to occur in waves and in some instances the newly regenerated epithelium in its turn undergoes coagulative necrosis. Thus layers of intact epidermis appear to be sandwiched between layers of necrotic epidermis. In the Stevens–Johnson syndrome any or all of the histological pictures described can be encountered. Cases which begin as Stevens–Johnson syndrome may in rare instances run a rapid and fatal course, with death due to generalised polyarteritis nodosa. Toxic epidermal necrolysis (TEN) is considered to be a severe variant of erythema multiforme.

Dermatitis herpetiformis

This intensely itchy, chronic, blistering disorder is characterised by small clusters of blisters which have a predilection for certain sites—the scapular areas, the elbows and the sacral area. As the lesions heal they may leave small pigmented scars.[10]

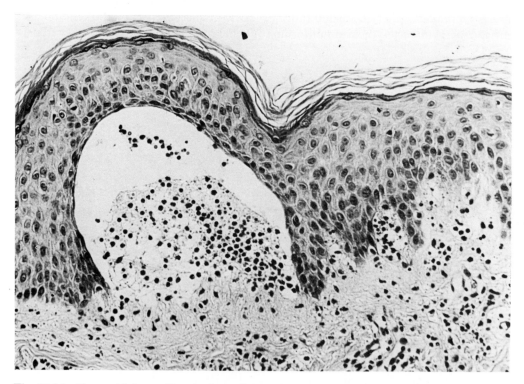

Fig. 12.16 Dermatitis herpetiformis. A small subepidermal blister is seen containing serous exudate and inflammatory cells. Early papillary abscesses can be seen in the dermal papillae to the right of the blister.

Histological examination of a small lesion shows one or several subepidermal blisters containing serous exudate with a few neutrophil and eosinophil leucocytes (Fig. 12.16). As with other subepidermal bullae the formation of the blister is rapid and it is not unusual to have sweat ducts or pilosebaceous follicles torn across at the dermo-epidermal junction. Aggregates of neutrophil polymorphonuclear leucocytes are frequently found in the dermal papillae adjacent to the blisters (Figs. 12.17 and 12.18). These abscesses are of considerable diagnostic value. The epidermis which overlies the papilla containing an abscess may be

Fig. 12.18 (opposite)   Dermatitis herpetiformis. Higher power view than Fig. 12.17 to show detail of papillary abscesses. Many of the eosinophil leucocytes show pyknosis and fragmentation of their neuclei. In this example the epidermis over the abscess has separated from the papilla.

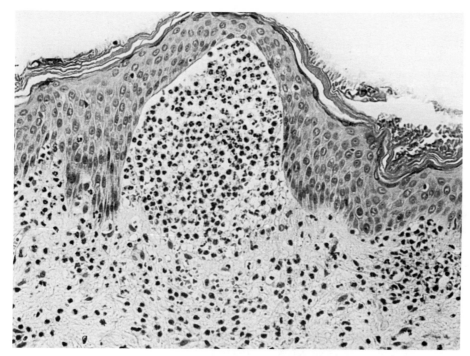

Fig. 12.17 Dermatitis herpetiformis. The dermal papilla contains numerous polymorphonuclear leucocytes (mainly eosinophils). There is some oedema of the papillary dermis and a diffuse inflammatory infiltrate in which eosinophils predominate.

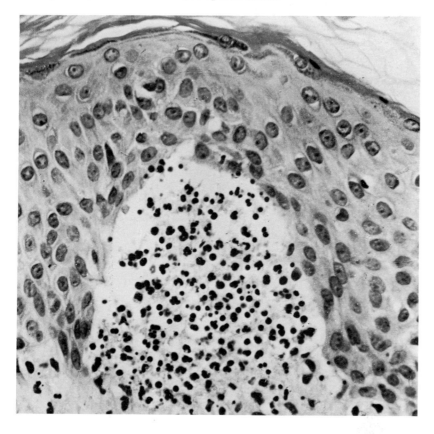

separated from the tip of the papilla by oedema fluid. Papillary lesions may not be found in every section but if dermatitis herpetiformis is suspected it is advisable to sample the block of tissue at different levels in an attempt to find them. Dermal inflammatory infiltrate is considerable, even in early lesions, and consists of lymphocytes, histiocytes, neutrophils and eosinophil leucocytes.

Immunopathology of dermatitis herpetiformis[11]   Examination of skin either from a perilesional site or from a site distant from any lesion will reveal in the majority of cases

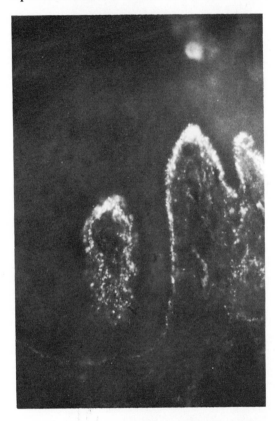

Fig. 12.19   Dermatitis herpetiformis. Direct immunofluorescence (IgA) shows granular deposits most marked in the tips of the dermal papilla.

granular deposits of IgA in the papillary dermis (Fig. 12.19). This is usually associated with C3 deposits and may be patchy, necessitating cutting in on the frozen block or repeated biopsy for its identification. In a small subset of patients (10–20 per cent, depending on the geographic area) the deposit of IgA is not clumped but in a linear configuration along the dermo-epidermal junction. Immunoelectron microscopy has demonstrated two distinct types of this linear IgA dermatitis herpetiformis variant with differing sites of deposition of immunoprotein within the basement membrane. No circulating antibody is used as a diagnostic test, although some 20 per cent of dermatitis herpetiformis patients have circulating antireticulin antibody.

Bullous pemphigoid[11]

The early lesion of bullous pemphigoid is a rather innocuous-looking subepidermal bulla containing only a little serous exudate. There is remarkably little dermal inflammation (Fig.

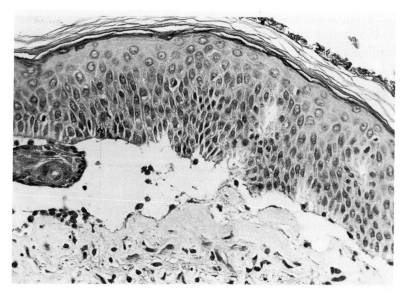

Fig. 12.20 Bullous pemphigoid. Note the clean split on the dermo-epidermal junction with an apparently normal overlying epidermis (cf. Fig. 12.14).

12.20). Histologically, bullous pemphigoid may be impossible to distinguish from some types of erythema multiforme. As the blister ages, marked inflammatory changes appear in the dermis, adding further to the similarity with erythema multiforme. In late (24–48 hours) blisters of bullous pemphigoid, abscesses composed of eosinophil leucocytes similar to those seen in dermatitis herpetiformis may be seen in the dermal papillae adjacent to the bullae. As these papillary abscesses are not seen in early lesions, the selection for biopsy of a blister

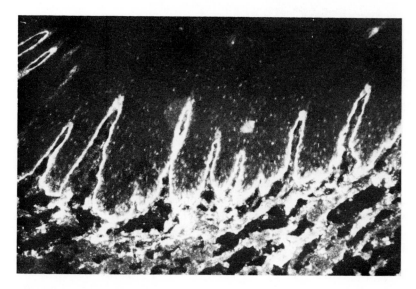

Fig. 12.21 Bullous pemphigoid in direct immunofluorescence (IgG), showing clear linear staining on primate oesophagus.

of not more than 12 hours' duration will obviate any confusion with dermatitis herpetiformis. Some types of porphyria show bullae which might on histological examination be confused with those of bullous pemphigoid. Biochemical estimation of urinary, faecal and erythrocyte porphyrins and immunofluorescent staining are necessary in order to differentiate between the two conditions.

Immunopathology of bullous pemphigoid   Immunopathological tests on perilesional skin reveal a smooth, regular linear deposit of IgG and C3 in the basement membrane zone. Serological tests also reveal an antibody directed against this site circulating in the patient's peripheral blood (Fig. 12.21).

Eosinophilic spongiosis[12]

In a small proportion of biopsies taken from patients with the early stages of pemphigus, pemphigoid or dermatitis herpetiformis the only abnormality is a gross epidermal infiltrate of eosinophils observed in association with intercellular oedema. This picture is thus termed

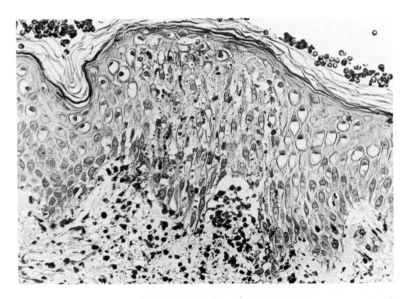

Fig. 12.22   Eosinophilic spongiosis. Note the eosinophils in granules from disrupted eosinophils within the epidermis.

eosinophilic spongiosis (Figs. 12.22 and 12.23). This pattern may also be seen at the edge of fully developed lesions of pemphigus. Eosinophils may also be present in the underlying dermis but the tissue eosinophilia is not associated with changes in the peripheral blood. The appearance is almost certainly due to the presence of components of the activated complement cascade which are chemotactic for eosinophils. The picture is thus not specific for any one of the immunobullous disorders and further pathological or immunopathological features must be sought.

Cicatricial pemphigoid (scarring pemphigoid, benign mucosal pemphigoid)[13]

This variant of bullous pemphigoid attacks the mucosal surfaces of the alimentary tract, the conjunctivae, the genitalia and even the inner ear. Cutaneous lesions are occasionally seen

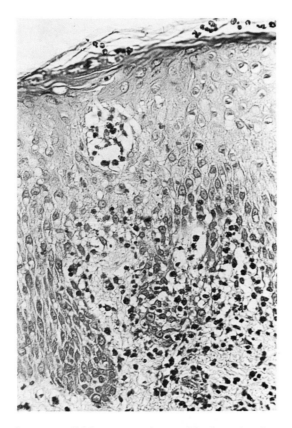

Fig. 12.23 Eosinophilic spongiosis. Note the microabscess of the eosinophils within the epidermis.

but are mild by comparison with the relentless painful activity on mucosal surfaces which may culminate in scarring, stricture formation and blindness. In contrast to bullous pemphigoid proper, this disease responds poorly to systemic steroid therapy.

Biopsy of a blister from a fresh lesion shows a subepidermal blister with an appearance indistinguishable from bullous pemphigoid.

Immunopathological tests usually reveal a linear band of tissue-fixed antibody and complement in the basement membrane zone are but no circulating antibody.

Herpes gestationis[14]

This rare condition occurs in pregnancy and tends to recur with increasing severity with each subsequent pregnancy. Blisters arise on areas of pruritic inflamed skin. The condition tends to deteriorate initially after delivery, and then clear spontaneously. Immunopathological and ultrastructural studies have indicated that this condition is more closely associated with bullous pemphigoid than with dermatitis herpetiformis. The histological appearance of the blister is identical to that seen in bullous pemphigoid.

Immunopathological studies reveal a coarse and characteristic linear deposit of complement components at the dermo-epidermal junction. This is not associated with immunoglobulin deposits. In a small number of patients a circulating complement-fixing IgG antibody can be detected by the indirect complement test. This is called herpes gestationis (HG) factor and its presence has been reported in cord blood of infants born to mothers with herpes gestationis.

Chronic benign bullous dermatosis of childhood[15]

Chronic blistering disorders in children are bedevilled by confusion over terminology. They are rare, and numerous names have been offered. Children rarely develop pemphigus, with the exception of fogo selvagem or Brazilian pemphigus, but they may develop bullous pemphigoid or dermatitis herpetiformis which is quite indistinguishable from the condition as it presents in the adult. In addition, however, a distinct childhood bullous dermatosis is recognised, named chronic benign bullous dermatosis of childhood (CBBDC). This tends to present between the ages of 3 and 8 years with pruritic clustered blisters, often maximal in the region of the genitalia. The lesions heal with crusting, and fresh crops appear intermittently. It is usually self-limiting after a period of months or even years. Recent studies would suggest that the condition is linked more closely to bullous pemphigoid than to dermatitis herpetiformis but this is still an area of controversy.

This consistent immunopathological finding is of a linear band of IgA at the dermo-epidermal junction. While this finding might tend to favour an association with the linear IgA dermatitis herpetiformis variant, the children affected have an excess incidence of HLA antigens A1 and B8. This immunogenetic association is not seen in the linear IgA variant of dermatitis herpetiformis of adults.

Porphyria

In the course of congenital erythrocytic porphyria, cutaneous hepatic porphyria and erythropoietic protoporphyria, blisters may arise on the skin following exposure to sunlight. Such blisters are again subepidermal bullae remarkably lacking in inflammatory changes. If the blister occurs on a part of the skin such as the hand where there are well-marked dermal papillae, these project into the cavity like the fingers of a glove (Fig. 12.24). This striking appearance seems to result from separation above the basal lamina so that the papillae are held rigid by the basal lamina itself (Fig. 12.25). This feature is most frequently encountered in porphyria, and if seen it should prompt the histologist to suggest the estimation of faecal, urinary and erythrocyte porphyrins.

In erythropoietic protoporphyria, even in the absence of blistering there are always present on the light-exposed skin histological features which are characteristic of porphyria. Dermal vessels are surrounded by a mantle of thick hyaline material (Fig. 12.26) which stains strongly with periodic acid–Schiff even after diastase. It also stains with Sudan black and exhibits metachromasia with toluidine blue. The histochemical reactions suggest that this substance is an acidic carbohydrate–protein–lipid complex, and is possibly derived from a combination of perivascular collagen fibres with a degradation product of porphyrin. Similar perivascular deposits have occasionally been reported in the skin from covered areas in patients with cutaneous hepatic porphyria.

Transient acantholytic dermatosis[16]

In the early 1970s an entity named transient acantholytic dermatosis (TAD) was reported, chiefly from New York city. The lesions were transient small bullae and the condition cleared spontaneously after 4–6 weeks. Histologically, striking acantholysis was present in some cases, and the picture resembled pemphigus vulgaris. The benign self-limiting clinical course and negative immunofluorescent studies for pemphigus antibody suggested, however,

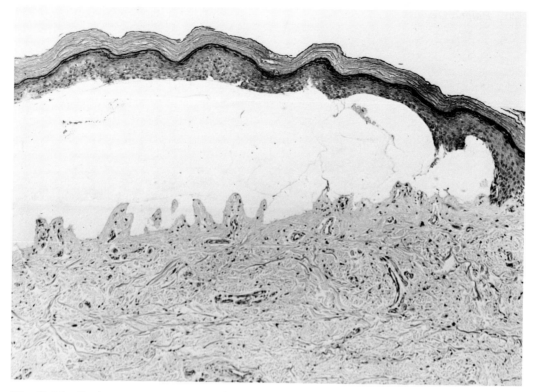

Fig. 12.24 Cutaneous hepatic porphyria. This section from the skin of the hand shows a subepidermal bulla containing a small amount of serous exudate. The dermal papillae project into the cavity bf the bulla.

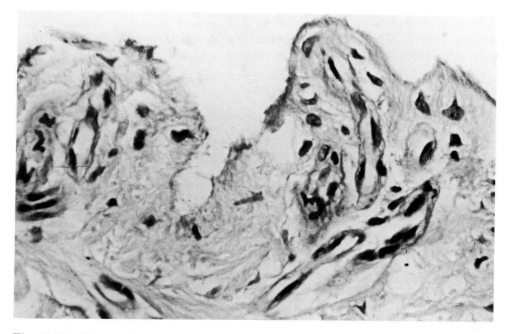

Fig. 12.25 Cutaneous hepatic porphyria. This shows the basal lamina attached to the dermal papilla in the floor of the blister cavity.

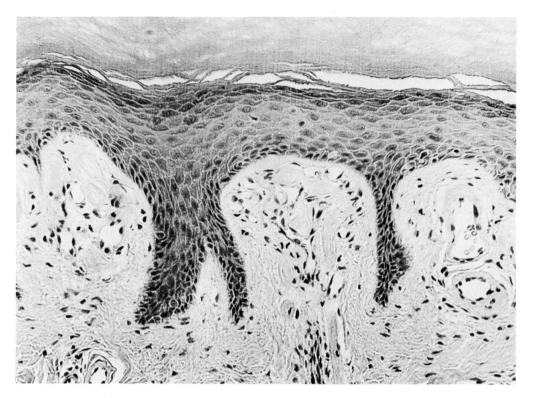

Fig. 12.26 Congenital erythropoietic protoporphyria. This section from the dorsum of the finger shows the characteristic mantling of hyaline material around the vessels in the papillary dermis.

that it is a clinically distinct condition. Variants with pathological features similar to Darier's disease, Hailey–Hailey disease and spongiotic dermatitis have also been reported.

References

1. Beutner EH, Jordon RE, Chorzelski TP. The immunopathology of pemphigus and bullous pemphigoid. *J Invest Dermatol* 1968; **51**: 63–80.
2. Lever WF. *Pemphigus and Pemphigoid*. Springfield, Illinois: Charles C Thomas, 1965.
3. Jablonska S, Chorzelski TP, Blaszczyk M *et al.* Pathogenesis of pemphigus erythematosus. *Arch Dermatol Res* 1977; **258**: 135–40.
4. Turbitt ML, MacKie RM, Young H, Campbell I. The use of paraffin-processed tissue and the immunoperoxidase technique in the diagnosis of bullous diseases, lupus erythematosus and vasculitis. *Br J Dermatol* 1982; **106**: 411–18.
5. Beutner EH, Chorzelski TP, Bean SF. *Immunopathology of the Skin*. 2nd ed. New York: Wiley Medical, 1979.
6. Petrali SP, Hinton DM, Moriaty AC, Sternberger LA. The unlabelled antibody enzyme method of immunocytochemistry. Quantitative comparison of sensitivities with and without peroxidase-antiperoxidase complex. *J Histochem Cytochem* 1974; **22**: 782–6.
7. Beutner EH, Lever WF, Witebsky E, Jordon R, Chertock B. Autoantibodies in pemphigus vulgaris. *JAMA* 1965; **192**: 682–8.
8. Chorzelski TP, von Weiss JF, Lever WF. Clinical significance of autoantibodies in pemphigus. *Arch Dermatol* 1966; **93**: 570–6.

9. Sneddon IB, Wilkinson DS. Subcorneal pustular dermatosis. *Br J Dermatol* 1956; **68:** 385–94.

10. Pierard J, Whimster I. The histological diagnosis of dermatitis herpetiformis, bullous pemphigoid and erythema multiforme. *Br J Dermatol* 1961; **73:** 253–66.

11. Chorzelski TP, Beutner EH, Jablonska S *et al*. Immunofluorescence studies in the diagnosis of dermatitis herpetiformis and its differentiation from pemphigoid. *J Invest Dermatol* 1971; **56:** 373–80.

12. Emmerson RW, Wilson Jones E. Eosinophilic spongiosis in pemphigus. *Arch Dermatol* 1968; **97:** 252–7.

13. Bean SF. Cicatricial pemphigoid. Immunofluorescent studies. *Arch Dermatol* 1974; **110:** 522–4.

14. Bushkell LL, Jordon RE, Goltz RW. Herpes gestationis—new immunological findings. *Arch Dermatol* 1974; **110:** 65–9.

15. Marsden RA, McKee PH, Bhogal B, Black MM, Kennedy LA. A study of benign chronic bullous dermatosis of childhood and comparison with dermatitis herpetiformis and bullous pemphigoid occurring in childhood. *Clin Exp Dermatol* 1980; **5:** 159–72.

16. Grover RW. Transient acantholytic dermatosis. *Arch Dermatol* 1970; **101:** 426–34.

13
Cutaneous Lymphocytic Infiltrates—Benign and Malignant

A large number of cutaneous disorders show evidence of an incidental lymphocytic infiltrate which is a part of a more specific disease process. Examples of this are the mixed band-like infiltrate seen in the papillary dermis in lichen planus and the infiltrate seen associated with spongiosis in acute dermatitis.

This chapter will deal with more specific situations in which a lymphoid infiltrate, either benign or malignant, is the salient histological feature. Conditions which in some situations appear to be precursor states to the development of malignant lymphoid infiltrates will also be considered.

New techniques in *in situ* identification of lymphoid cells

The past decade has seen rapid advances in our ability to identify subsets of lymphocytes which have distinctive morphological and functional characteristics. From the simple distinction between T (thymus associated) and B (bursa-equivalent associated) lymphocytes we can now subdivide T lymphocyte subsets into those with 'helper' and 'cytotoxic/suppressor' functions, and also identify immature T cell subsets during their intrathymic maturation process. These advances in identification have been made largely as a result of the development of the hybridoma technique for the synthesis of monoclonal antibody and subsequent use of these monoclonal antibodies raised against T cell subsets both on lymphocytes in suspension and on tissue sections.[1] The use of enzyme techniques such as non-specific esterase and alpha-naphthyl acetate esterase (ANAE) has also facilitated this type of approach.[2]

At the time of writing both antibody and histochemical techniques can be applied to frozen sections from skin biopsies. Personal experience would suggest that the monoclonal antibody technique and the immunoperoxidase system comprise a reproducible and accurate method of identifying T cell membrane markers. These techniques at present are used mainly in research studies, and over the next three to four years their place in diagnostic dermatopathology will become established. An important point to be borne in mind is the fact that at present fresh snap-frozen material is required both for monoclonal antibody studies of T lymphocyte membrane markers and for enzyme histochemistry. This requires foresight and the snap-freezing of a representative portion of the lesion at the time of skin biopsy. This is in contrast to the situation in which immunoperoxidase techniques are used to identify cytoplasmic immunoglobulins such as kappa and lambda light chains in the differentiation between monoclonal and polyclonal lymphoid infiltrates. In this situation retrospective studies on paraffin-processed material are possible.

The use of 'thin sections' (1 μm) in the assessment of cutaneous lymphoid infiltrates is already well established in many departments. This technique greatly improves visualisation of cellular detail. The choice of epoxy resin for embedding and stains used depend on personal preference; in this department we find routine haematoxylin and eosin staining and toluidine blue of value.

Two morphological approaches to the study of lymphoid infiltrates and in particular to differentiation between reactive and malignant cells are DNA cytophotometry[3] and measurement of the nuclear contour index.[4] The former method assesses total DNA content of individual cells and identifies hypertetraploid cells as being malignant. Prospective studies using this method have shown a good correlation between this measurement and the subsequent clinical course of the patient. Until recently, use of this method has been restricted to a very few centres because of the need for expensive equipment, but the greater availability of cell sorters should make it more widely available. The latter technique, measurement of nuclear contour index (NCI), is the figure obtained by dividing the perimeter of the cell by the area. It would appear that malignant lymphoid cells are more convoluted and therefore have a higher NCI than benign cells. This method requires further prospective correlative clinical studies but appears to be a promising and relatively simple approach.

T and B cell patterns and the skin

For many years it has been suggested that a subset of lymphocytes may traffic regularly through the epidermis.[5] Evidence for such a subset is largely circumstantial, but many observations suggest that T lymphocytes, and possibly a select subset of T lymphocytes, may have a particular affinity for the epidermis. The phenomenon of lymphocytes preferentially seeking out the epidermis is termed 'epidermotropism', and this feature has given rise to the concept of T lymphocyte and B lymphocyte patterns of infiltration in the skin. The T lymphocyte pattern is one in which the epidermis and the papillary dermis are preferentially involved with relative sparing of the deeper reticular dermis, while the B lymphocyte pattern is that of circular aggregates of lymphoid cells with or without germinal centre formation and is found deeper in the reticular dermis (Fig. 13.1). This type of pattern appears to hold good for many situations, but it is not an absolute guide to the type of

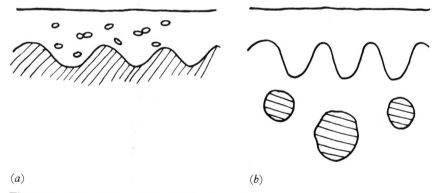

(a)   (b)

Fig. 13.1 Illustration of the distribution of lymphocytic infiltrates of the epidermis and dermis described as 'T' and 'B' patterns. (a) The T pattern involves lymphocytes within the epidermis and an infiltrate occupying the papillary dermis up to the dermo-epidermal junction. (b) The B pattern involves relative sparing of the epidermis and circular lymphocytic infiltrates with or without germinal centres situated more deeply in the dermis with obvious sparing of the dermo-epidermal junction zone.

lymphocytes involved, as in the case of malignant lymphoid cells some of the characteristics of the benign cells from which they were originally derived appear to be lost with disease progression. This is well illustrated in mycosis fungoides (MF) because in the early lesion the lymphoid infiltrate, which is predominantly composed of T lymphocytes with T helper functional capacity, does indeed show this T lymphocyte distribution whereas in later stages of the disease the aggressively neoplastic T cells which have lost some of their surface membrane markers form nodules deep in the dermis and the epidermotropism is lost.

'Benign' lymphocytic infiltrates with a B lymphocyte distribution

Terminology in this group of disorders is bedevilled by multiple names and eponyms. In general, two broad subdivisions can be identified—those with and those without evidence of germinal centre formation. Alternative names for the former include Spiegler–Fendt sarcoid, lymphadenosis benigna cutis (Bäfverstedt) and disseminated or miliary lymphocytoma. A lesion in which no clear evidence of germinal centre formation is seen is usually termed lymphocytic infiltration of Jessner and Kanof. It is suggested that *cutaneous lymphocytoma with (or without) evidence of germinal centre formation* accurately describes both groups of lesions. However, even this classification may present problems because, in situations in which multiple nodules are present, a mixture of germinal centre and non-germinal centre lesions may coexist. The majority of these lesions would appear to be composed predominantly of B lymphocytes, and recent publications on the development of lymphoid malignancies in the region of such areas of preceding apparently benign lymphoid hyperplasia are of importance. At least eight such reports are now in the literature and refer to lymphocytic hyperplasia with and without germinal centre formation.[6] This strongly suggests that in some instances these apparently benign lymphoid aggregates are premalignant, and it is therefore important that patients with such lesions are on long-term follow-up.

Cutaneous lymphocytic infiltrate with germinal centre formation (Spiegler–Fendt sarcoid)

This condition may be a group of discrete, almost translucent papules or a more widely disseminated sheet of lesions. In the majority of cases reported lesions are on the face and an element of light sensitivity may coexist, causing exacerbation in the spring and summer. The lesions tend to regress and recur spontaneously but also respond well to x-ray therapy.

   Biopsy shows a narrow band of normal papillary dermis (Grenz zone) beneath a normal epidermis (Fig. 13.2). The deeper parts of the dermis are heavily infiltrated with a diffuse and uniform lymphocytic infiltrate. Germinal centres are most easily identified at lower magnifications, and there is no destruction of skin appendages. The cells do not invade the subcutis and there are few hyperchromatic cells or mitotic figures, both features of importance in the differentiation from malignant lymphoid infiltrates. Superficial ulceration and destruction of vascular walls or adnexal structures in the dermis are not seen in association with B lymphocyte reactive lesions. Their presence should suggest a true B lymphocyte malignancy.

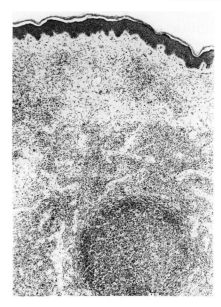

Fig. 13.2 Spiegler–Fendt sarcoid. A nodule of mature lymphoid tissue with a germinal centre can be seen in the dermis. Surrounding this nodule is an infiltrate composed of lymphocytes, histiocytes and eosinophils. In this particular example the infiltrate surrounding the lymphoid nodules is more extensive than is usually seen.
(Section by courtesy of Dr J.M. Anderson, Greenock.)

Cutaneous lymphocytic infiltrate without germinal centre formation

These lesions are macular or slightly raised, reddish-brown plaques which occur predominantly on the face. Scaling and follicular plugging are absent (cf. lupus erythematosus, Chapter 11). In common with the germinal centre associated variety, there is a tendency for lesions to be initiated or aggravated by sun exposure, and spontaneous resolution and recurrence are also common. The lesions are asymptomatic and respond poorly to therapy.

Histologically the picture is that of well-circumscribed, densely packed nodules of mature lymphocytes scattered at all levels of the dermis (Fig. 13.3). The lymphocytes are normal in appearance and lack mitotic figures. The use of a dilute Giemsa stain will usually greatly assist careful examination of cellular detail at higher magnifications. These lesions should alert the physician to examination of the peripheral blood and sternal marrow, and biopsy of palpable lymph nodes if present. Only after negative results of these tests have been obtained should the diagnosis of benign cutaneous lymphocytic infiltrate be made. Even then, long-term follow-up of these patients is necessary.

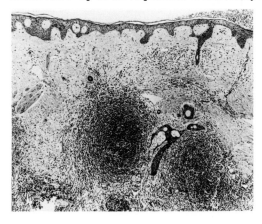

Fig. 13.3 Lymphocytoma cutis. Sharply circumscribed nodules of mature lymphocytes are scattered throughout the mid dermis. These nodules have no germinal centres (cf. Spiegler–Fendt sarcoid, Fig. 13.2).

'Pseudo'-malignant and possibly premalignant cutaneous infiltrates

Over the past decade several conditions have been described in which, although the histological features of the lymphoid infiltrate are suggestive of malignancy, the clinical course is non-progressive. Conditions in this category include actinic reticuloid, lymphomatoid papulosis and lymphomatoid pityriasis lichenoides. While these conditions may initially be a benign and reactive host response to antigenic stimulation, there are now several reports of progression to true lymphoid malignancy in each of these situations, indicating that if any of these histological diagnoses is considered, discussion with the clinician in charge of the patient should take place and the patient be carefully assessed and followed up.

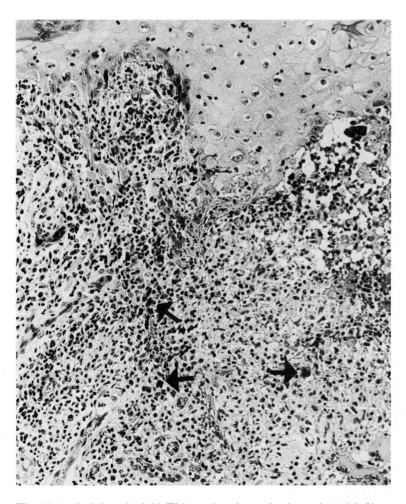

Fig. 13.4   Actinic reticuloid. This section shows the dense dermal infiltrate which extends up to and invades the stratum basale of the epidermis. The infiltrate is pleomorphic in character and contains a number of large aberrant-looking cells with clumped hyperchromatic nuclei (arrowed). Histologically this picture is indistinguishable from a lymphoid neoplasm of mycosis fungoides type.
(Section by courtesy of Dr J. O'D. Alexander, Glasgow.)

Actinic reticuloid[7]

This condition has been described mainly in males. A history of photosensitive dermatitis precedes the development of acute, severe and persistent light sensitivity. The patient develops infiltrated nodules and grossly thickened plaques on exposed sites. Biopsy of these lesions reveals a dense, mixed, predominantly lymphocytic infiltrate which extends from the basal layer of the epidermis deep into the dermis and subcutis. Among the lymphocytic cells are large atypical cells with hyperchromatic nuclei and abnormal mitotic figures (Fig. 13.4). Upward movement of lymphoid cells into the epidermis (epidermotropism) is not common by comparison with mycosis fungoides. Treatment consists of total sun avoidance, and even then the lesions may be remarkably persistent.

Lymphomatoid papulosis[8]

This condition is characterised by the appearance of a crop of papules, some of which may be very large and progress to ulceration and subsequent scarring. The papules heal slowly, leaving residual pigmentation, and are followed after a variable interval of time by a fresh crop of similar lesions. This process may repeat itself over many years and even decades, but

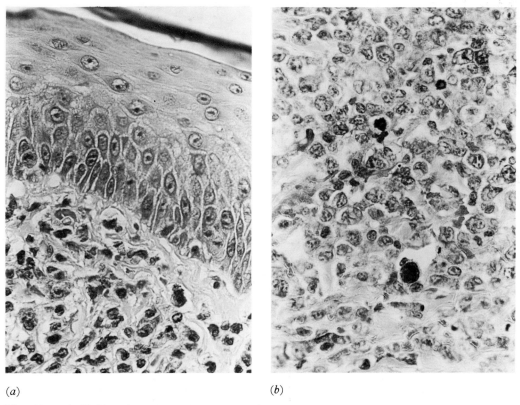

(a)   *(b)*

Fig. 13.5   (*a*) Epidermis and papillary dermis of a patient with a 15-year history of lymphomatoid papulosis. Note the relatively normal epidermis overlying a dense infiltrate abutting the dermo-epidermal junction. Cells in this infiltrate are clearly abnormal with atypical nuclei, but epidermotropism is not seen.   (*b*) Section from a deeper part of the same biopsy, showing grossly abnormal mitoses in the deeper infiltrate of this lesion.

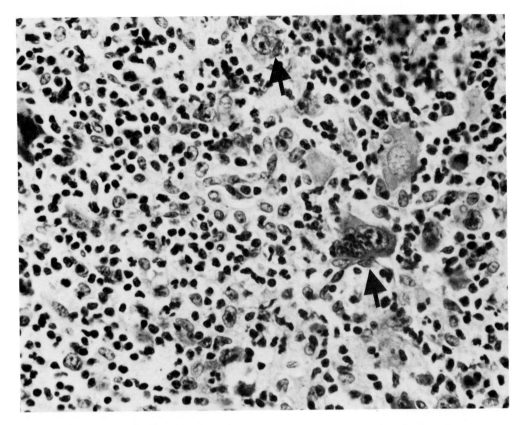

Fig. 13.6 Hodgkin's disease. The dermis is diffusely infiltrated by a pleomorphic infiltrate composed of lymphocytes, histiocytes, eosinophil leucocytes, an occasional plasma cell and aberrant reticulum cells. Some of the latter have the characteristic mirror image nuclei (arrowed) of the Reed–Sternberg cells. This is an unusually florid example of Hodgkin's disease of the skin. The majority of cases contain fewer Reed–Sternberg type cells.

the reports of progression to frank mycosis fungoides, and the coexistence with mycosis fungoides, indicate that this also is a condition which requires careful monitoring once the diagnosis has been made.

The histological features include the presence of a mixed but predominantly lymphocytic infiltrate together with atypical histiocytic cells. Abnormal mitotic figures and nuclear hyperchromatism are frequent, and free red cells are usually present (Fig. 13.5). The polymorphic nature of the infiltrate may be such that cutaneous Hodgkin's disease has to be considered in the differential diagnosis (Fig 13.6). The diagnosis should not be made without clinicopathological consultation, and the patient should thereafter be on regular review.

Lymphomatoid pityriasis lichenoides[9]

This condition shares many features with lymphomatoid papulosis. Clinically the patient presents with crops of recurrent plaques, papules and purpuric patches which prove on biopsy to contain a proportion of large atypical cells with hyperchromatic nuclei and atypical mitotic figures. Free red cells are said to be a valuable diagnostic sign in both this and the

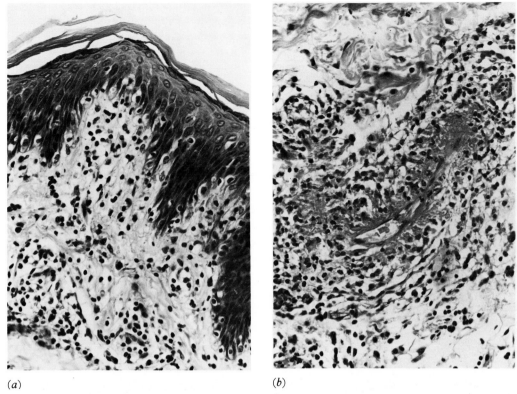

(*a*)   (*b*)

Fig. 13.7   (*a*) Biopsy from a patient with a 6-year history of lymphomatoid pityriasis lichenoides. Note some epidermotropism and the presence of a lymphocytic infiltrate with some large and atypical cells in the papillary dermis.   (*b*) Deeper section from the same biopsy. Note the gross infiltration of a deep dermal blood vessel with considerable fibrin seepage.

more benign variety of pityriasis lichenoides. A significant degree of vasculitis and vessel swelling is a constant feature of both the benign and the lymphomatoid varieties of pityriasis lichenoides (Fig. 13.7).

Cutaneous lymphoma

At present four major classifications of the lymphomata have been offered. The Kiel classification[10] divides lymphomata into low- and high-grade malignancies, while the classification developed by Lukes and Collins[11] uses broad T and B lymphocyte subdivisions. The WHO classification[12] is on a broader morphological base and includes Hodgkin's disease, plasmacytoma and reticulosarcoma as well as 'lymphosarcomata'. The British Lymphoma Group's classification[13] divides broadly into follicular and diffuse lymphoma types and also histiocytic and plasma cell tumours.

All of the types of lymphoma covered in these classifications may on occasion be found in the skin but the occurrence of each variety is rare by comparison with mycosis fungoides, the cutaneous T cell lymphoma most frequently found in the skin. At present the gulf between lymphoma pathologists and dermatopathologists is wide, as is illustrated by the fact that mycosis fungoides is specifically classified only in the WHO publication. In the other three classifications it is relegated to the ranks of 'other', 'unclassifiable' or 'miscellaneous'. It is to be hoped that the current interest in immunological typing of cells in cutaneous lymphoid infiltrates and particularly in mycosis fungoides will lead to greater collaboration and integration between the two subspecialties.

Mycosis fungoides (MF)

This is a chronic, persistent pruritic condition considered by some to be initially a reactive response to an unidentified allergen and by others to be a T lymphocyte malignancy *ab initio*. Recent identification of a retrovirus in a subset of patients with severe MF and also in adult T cell leukaemia in Japan has stimulated interest in a possible viral aetiology of the condition.[14]

The early clinical features of MF include the presence of pruritic raised plaques on any body site. In more advanced disease the plaques become more extensive, covering over 10 per cent of the cutaneous surface, and many progress to raised nodules which ulcerate—tumour stage MF. A proportion of patients eventually develop lymphadenopathy, histological involvement of the lymph nodes in the MF process, and disseminated disease. This

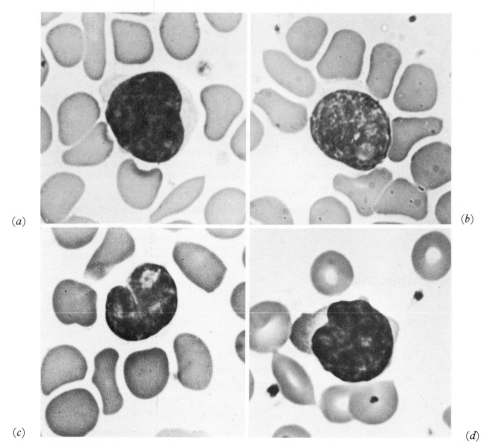

(a)   (b)

(c)   (d)

Fig. 13.8 Sézary syndrome. These cells from the peripheral blood show the characteristic large mononuclear cells with pale convoluted nuclei (Sézary cells). (By courtesy of Dr H.E. Hutchinson, Glasgow.)

proportion appears at present to be substantially higher in North America than in European studies. Relative sparing of the bone marrow is a feature of MF. A subset of MF patients present with an erythrodermic variant of the condition *ab initio*, and this appears to carry a poorer prognosis than the plaque and nodule variety.

Sézary syndrome   The Sézary syndrome[15] as originally described comprised the triad of generalised erythroderma, clinical lymphadenopathy and the presence in the peripheral blood of atypical mononuclear cells (Fig. 13.8). Over the years the term has tended to be

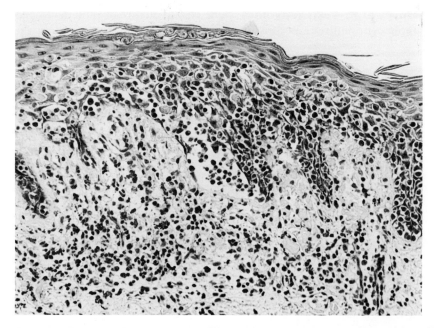

Fig. 13.9 Woringer-Kolopp disease. The epidermis is diffusely infiltrated by cells of the lymphoid series, giving an appearance reminiscent of Paget's disease or carcinoma in situ. There is also a dense infiltrate of the papillary dermis by smaller cells of the lymphoid series. (Section by courtesy of Dr C.E. Stuart, Wakefield.)

used more loosely, and currently it is frequently employed to describe the combination of cutaneous lesions of the MF type and circulating atypical mononuclear cells. While many dermatologists consider that the Sézary syndrome is a variant of MF, this view should be considered with caution because by no means all MF patients proceed to the Sézary syndrome and many cases of Sézary develop without preceding MF. Unfortunately, the rarity of the condition delays accurate classification of the Sézary syndrome.

Woringer-Kolopp disease   Woringer-Kolopp disease,[16] or epidermotropic lymphoblastoma, is a rare variant of MF characterised by the presence of one or more isolated plaques, usually on the lower legs (Fig. 13.9). The condition persists unchanged for many years and appears to be curable by local excision or radiotherapy.

It will be seen from this brief description of the varying names and eponyms used in this complicated field that simplification and a unifying concept are needed. This led Edelson to propose the term 'cutaneous T cell lymphoma (CTCL).[17] This is now widely used in North America and has much to recommend it.

Therapeutic approaches to MF depend on the clinician's philosophy. Those who consider MF a T cell malignancy *ab initio* believe in early, radical and intensive therapy with radiation and systemic cytotoxic therapy, while those who believe that initially it may be a benign reactive condition believe in less aggressive approaches with photochemotherapy (PUVA) or topical nitrogen mustard. There is as yet no convincing evidence of significant differences in mortality or morbidity in patients treated with these two approaches.

Histological features of mycosis fungoides   The classic picture of fully developed MF is that of a lymphocytic infiltrate occupying the papillary dermis and invading the

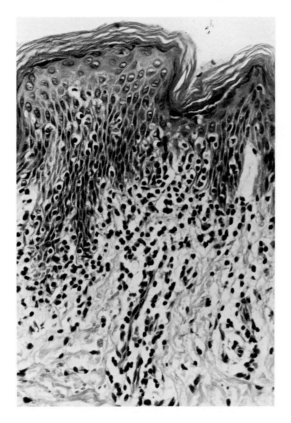

Fig. 13.10 Mycosis fungoides showing generalised infiltration of the epidermis with convoluted lymphoid cells. This pattern of epidermotropism is distinct from Pautrier abscesses but a common feature of mycosis fungoides.

epidermis (Fig. 13.10). This is the so-called 'T lymphocyte zone', and the majority of cells in this infiltrate have indeed been shown to be T lymphocytes and to have membrane markers of T helper lymphocytes. Within the epidermis, the lymphocytes may be situated singly or in clusters—Pautrier microabscesses (Fig. 13.11). Examination of these lymphocytes under high power and on epon sections shows that many of the lymphoid cells have an unusually cerebriform indented and infolded nucleus, and ultrastructural studies will show this characteristic strikingly. This is the so-called Lutzner cell or MF cell. Spongiosis and intercellular oedema are not striking and regular features of MF. Their presence should suggest a dermatitis reaction.

Much more difficult to diagnose is the early stage of MF in which a rather mixed but predominantly lymphocytic infiltrate in the papillary dermis shows occasional cells with large hyperchromatic nuclei and a few individual lymphoid cells situated singly in the epidermis (Fig. 13.12). Thin sections and dilute Giemsa stains may be of value in this situation, but in many cases even after consultation with clinical colleagues the diagnosis cannot be confirmed histologically and the pathologist is obliged to use a phrase such as 'suggestive but not diagnostic of MF' after describing the features observed. In such cases careful clinical supervision and a repeat biopsy after 3–6 months may confirm the diagnosis. Several clinicopathological correlative studies have suggested that there is a mean duration of 3 years between the development of clinical suspicion and histological confirmation of MF.

The differential diagnosis at this early stage includes a dermatitis reaction ('lymphomatoid'

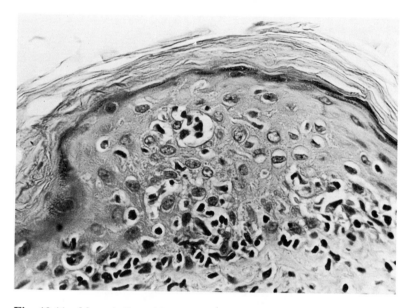

Fig. 13.11 Mycosis fungoides showing a Pautrier abscess and hyperkeratosis but no parakeratosis.

contact dermatitis), reactions to retained parts of parasites such as the scabies mite or *Cheyletiella*, and lymphoid reactions to ingested drugs. A careful history will help to rule out each of these possibilities, and the use of crossed prisms may identify residual parts of the scabies mite or *Cheyletiella*.

In advanced MF the epidermotropic quality of the infiltrate is lost and there is a tendency for the nodules of lymphoid cells to be situated in the mid dermis with less T zone involvement than in the early cases. Abnormal mitotic figures are frequent within the cells and the nuclear/cytoplasmic ratio is high. The differential diagnosis in this situation is from other non-epidermotropic varieties of lymphoma, and once again careful clinicopathological correlation is essential. Palpable lymph nodes should be biopsied but 'blind' lymph node biopsy of non-palpable nodes has a low yield of useful information. Some cases of lymphadenopathy show definitive infiltration with MF cells. The true nature of dermatopathic lymphadenopathy is at present under investigation. The process would appear to involve an increase in the number of dendritic cells in the nodes carrying Ia (immune-associated)

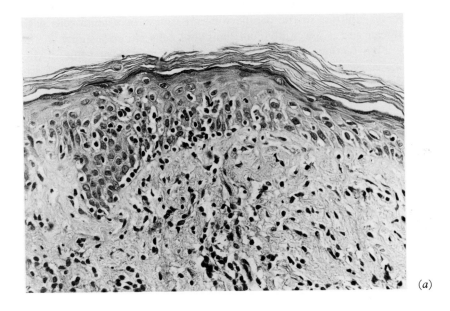

(a)

(b)

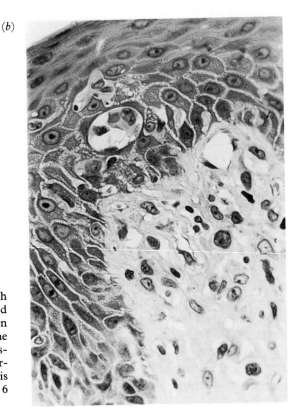

Fig. 13.12 (a) Biopsy from a patient with possible mycois fungoides, showing scattered small areas of epidermotropism. (b) Epon (1 μm) section from a biopsy taken from the same patient at the same time. Note the presence of obviously atypical cells in Pautrier-abscess-like lesions in the epidermis. This patient developed classic mycosis fungoides 6 months after this biopsy.

antigen.[18] Clinical studies suggest that even this degree of nodal change is associated with a poorer prognosis.

Premycotic lesions

A premycotic condition can be defined as one in which a significant number, if followed over a number of months or years, progress to definitive mycosis fungoides. This term has been used for three main groups of lesions: **parapsoriasis en plaques, poikiloderma** and **follicular mucinosis**.

The term **parapsoriasis en plaques** is used to describe raised pruritic plaques which, although clinically suspicious of MF, are not histologically proven MF on biopsy. The histology is generally that of a lymphocytic infiltrate of varying intensity around vessels and in the papillary dermis (Fig. 13.13). The epidermotropism and Pautrier abscesses of fully developed MF are absent. This type of biopsy strongly suggests that, given time, true MF will develop. The clinical differential diagnosis of this type of lesion includes a benign chronic plaque type of dermatitis which may be called chronic superficial dermatitis, digitate dermatosis or xanthoerythrodermia perstans. The aetiology is unknown, and the condition

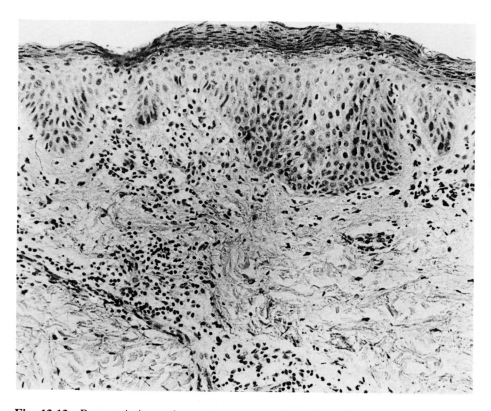

Fig. 13.13 Parapsoriasis en plaques (early mycois fungoides). There is a patchy acanthosis of the epidermis associated with some loss of the stratum granulosum and parakeratois. There is a moderate perivascular cellular infiltrate which extends deep into the reticular dermis. The depth to which this perivascular infiltrate extends, no matter how banal it appears, should always arouse suspicion of a malignant reticulosis.

tends to persist unchanged for many years. Histologically, a very mild dermatitis reaction is seen and progression to MF does not occur, although MF and chronic superficial dermatitis may co-exist.

An undetermined number of patients with **poikiloderma** progress to frank mycosis fungoides. These patients present clinically with a 'dappled' skin pattern of alternating increase and decrease in melanin pigmentation on an erythematous background. The essential histological features are those of epidermal atrophy, liquefaction degeneration of the basal layer, and free red cells in the underlying dermis (Fig. 13.14). These histological features are

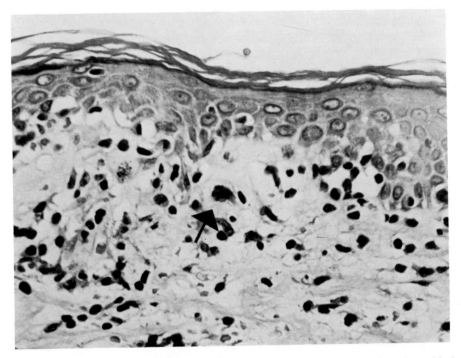

Fig. 13.14 Parapsoriasis en plaques—poikilodermatous type (early mycosis fungoides). The epidermis shows a patchy thinning and there is liquefaction degeneration of the cells of the stratum basale. Erythrocytes can be seen between the collagen fibres of the papillary dermis. The cellular infiltrate in the dermis, although not great in quantity, shows some pleomorphism, nuclear pyknosis and an occasional large cell of the reticulum series with scant cytoplasm and large irregular hyperchromatic nucleus (arrowed). Patchy replacement of basal cells by cells of the lymphoid series can be seen.

also common to the other clinical conditions in which poikiloderma may be a feature—lupus erythematosus, dermatomyositis and certain drug eruptions. Only after exclusion of this triad can the diagnosis of pre-MF poikiloderma be considered. As with 'parapsoriasis', it is essential that the patient be kept under regular review and biopsies repeated at regular intervals.

Follicular mucinosis (alopecia mucinosa) has in the past been divided into two types—one associated with subsequent development of MF, and the other with no such association. It has been said that multiple nodular lesions of follicular mucinosis on the head and neck are not associated with MF, but personal experience indicates that this is not an invariable rule. It is therefore advised that all cases of follicular mucinosis be followed carefully.[19,20]

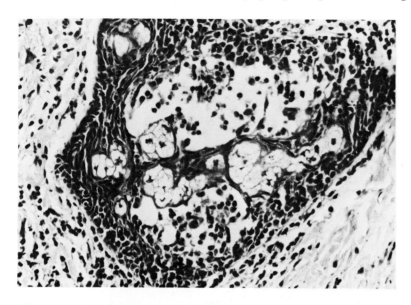

Fig. 13.15 Follicular mucinosis. This biopsy was taken from a patient with classic mycosis fungoides and, in addition, follicular mucinosis. Note the obvious destruction of hair follicle epithelium with a dense lymphocytic infiltrate in and around the follicular and the sebaceous gland elements. Specific stains for tissue mucin were strongly positive in this case.

These patients present with one or more raised boggy plaques on any body site. The lesions may be extremely moist and those on the scalp or eyebrow may be associated with significant hair loss. The striking histological feature is of damaged pilosebaceous follicles and degeneration of the hair shaft (Fig. 13.15). Tissue mucin stains are strongly positive in the hair follicle cells. The condition appears to be specific for the pilosebaceous follicle, and other skin appendages are not similarly affected.

Letterer–Siwe disease

This rare disorder is an example of proliferation of the epidermal Langerhans cell. As the condition was generally fatal, it has until recently been considered a malignant proliferation of these cells, but there are currently suggestions that a failure of maturation or a reactive state is more appropriate terminology. This view is strengthened by early reports of excellent clinical response to therapy with thymus extracts.[21]

The condition usually presents in the first year of life as greasy papules on the face, scalp and trunk. The underlying skin may be purpuric, and crusting and haemorrhage may develop. On biopsy the epidermal basal cells appear to be replaced by large pale cells which contain the ultrastructural hallmark of the Langerhans cell, the Birbeck granule (Fig. 13.16).

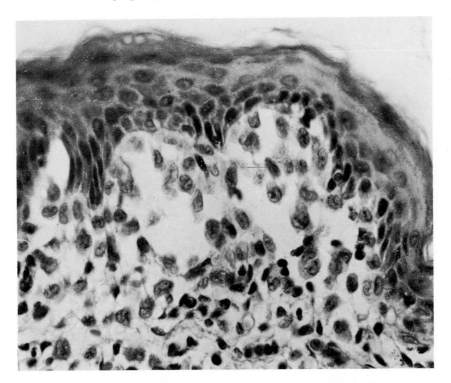

Fig. 13.16 Letterer–Siwe disease. The upper dermis is extensively infiltrated by large pale histiocytes with indented vesicular nuclei. The reduction of the nuclear/cytoplasmic ratio indicates a degree of immaturity. The quantity of infiltrate in the papillary dermis has resulted in a separation at the dermo-epidermal junction of this infant skin.

Histiocytic tumours

The availability of monoclonal antibodies raised against a variety of T lymphocyte differentiation markers and of specific B lymphocyte markers has greatly reduced the number of cutaneous neoplasms considered to be of histiocytic origin, as it is now well established that many lesions previously included in this category are neoplasms of the B lymphocyte maturation pathway. True histiocytic tumours in the skin are rare and present as non-specific nodular lesions occupying the mid and deep dermis. Overlying epidermal ulceration may be present. On haematoxylin and eosin or Giemsa staining, large pale-staining cells are seen with multiple bizarre mitotic figures (Fig. 13.17). An associated, lymphocytic reaction may be present and confuse the diagnosis. Positive identification of histiocytic origin may be obtained at light microscopic level by demonstration of lysozyme, α-antitrypsin and α-antichymotrypsin in the cytoplasm.

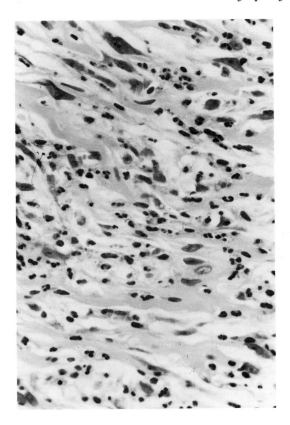

Fig. 13.17 Histiocytic tumour with large, pale-staining histiocytes admixed with reactive cells. Specific staining for lysozyme and for antichymotrypsin were both strongly positive in this case.

References

1. MacKie RM, Turbitt ML. The use of a double-label immunoperoxidase monoclonal antibody technique in the investigation of patients with mycosis fungoides. *Br J Dermatol* 1982; **106:** 379–84.
2. Leder LD. The chloroacetate esterase reaction. *Am J Dermatopathol* 1979; **1:** 39–42.
3. van Vloten WA, van Duijn P, Schaberg A. Cytodiagnostic use of Feulgen–DNA measurements in cell imprints from the skin of patients with mycosis fungoides. *Br J Dermatol* 1974; **91:** 365–71.
4. Meijer CJL, van der Loo E, van Vloten WA. Early diagnosis of mycosis fungoides and the Sézary syndrome by morphometric analysis of lymphoid cells in the skin. *Cancer* 1980; **45:** 2864–71.
5. Streilein JW. Lymphocyte traffic, T-cell malignancies and the skin. *J Invest Dermatol* 1978; **71:** 167–71.
6. Shelley WB, Wood MG, Wilson JF, Goodman R. Premalignant lymphoid hyperplasia. *Arch Dermatol* 1981; **117,** 500–3.
7. Ive FA, Magnus IA, Warin RP, Wilson Jones E. Actinic reticuloid. *Br J Dermatol* 1969; **81:** 469–85.
8. Macauley WL. Lymphomatoid papulosis. A continuing self-healing eruption, clinically benign—histologically malignant. *Arch Dermatol* 1968; **97:** 23–30.
9. Black MM, Wilson Jones E. 'Lymphomatoid' pityriasis lichenoides. A variant with histological features simulating a lymphoma. *Br J Dermatol* 1972; **86:** 329–47.

10. Lennert K. *Malignant Lymphomas other than Hodgkin's Disease*. New York: Springer-Verlag, 1978.
11. Lukes RJ, Collins RD. New approaches to the classification of lymphoma. *Br J Cancer* 1975; **31:** 1.
12. Mathé G, Rappaport H. *Histological and Cytological Typing of Neoplastic Diseases of Haemopoietic and Lymphoid Tissues*. Geneva: World Health Organization, 1976.
13. Bennet MH, Farrer-Brown G, Henry K, Jelliffe AM. A classification of non-Hodgkin's lymphomas. *Lancet* 1974; **ii:** 405-6.
14. Poiesz BJ, Ruscetti FW, Gazdar AF *et al*. Detection and isolation of C type retrovirus particles from fresh and cultured lymphocytes of a patient with cutaneous T-cell lymphoma. *Proc natlAcad Sci USA* 1980; **77:** 7415-19.
15. Winkelmann RK. Symposium on the Sézary cell. *Mayo Clin Proc* 1974; **49:** no. 8.
16. Geerts ML, Kaiserling E, Kint A. The microenvironment of Woringer–Kolopp disease. *Dermatologica* 1982; **164:** 15-29.
17. Lutzner M, Edelson R, Schein P *et al*. Cutaneous T cell lymphomas. The Sézary syndrome, mycosis fungoides and related disorders. *Ann Intern Med* 1975; **83:** 534-46.
18. Lampert IA, Pizzolo G, Thomas JA, Janossy G. Immunohistochemical characterisation of cells involved in dermatopathic lymphadenopathy. *J Pathol* 1980; **131:** 145-56.
19. Emmerson RW. Follicular mucinosis. A study of 47 patients. *Br J Dermatol* 1969; **81:** 395-413.
20. Coskey RJ, Mehregan AJ. Alopecia mucinosa. A follow-up study. *Arch Dermatol* 1970; **102:** 193-4.
21. Osband ME, Lipton JM, Lavin P *et al*. Histiocytosis X. Demonstration of abnormal immunity I cell histamine H_2 receptor deficiency and successful treatment with thymic extract. *N Engl J Med* 1980; **304:** 146-53.

14
Epithelial Skin Tumours

Epithelial skin tumours can arise from both the epidermis and the adnexa derived from it. The number of tumour types is large and it is beyond the scope of this book to review them all. Those which arise mainly from the epidermis will be discussed in this chapter.

For histological diagnosis an excisional biopsy is desirable, but if an incisional biopsy only can be provided it should include the advancing edge of the tumour and if possible its deepest infiltrating part. If the tumour presents with an unusual clinical appearance, small pieces of the tumour should be fixed in glutaraldehyde in case ultrastructural examination is needed to confirm the diagnosis.

Hamartomata

Lesions produced by hamartomatous malformation of the surface or adnexal epithelium are often grouped under the heading of epithelial naevi. While epidermal naevi are more common, malformations of the different adnexa have also been recorded.

Epidermal naevus (hard epidermal naevus, soft epidermal naevus, naevus unius lateralis, ILVEN)

The descriptive terms used for epidermal naevi are derived from their clinical appearances. In general, epidermal naevi have a linear distribution and appear clinically as warty thickenings of the surface of the skin. The basic lesion consists of localised acanthosis associated with a variable amount of hyperkeratosis. The epidermal naevus which is hard, shows considerable hyperkeratosis, while the soft epidermal naevus shows relatively little. Because the acanthosis of the epidermis occurs between fixed points the surface tends to be thrown into folds which may produce a complex pattern, pulling up the related dermis and giving rise on section to elongated and rather prominent dermal papillae (Fig. 14.1). Soft epidermal naevi may at times histologically mimic basal cell papilloma, and only the age of the patient and the shape of the lesion indicate its true nature.

In some linear naevi the various phases of the dermatitis reaction may be superimposed, and the lesion is then known as an inflammatory linear verrucous epidermal naevus (ILVEN). When this occurs, the spongiosis of the epidermis interferes with keratinocyte metabolism resulting in loss of the granular layer and parakeratosis. Occasionally the acanthosis, elongation of the dermal papillae and parakeratosis may simulate psoriasis. In such cases a histological diagnosis may only be possible when considered in conjunction with the linear distribution and the lack of response to therapy.

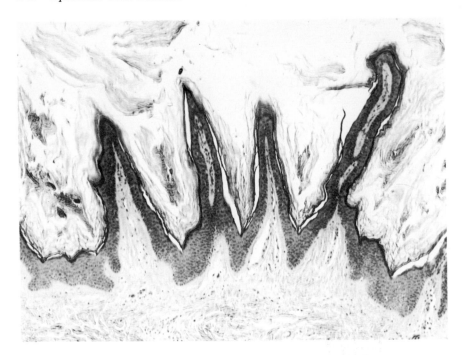

Fig. 14.1 Epidermal naevus (hard variety). There is marked hyperkeratosis and the overgrowth of the epidermis has thrown it into folds with resulting elongation of the dermal papillae.

Organoid naevus

This lesion is discussed in this chapter with the other hamartomata although more than one element of the skin is malformed, the epidermis, hair follicles and sebaceous, apocrine and eccrine glands all being involved in different proportions, often in association with an overgrowth of connective tissue. The most common site is the scalp but the lesion may occur on the face and neck, and rarely elsewhere.

There are three stages in its evolution.[1] Before puberty it presents as a hairless papillomatous area of skin. Histologically there is hyperplasia of the epidermis associated with malformed and often underdeveloped pilosebaceous follicles. At puberty, as part of general sexual maturation, there is growth of the sebaceous glands in the lesion; when this is marked and there are numerous glands the appearances then give rise to the original terminology of naevus sebaceous of Jadassohn. Some organoid naevi may show only hyperplasia of the epidermis associated with a few malformed pilosebaceous follicles and apocrine glands (Fig. 14.2). The third stage in development is the tumour stage.

Approximately 10 per cent of organoid naevi develop basal cell carcinoma, this hamartoma providing the background to most basal cell carcinomata occurring in young adults. Small lesions are seen as atypical basal cell proliferation which may in fact represent aborted hair follicles,[2] but frank basal cell carcinoma is seen (Fig. 14.3). Other tumours of both the adnexa and the epithelium may also develop, and of these the commonest is syringocystadenoma papilliferum.

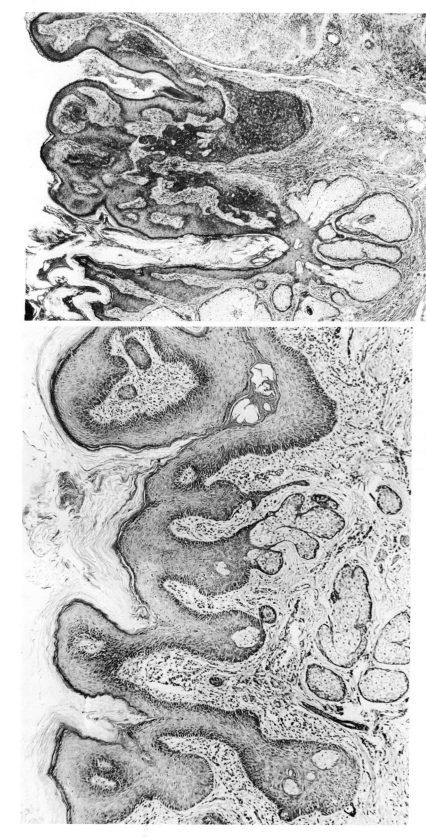

Fig. 14.2 Organoid naevus. There is a papillomatous epidermis with hyperkeratosis and acanthosis. Abnormal hair follicles and sebaceous glands are present.

Fig. 14.3 Basal cell carcinoma, occurring in an organoid naevus. There is a large, abnormal pilosebaceous follicle and a papillomatous epidermis from which the basal cell carcinoma is arising.

Benign tumours of the epidermis

Basal cell papilloma (seborrhoeic keratosis)

This is one of the commonest benign tumours arising from the epidermis. It is often heavily pigmented and may be clinically misdiagnosed as a malignant melanoma. Three main histological types are encountered: a solid type, a verrucous type and a reticular type. Tumours with combinations of the different types are frequently seen.

Histological examination of a basal cell papilloma shows that its base is on the same level

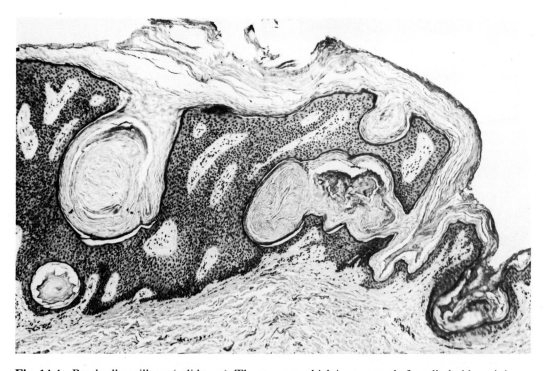

Fig. 14.4   Basal cell papilloma (solid type). The tumour, which is composed of small, darkly staining, basal-like cells, is raised above the level of the surrounding normal epidermis. The characteristic concentric layers of keratin (horn cysts) can be seen at all levels of the tumour. Some of these can be seen opening on to the surface and contributing to the hyperkeratotic stratum corneum which covers the tumour.

as the surrounding epidermis and so the major part of the tumour is raised above the skin, giving the tumour its clinical 'stuck on' appearance. It is formed largely of small darkly staining cells which resemble the basal cells of the epidermis. A few, more mature, keratinocytes are also present. Characteristically, horn cysts are present at all levels within these lesions. The cysts are formed of concentric, roughly circular layers of keratin and there is abrupt transition from the basal-cell-like elements to the delicate concentric rings of keratin (Fig. 14.4). Many of these cysts open on to the surface, and these keratin plugs combined with the hyperplastic epithelium thrown into folds give the lesion its cerebriform appearance clinically. The degree of melanin pigmentation varies, but is usually quite marked. Melanocytes are present among the basaloid cells, and melanin is found both in the cytoplasm of these basiloid cells and in the macrophages in the tumour stroma.

The reticular type of basal cell papilloma consists of connected thin strands of basiloid cells which contain abundant melanin. These strands form a lace-like network in the papillary dermis (Fig. 14.5). Horn cysts are scattered throughout the lesions in varying numbers.

If a basal cell papilloma is irritated, either by mechanical irritation or by inflammation, areas of keratinocyte maturation are seen and these form squamous eddies (Fig. 14.6). In severely irritated basal cell papillomata the appearances may mimic a squamous carcinoma, but the presence of horn cysts and the sharp demarcation of the lesion should help to make the correct diagnosis.

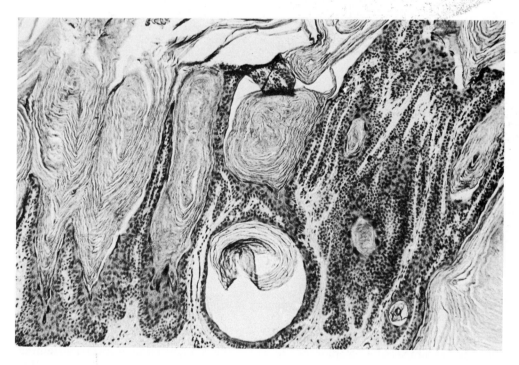

Fig. 14.5 Basal cell papilloma (reticular type). The thin lace-like strands of 'basal' cells form a network in the papillary dermis. There is marked surface hyperkeratosis, and both horn cysts and small 'squamous eddies' can also be seen.

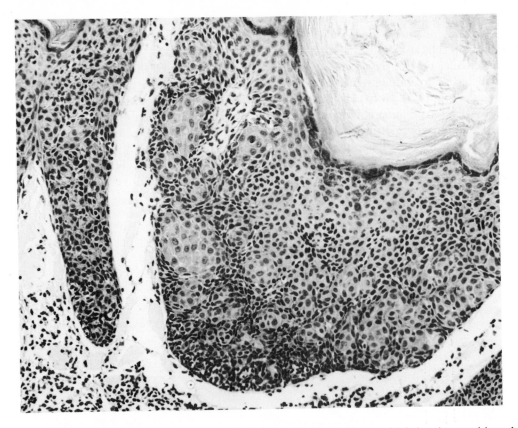

Fig. 14.6 Basal cell papilloma (irritated). This basal cell papilloma which has been subjected to irritation by clothing shows the circular areas of paler-staining keratinocytes ('squamous eddies') among the darkly staining basal cells.

Inverted follicular keratosis

This lesion is essentially similar to a basal cell papilloma but arises in the infundibulum of the hair follicle. Instead of having the 'stuck on' appearance of a basal cell papilloma it grows downwards into the dermis. As these lesions are often 'irritated', squamous eddies are prominent. Hair follicles can sometimes be seen entering the lower part of the tumour.

Clear cell acanthoma of Degos

Although this condition is probably inflammatory in origin, it presents clinically as a solitary small tumour.

Sections through the edge of such a lesion (Fig. 14.7) show an abrupt transition from normal epidermis to acanthotic epidermis in which the cells are swollen and pale staining. This swelling and pallor of the keratinocytes is due to an increased glycogen content. The importance of the lesion lies in its differential diagnosis from an early carcinoma in situ of Bowen's type.

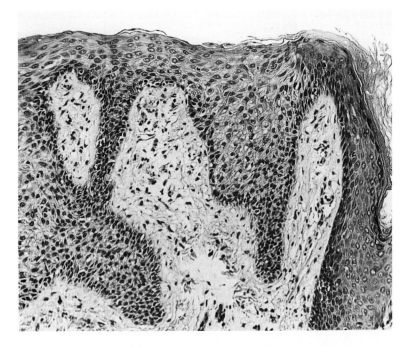

Fig. 14.7 Clear cell acanthoma of Degos. There is an abrupt transition from the normal epidermis to the acanthotic epidermis composed of swollen pale-staining keratinocytes containing glycogen.

Pseudotumours

Keratoacanthoma

This is a self-healing lesion which may, during its growth phase, resemble a squamous carcinoma. It was brought to general attention by McCormac and Scarff.[3] They called it molluscum sebaceum, but the term 'keratoacanthoma' is now generally accepted.[4] Clinically it presents as a nodule in previously normal skin—most often on an exposed site—which rapidly increases in size, usually over a period of 6–8 weeks, and forms a central keratin plug. In its fully developed state it has the appearance of a 'button epithelioma', the lesion for which it was originally mistaken. Untreated, the keratin plug is extruded and the lesion heals to leave a shallow, flat, circular scar in a further 6–8 weeks.

Histologically the lesion is cup shaped, with a well-marked shoulder, and the related epidermis is normal (Fig. 14.8). It passes through three stages. There is an early epithelial proliferative phase with invasion and destruction of the dermis, followed by a keratinising phase with formation of the keratin plug, and finally a healing phase in which the keratin plug is extruded, leaving a depressed area with scarred dermis in which an occasional foreign body giant cell reaction to keratin remnants can be seen, the overlying epidermis having reverted to normal.

During the growth phase the strands of proliferating squamous epithelium invade the dermis with blunt pushing margins in which mitoses are present only in the outermost layers. The cells have eosinophilic cytoplasm and may be larger than usual but have a

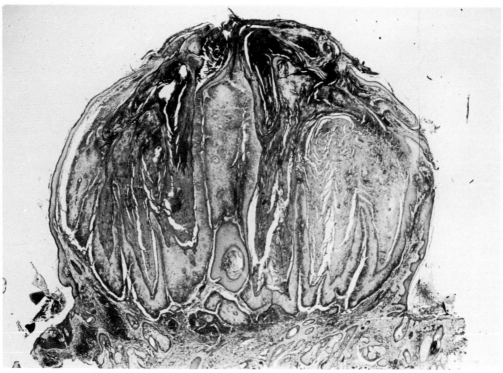

Fig. 14.8   Keratoacanthoma (fully formed lesion). The cup-shaped mass of proliferating epithelial cells has produced a central core of keratin. The surrounding normal epidermis has been drawn upwards around the lesion to produce the characteristic shoulder. There are patches of dense inflammatory infiltrate at the base of the lesion. Note the symmetry of the lesion and that it has not extended beyond hair follicle level.

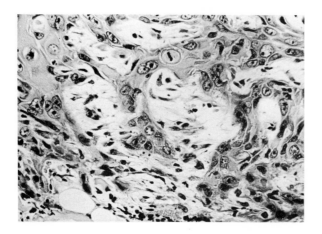

Fig. 14.9 Keratoacanthoma (early lesion). Fragmentary poorly orientated biopsy, showing branching strands of infiltrating squamous epithelium indistinguishable from a squamous carcinoma. The cells are large with eosinophilic cytoplasm and open vesicular nuclei, except at the periphery of the branches where the nuclei are hyperchromatic or undergoing mitois.

relatively normal nuclear/cytoplasmic ratio (Fig. 14.9). There is an absence of dyskeratosis with mainly orthokeratotic maturation of the cells towards the centre as the lesion progresses. These lesions do not invade beyond the level of hair papillae.

At a later stage the strands of epithelium may be infilatrated by polymorphs (Fig. 14.10) and other inflammatory cells, a feature not usually seen in squamous carcinoma except when it arises in a mucous membrane.

Extremely important in diagnosis is the time scale of evolution—6–8 weeks' growth phase and a 6–8-week period of resolution; while this is not invariably the case, a lesion of 3

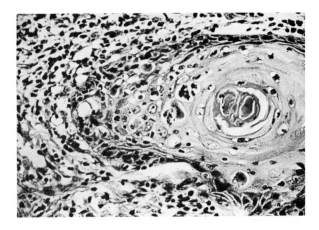

Fig. 14.10 Keratoacanthoma (regressing lesion). A finger-like process of aberrant keratinocytes containing an 'epithelial pearl' is being infiltrated by inflammatory cells (neutrophils, lymphocytes and histiocytes).

months' duration which has not healed or is not showing evidence of resolution should be treated as a squamous carcinoma. A keratoacanthoma should not be diagnosed in the absence of an adequate clinical history.

In addition to the overall morphology the histological criteria of greatest diagnostic importance are the presence of a shoulder and the depth of invasion. Any biopsy should therefore include the edge of the lesion and the deepest infiltrating part in its centre. A small fragmentary biopsy will show invading strands of aberrant squamous epithelium which are indistinguishable from infiltrating squamous carcinoma. Even with a full history it may still be difficult to make a definite diagnosis.

Familial self-healing squamous carcinoma (Ferguson-Smith disease)

This condition is a distinct clinical and pathological entity and should not be confused with multiple keratoacanthoma. It is discussed in Chapter 5.

Premalignant lesions of the epidermis

Under this heading are considered lesions which are regarded as having invasive potential. In the UK literature, two of them—actinic keratosis and Bowen's disease—tend to be grouped under the general term 'carcinoma in situ', but they are distinct in their clinical features, histological characteristics and prognosis.

Actinic keratosis

Actinic keratosis is a focal lesion which arises on a background of actinically damaged skin. It is frequently multiple and most strikingly concentrated on the exposed surfaces. In men the face, ears, hands and forearms are the commonest sites; in women the face, legs and, occasionally, hands and forearms. There is clearly a genetic factor in its aetiology in that it presents in its most widespread form in the fair-skinned, reddish-haired individual, whose skin does not tan easily.

The histological signs of actinic damage are present in both epidermis and dermis. The epidermis as a whole is rather atrophic and there are early signs of dysplasia in the basal

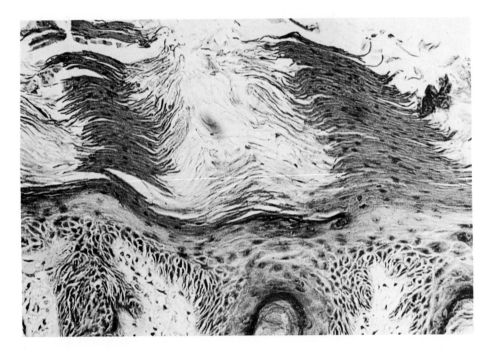

Fig. 14.11   Actinic keratosis. This photomicrograph illustrates the hallmark of actinic keratosis. On the surface there are alternating columns of hyperkeratosis and parakeratosis. Beneath the parakeratotic columns there is no granular layer. The hyperkeratosis is confined mainly to the region of the openings of pilosebaceous follicles, while the parakeratois is seen covering the epidermis between the follicles. Dysplastic changes, as evidenced by loss of polarity and hyperchromatism of the keratinocyte nuclei, are seen particularly in the lower layers of the epidermis.

layers. The melanocytes are increased in number and show dysplastic changes. Elastosis is present in the dermis.

The hallmark of fully developed actinic keratosis is the presence of alternating columns of hyperkeratosis and parakeratosis, the hyperkeratosis occurring over the ostia of the hair follicles and sweat glands, the parakeratosis overlying the epithelium between the adnexa (Fig. 14.11). The epithelium which underlies the column of parakeratosis is markedly disorganised, showing the features of *in situ* squamous carcinoma, with loss of polarity and maturation of the cells, hyperchromatism and pleomorphism of the nuclei. The nuclear/cytoplasmic ratio is usually increased although the cells of the prickle cell layer may show an

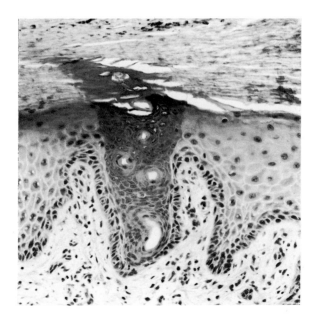

Fig. 14.12 Actinic keratosis from back of hand, showing the normal periappendicular epithelium around a sweat duct and the overlying orthokeratin. The increase in size of the abnormal keratinocytes can be seen in the related epidermis. The dysplastic changes are also extending into the basal layer around the sweat duct.

increase in the amount of cytoplasm as well as an increase in the size of the nucleus (Fig. 14.12).

In the early stages of the lesion the epidermis is usually atrophic and shows foci of dysplasia in the basal cells with either orthokeratosis or hyperkeratosis of the overlying horny layer. As the dysplasia increases in severity the cellular atypia, hyperchromatism and nuclear pleomorphism extend upwards to involve the entire thickness of the epidermis. The cells no longer mature and keratinise properly, there is a loss of the granular layer and parakeratosis replaces the hyperkeratosis.

As the lesions progress, further dysplastic changes become marked with more obvious pleomorphism and loss of polarity of the cells, and downgrowths of these cells into the dermis are seen. Dysplastic changes also extend down the adnexa, involving the basal layers (Fig. 14.12). Despite the apparent invasion of the dermis, an appearance which can be accentuated by obliquity of cut, the lesion is still contained by a 'basement membrane',

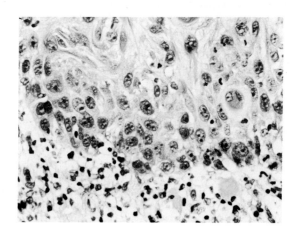

Fig. 14.13 Early infiltrating squamous carcinoma. Note the frayed appearance and lack of basal lamina along the base of the abnormal keratinocytes.

possibly manufactured by the tumour cells, and is still referred to as carcinoma in situ. Breakdown of basement membrane synthesis produces a frayed appearance (Fig. 14.13) and finally frank invasive squamous carcinoma becomes apparent. Actinic keratoses have a long natural history and it is probably only a very small proportion which progress to invasive squamous carcinoma. Even where the lesion is invasive the hallmark of hyperkeratosis and parakeratosis may still remain.

Certain problems of nomenclature have arisen because a comparable pathological sequence occurs in the cervix and the terms used in the two anatomical sites are different even though the histological pictures are similar. When the basal layers alone show evidence of neoplasia and the pattern of maturation is relatively normal the gynaecological pathologist describes the appearance as 'CIN I' (cervical *in situ* neoplasia), taking the view that the basal cells are irrevocably committed to neoplasia and the tumour is well differentiated.

In the skin it is conventional to reserve the term 'carcinoma in situ' for obvious full-thickness involvement of the epithelium, an appearance the gynaecological pathologist would label CIN III. Indeed some pathologists retain the term 'actinic keratosis' as long as the epithelial cells remain within the basement membrane, using the term 'carcinoma' only when there is evidence of invasion.

Variants of actinic keratosis are sometimes encountered. In one the neoplastic cells lose their adhesive properties, the process being referred to as malignant acantholysis, producing

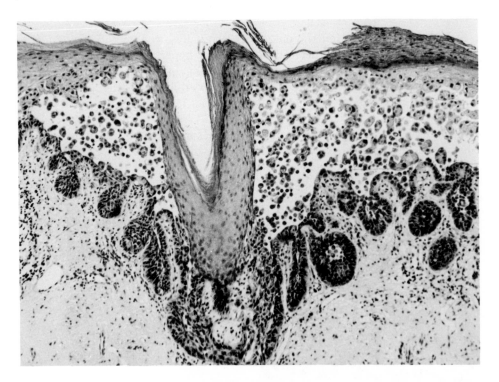

Fig. 14.14   Actinic keratosis. Surrounding a pilosebaceous follicle there is a microscopic vesicle containing dysplastic acantholytic cells. Note the budding of the dysplastic basal layer which is contained by a basal lamina and is regarded as still being an *in situ* carcinoma. Extension of the acantholysis into these buds gives the lesion an adenomatous appearance.

bullae or an adenomatous pattern (Fig. 14.14). In some instances true bullae are not formed; instead one sees small foci of suprabasilar acantholytic cleft formation. Such lesions can be mistaken for Darier's disease or early pemphigus vulgaris.

Another variant, seen more often on the face than elsewhere, is the so-called Bowenoid type of actinic keratosis. In this variant the alternating columns of hyperkeratosis and parakeratosis are retained but there are in addition large individually keratinising cells reminiscent of those seen in Bowen's disease in the midst of a dysplastic epithelium which is often thicker than usual.

A rare variant is *warty dyskeratoma*. This shows the features seen in Darier's disease but it is a solitary lesion.

Bowen's disease

This type of carcinoma in situ is found most often on the lower limbs but may also occur on the trunk. It presents clinically as a slowly enlarging, slightly raised, well-demarcated, scaly plaque, often thought by the patient to be a solitary patch of psoriasis or dermatitis, hence its original name, precancerous dermatosis. If infiltrative squamous carcinoma supervenes at all, it does so after 15–25 years.

Histological examination shows parakeratotic scaling and marked acanthosis of the epidermis with compression and distortion of the dermal papillae. The structure of the epidermis is completely disorganised. The cells are large and there is a general increase in the

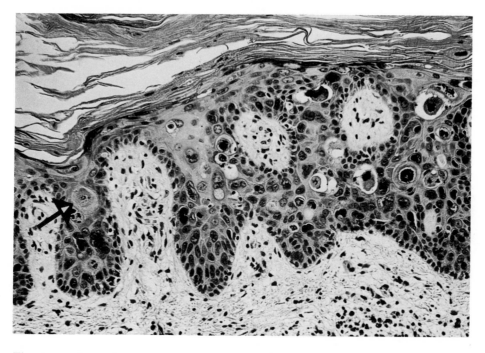

Fig. 14.15 Bowen's disease. The epidermis is thickened, disorganised and shows numerous large atypical cells with irregular hyperchromatic nuclei. Some cells are multinucleated, others show very abnormal mitoses and others are undergoing premature keratinisation and have deeply eosinophilic cytoplasm. The cell (arrowed) shows the pallor of the cytoplasm of some of the large cells.

nuclear/cytoplasmic ratio, some cells being multinucleated. Numerous, very large cells with clear cytoplasm are present with either large irregular nuclei or grossly abnormal mitoses. Some of these large cells show premature keratinisation and other dyskeratotic cells are seen throughout the epidermis (Fig. 14.15). A marked inflammatory infiltrate composed of lymphocytes, histiocytes and some plasma cells is present in the upper dermis. The lesions are usually well demarcated. As the lesion progresses the epidermis becomes greatly thickened. On the very rare occasion when a squamous carcinoma does develop, it is described as retaining the features of the *in situ* lesion.

Leucoerythroplakia

'Leucoplakia' is a term which clinicians use to describe a white patch on the mucous membrane of the mouth or vulva. Such a patch results from the presence of a horny layer on the mucosal surface which turns white in the moist environment. Any condition which gives rise to keratosis, such as chronic irritation and trauma, lichen planus, lichen sclerosis et atrophicus, and lupus erythematosus, when it occurs in the oral or vulvar mucosa, will give rise to a 'white patch'. Leucoplakia does of course occur also in certain premalignant states. In any such patch candidosis should always be excluded as an underlying cause of the white patch or as a superadded infection.

Most biopsies are taken in order to establish whether or not the patch of leucoplakia represents a premalignant condition. It cannot be stressed too strongly that 'leucoplakia' is a clinically descriptive term and has no pathological counterpart. It should have no place in the histological vocabulary of the pathologist. If he considers the lesion to be premalignant he should define it as such with a clear indication of the amount of cellular atypia and loss of maturation. These premalignant lesions in any case usually present clinically as leucoerythroplakia rather than solely as leucoplakia. Any biopsy should include a red area, since these are the areas that have progressed furthest towards invasion.

Premalignant fibroepithelial tumour

A rare but easily recognised tumour is the premalignant fibroepithelial tumour of Pinkus.[5] This is a pedunculated lesion which occurs mainly on the lower trunk and thighs.

Histologically it is composed of interlacing strands of 'basal' cells enclosing in their

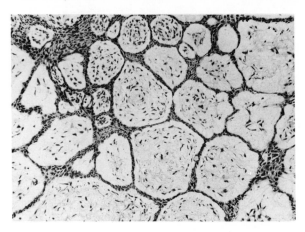

Fig. 14.16 Pre-malignant fibroepithelial tumour of Pinkus. The microphotograph shows part of a pedunculated lesion. Interlacing strands of 'basal' cells enclose areas of loose, oedematous, cellular connective tissue, in which the fibroblast nuclei have a stelate shape.

network areas of loose connective tissue (Fig. 14.16) similar in appearance to the stroma of a fibroadenoma of the breast. These tumours may progress to basal cell carcinoma.

Malignant epithelial tumours

Basal cell carcinoma

Basal cell carcinoma is the commonest malignant neoplasm found in the skin. Although usually locally invasive only, it metastasises on rare occasions and is classified with the malignant tumours.

It occurs mainly on the face, the proportion on the head and neck region being as high as 91 per cent in some series.[6] With increased exposure to the sun there is an increasing incidence in the population, particularly in fair-skinned, blue-eyed, reddish-haired individuals often of Scottish or Irish descent. Although in the UK basal cell carcinoma is found mainly in the fifth, sixth and seventh decades, it occurs in younger age groups in such countries as Australia and the USA. In addition, with changing fashions in clothing the percentage of basal cell carcinomata arising on the trunk and limbs is increasing, being as high as 34 per cent in a recent series from Queensland.[7] This is an extreme situation, however, the majority of extrafacial basal cell carcinomata being unrelated to sun exposure.

In spite of its name, the cell of origin is still in doubt but many of the lesions are thought to arise from the pluripotential cells of the basal layer of the epidermis or from the epithelium of hair follicles. Cells of the basal cell carcinoma have an ultrastructural morphology similar to the immature keratinocytes of the lower layers of the epidermis.

These locally invasive tumours vary in their aggressiveness, their clinical presentation and their morphology.

Histologically the lesions consist of islands or cords of tumour cells with oval basophilic

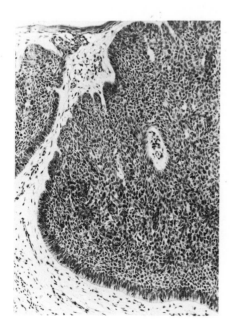

Fig. 14.17 Basal cell carcinoma. Part of a circumscribed lesion, composed of clumps of small darkly staining basal cells with the characteristic palisading around the periphery.

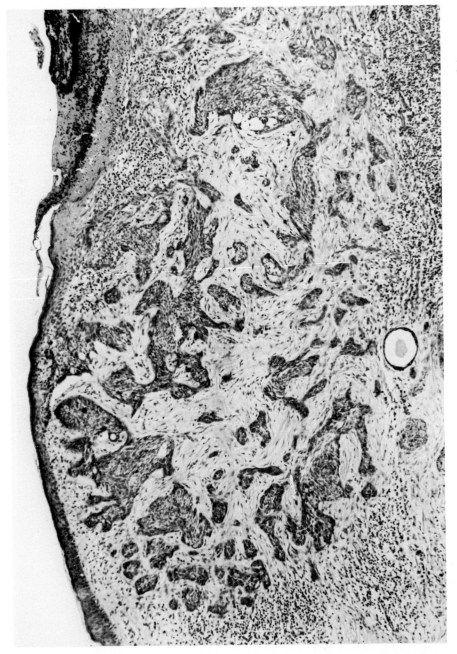

Fig. 14.18 Basal cell carcinoma (rodent ulcer variant). This shows ulceration in the centre and infiltration of the tumour laterally to produce the characteristic rolled margin seen clinically. This lesion has a more obvious stroma and more infiltrative pattern. There is an inflammatory infiltrate around the periphery of the lesion.

nuclei and a scant cytoplasm, resembling the basal cells of the epidermis, a closely related fibrous tissue stroma, and a related inflammatory infiltrate consisting of plasma cells and lymphocytes. Pinkus drew attention to the importance of the stroma. It is the interaction of this stroma with the peripheral tumour cells which produces their characteristic palisading (Fig. 14.17) and the production of a basement membrane. The presence of this basement membrane may account for the usual absence of metastases from these lesions. As the stroma is an integral part of the tumour it is important to include it in any assessment of adequacy of excision. The proportion of stroma to epithelium in the different infiltrative patterns accounts for the different clinical appearances. Certain distinctive types of basal cell carcinoma are recognisable both clinically and histologically.

The *cystic* variant is a non-ulcerated well-circumscribed nodular tumour which may have either an 'adenomatous' or a cystic pattern, due in both instances to mucoid degeneration of the tumour cells.

Some lesions ulcerate centrally and when they do they create the classic picture of a *rodent ulcer*. Infiltration occurs laterally under the epidermis, producing the typical rolled margin (Fig. 14.18).

The tumour is described as *sclerotic* when the stroma is particularly marked. The pattern is one of diffuse infiltration. A variant of the sclerotic type is the *morphoeic* basal cell carcinoma in which the islands of tumour cells are small and sparse (Fig. 14.19). The importance of this variant lies in its relative radioresistance and the difficulty of estimating adequate clearance.

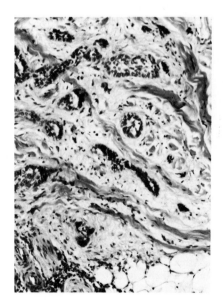

Fig. 14.19 Basal cell carcinoma (morphoeic type). Small islands of basal cells accompanied by their fibrous tissue stroma are seen infiltrating between the collagen bundle in the lower half of the dermis.

A further variant of basal cell carcinoma appears to spread peripherally while 'healing' centrally, though frequently incompletely, leaving a mixture of healed scarred skin and areas of residual basal cell carcinoma. At the advancing edge of such a lesion histology shows a multifocal tumour apparently arising mainly in relation to hair follicles. Nearer the centre, tumour is seen being destroyed by inflammatory cells, and in the centre the dermis is replaced by scar tissue in which the hair follicles are absent although the sweat glands are preserved. This type of basal cell carcinoma is referred to as *centrally healing* or *field-fire*.

Another form taken by multifocal basal cell carcinoma is the very superficial lesion, predominantly arising extrafacially, which appears clinically as a localised red scaly patch, and is frequently misdiagnosed clinically as Bowen's disease or psoriasis. Multiple foci of tumour cells appearing to bud from the basal layer of the epidermis or from hair follicles are characteristic of this type (Fig. 14.20).

Pigmentation is occasionally a marked feature of basal cell carcinoma, seen both in the islands of tumour and in the macrophages in the stroma. Differentiation can take other forms—trichoepitheliomatous, squamous and sebaceous.

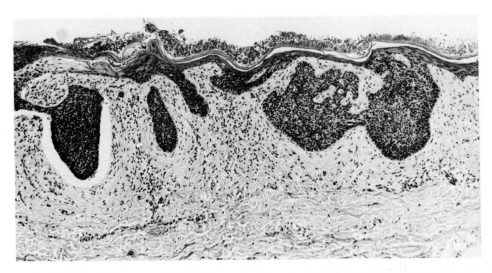

Fig. 14.20 Basal cell carcinoma (multifocal extrafacial type). Small islands of basal cell carcinoma appear to bud down from the lower layer of the epidermis. Note the associated fibrous tissue stroma and inflammatory infiltrate. The island of tumour on the left shows a shrinkage artefact often seen in basal cell carcinoma.

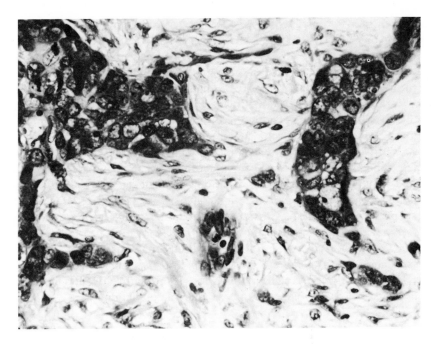

Fig. 14.21 Metatypical basal cell carcinoma. Irregular islands of cells with large open vesicular nuclei are embedded in a dense fibrous tissue stroma. Note the lack of palisading. Numerous mitotic figures are often present.

Basal cell carcinomata in general do not metastasise. There are, however, certain varieties which behave aggressively and may metastasise. One type is the *metatypical basal cell carcinoma*. This tumour has been defined by Farmer and Helwig[8] as 'a tumour having the features of a basal cell carcinoma with foci of squamoid differentiation. The characteristic cell has a polygonal shape, eosinophilic cytoplasm and a large, more open nucleus. The tumor lobule is more irregular and peripheral palisading is less pronounced, but focally present. Stromal proliferation is more prominent' (Fig. 14.21). In a recent series of metastatic basal cell carcinomata investigated by these authors, eight out of ten showed metatypical features in the primary lesion. The primary lesion itself also behaves aggressively and infiltrates deeply. This tumour has been given various names. One such was 'intermediate cell carcinoma' because the cells appeared to be half way between those seen in basal carcinoma and squamous carcinoma. For the same reason they were called 'basi-squamous carcinomata'. This term fell into disrepute because it was applied also to basal cell carcinomata showing merely squamous differentiation, and retaining the prognosis of basal cell carcinomata in general.

A tumour which requires to be distinguished from basal cell carcinoma, but which in its initial presentation may resemble basal cell carcinoma with an adenoid pattern, is **adenoid cystic carcinoma** arising probably from sweat glands. It behaves like any other adenoid cystic carcinoma, infiltrating widely and diffusely in tissue planes and along perineural spaces, with a typical lack of host response. These tumours may eventually metastasise.

A further tumour which may be misdiagnosed as a basal cell carcinoma is the **neuro-secretory tumour** which probably arises from Merkel cells (Fig. 14.22). This tumour can be diagnosed at the ultrastructural level by the demonstration of neurosecretory granules. It is locally aggressive and capable of rapid metastases to regional lymph nodes.

Common to all of the aggressive tumours properly or mistakenly diagnosed histologically as basal cell carcinoma is their infiltrative pattern. This fact justifies the simple classification of Headington[9] who has classified basal cell carcinomas into two main groups: those which are circumscribed with 'discrete or interanastomosing lobules of neoplasm with blunt pushing margins' and those 'with a diffusely infiltrative pattern, which can microscopically extend beyond the clinical detectable margins'. In view of its relevance to diagnosis and treatment this would seem to be a very rational general classification. In particular there are certain sites—the nasolabial folds, around the eyes, and the pinna—where basal cell carcinomata are often infiltrative, create problems of clinical assessment and are difficult to treat. Care should be taken in assessing clearance margins in such tumours.

In the *naevoid basal cell carcinoma syndrome*, multiple basal cell carcinomata of the skin are associated with jaw cysts and other skeletal abnormalities (see p. 77). The basal cell carcinomata which occur in this syndrome are, from their inception, similar to and just as aggressive as the basal cell carcinomata which arise in the general population.

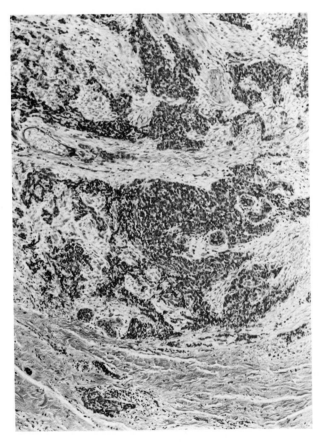

Fig. 14.22 Neurosecretory tumour. Islands of basophilic cells accompanied by a fibrous tissue stroma are infiltrating the dermis. These cells usually have a more open nucleus than those of a basal cell carcinoma and can resemble those of an oat cell carcinoma of bronchus. Note the lack of palisading.

Squamous carcinoma

This invasive and potentially metastasising tumour arises from the squamous epithelium of the skin, skin appendages and mucous membranes. It can also take origin from any epithelium which has undergone squamous metaplasia; e.g. endocervix, bronchus, gallbladder and urinary tract. In the skin it may arise apparently *de novo* but most arise on previously damaged epidermis. Actinic keratosis is the most frequent background, though arsenic, mineral oil, tar and radiation keratosis, or long-standing ulceration, occasionally provide the predisposing lesion.

Histologically, squamous carcinoma shows finger-like processes and strands of pleomorphic keratinocytes in varying stages of maturation invading the tissue. It is usually also possible to find single keratinocytes or columns of cells infiltrating between the collagen bundles. Care must be exercised in the distinction between true invasion and oblique cut of a rete ridge which is the seat of carcinoma in situ, and contained by a basement membrane. The less mature cells are small and dark with hyperchromatic nuclei; the more mature cells are larger with an open vesicular nucleus, a prominent nucleolus and eosinophilic cytoplasm. Some cells mature to produce orthokeratin; others are dyskeratotic (Fig. 14.23).

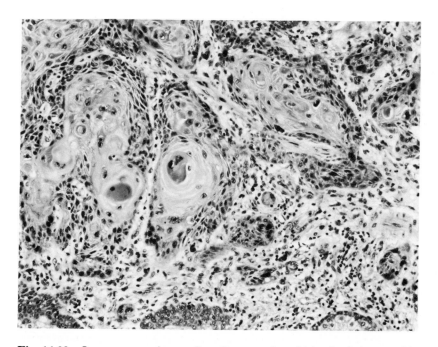

Fig. 14.23 Squamous carcinoma. Invading strands and islands of pleomorphic squamous epithelium in various stages of maturation are seen invading the dermis. The well-differentiated cells are larger with open vesicular nuclei; the less well differentiated cells are smaller with hyperchromatic nuclei. 'Epithelial pearls' are seen where the better differentiated cells are maturing to produce a central core of keratin.

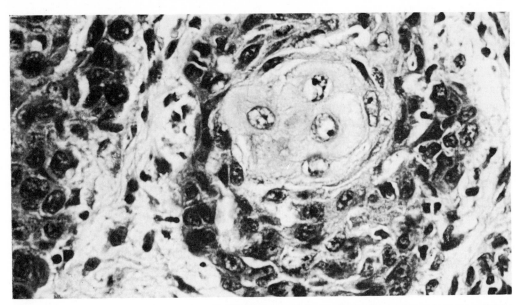

Fig. 14.24   Squamous carcinoma (poorly differentiated). Imperfectly formed 'epithelial pearls' in a squamous carcinoma. This tumour was composed of strands of epipithelial cells with hyperchromatic nuclei and numerous mitoses. Only a few areas showing squamous differentiation were found in the entire tumour.

No difficulty in diagnosis should be experienced with the well-differentiated squamous carcinoma where strands of keratincoytes are seen maturing towards the centre, often with the formation of an imperfect granular layer and a centre of keratin. The transverse sections of these strands of neoplastic epithelium constitute the 'epithelial pearls'. In less well-differentiated tumours, epithelial pearls may have to be searched for (Fig. 14.24) and are often imperfectly formed. In the poorly differentiated type the cells may be so anaplastic that only an occasional keratinised cell betrays its origin. Mitotic figures, often abnormal, are invariably found. In well-differentiated tumours these may be relatively sparse while in poorly differentiated tumours they are numerous.

The degree of maturation reflects the differentiation of the tumour and it is usual for the pathologist to comment on this in his report. Whether it has any relevance in terms of behaviour or prognosis is extremely doubtful.

References

1. Mehregan AH, Pinkus H. Life history of organoid nevi. *Arch Dermatol* 1965; **91**: 574–88.
2. Wilson Jones E, Heyl T. Naevus sebaceous: a report of 140 cases with special regard to the development of secondary malignant tumours. *Br J Dermatol* 1970; **82**: 99–117.
3. McCormac H, Scarff RW. Molluscum sebaceum. *Br J Dermatol* 1936; **48**: 624–6.
4. Rook A, Whimster I. Keratoacanthoma—a thirty year prospect. *Br J Dermatol* 1979; **100**: 41–7.
5. Pinkus H. Premalignant fibroepithelial tumors of skin. *Arch Dermatol* 1953; **67**: 598–615.
6. Brodkin RH, Kopf AW, Andrade R. Basal-cell epithelioma and elastosis. A comparison of distribution. In Urbach F, ed. *The Biological Effects of Ultraviolet Radiation*. Oxford: Pergamon Press, 1969: pp. 581–618.
7. Green AJ. Basal cell carcinoma in Queensland: a new trend. *Aust NZ J Surg* 1982; **52**: 63–5.
8. Farmer ER, Helwig EB. Metastatic basal cell carcinoma. *Cancer* 1980; **46**: 748–57.
9. Headington JT. Epidermal carcinomas of the integument of the nose and ear. In Batsakis JG. *Tumors of the Head and Neck*, 2nd ed. Baltimore: Williams & Wilkins, 1979; pp. 420–30.

15

Adnexal Tumours

A great deal of interest has been shown in recent years concerning the precise origin of adnexal growths. New research techniques have advanced our knowledge considerably but they have also resulted in a proliferation of terms and complex classifications. Although in their embryological origin, anatomy and function human eccrine and apocrine glands are different, they are often classed together as sweat glands,[1] thus adding to the confusion. Eccrine glands are sweat glands, whereas apocrine glands are derived from the pilosebaceous follicle.

Hashimoto and Lever[2] attempted to classify some of these tumours on the basis of their different enzymes, but neoplasms may not be sufficiently differentiated to produce enzymes, and the lack of agreement on how to classify certain tumours, particularly the syringoma, the spiradenoma, the syringocystadenoma, papilliferum and the cylindroma, remains. Certain tumours with a similar morphology such as the cystadenomata can be of both eccrine and apocrine origin and it may be that there are other tumours, possibly the spiradenoma and syringoma, which also arise in both glands. Certainly the various issues regarding origin are far from settled.

The difficulty in classifying adnexal tumours should be anticipated prior to biopsy, and the pathologist alerted so that he can obtain tissue for special studies. In particular, many histochemical studies for enzymes require fresh or frozen tissue and a portion of tissue should be snap-frozen at $-20°C$. Tissue should also be taken in 1 mm cubes and fixed in glutaraldehyde for ultrastructural study. Although there is considerable sampling difficulty, ultrastructural study may prove valuable in diagnosis.

Tumours of the pilosebaceous follicle

The pilosebaceous follicle consists of the hair follicle, the sebaceous gland and, in certain sites, the apocrine gland.

Hair follicle tumours

Trichofolliculoma

This name is given to a highly organised hamartoma derived from hair follicle (Fig. 15.1). Histologically it consists of one or more sinus tracks containing keratin, surrounded by a number of abortive and imperfectly formed hair roots (Fig. 15.1). Some of these produce defective hair filaments which protrude from the surface of the skin.

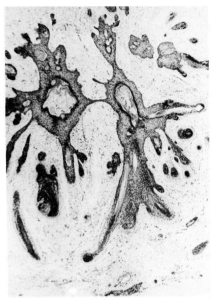

Fig. 15.1 Trichofolliculoma. Surrounding two epithelium-lined, keratin-filled sinus tracks are a number of abortive and imperfectly formed hair follicles and hair roots.

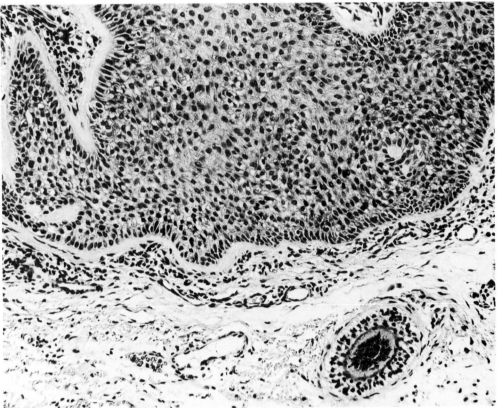

Fig. 15.2 Tricholemmoma. Part of a lesion showing a lobule of pale-staining glycogen-filled cells. The cells around the periphery are arranged perpendicular to a thick, sharply defined hyaline membrane.

Tricholemmoma

Tricholemmoma is the name applied to a benign tumour of outer sheath origin. It grows in close connection with the undersurface of the epidermis and is composed of lobular masses of large pale glycogen containing cells similar to those of the outer root sheath. At the periphery of the lobules, these cells are arranged perpendicularly to a thick hyaline membrane (Fig. 15.2).

Pilomatricoma (calcifying epithelioma of Malherbe)

A benign cystic lesion, until recently known as calcifying epithelioma of Malherbe, has now been identified as a tumour of hair matrix, and called pilomatricoma. This lesion is commoner in young people and occurs predominantly on the face and scalp. On histological examination the tumour, which is seen deep in the dermis, is surrounded by a condensed pseudocapsule of fibrous tissue. It consists of folded masses of small, darkly staining cells bearing a strong resemblance to the cells of the hair matrix. The nuclei are oval and hyperchromatic. These cells merge imperceptibly with larger, paler cells indistinguishable from epidermal keratinocytes which finally become empty keratinised 'shadow cells' devoid of nuclei (Fig. 15.3). Eventually calcium is deposited in the shadow cells. The stroma, which follows closely the epithelial infoldings, is composed of highly vascularised connective tissue which sometimes contains deposits of haemosiderin from previous haemorrhage. Numerous foreign body giant cells reacting to the keratin may also be present.

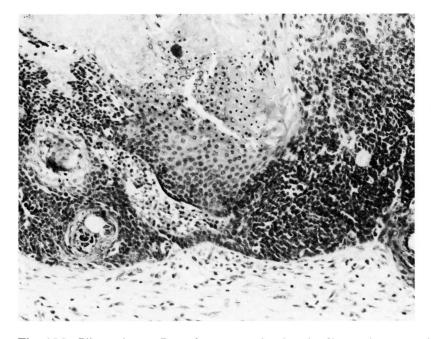

Fig. 15.3 Pilomatricoma. Part of a tumour showing the fibrous tissue capsule. The cells at the periphery, which are small and very darkly staining with oval nuclei, resemble the cells of the hair matrix. These dark cells merge with larger paler cells which are indistinguishable from keratinocytes, and these in turn merge into empty ghost cells devoid of nuclei.

Trichoepithelioma

Trichoepithelioma may occur singly or as multiple tumours when they are dominantly inherited and the condition is known as epithelioma adenoides cysticum. In this condition multiple lesions occur predominantly on the face and upper chest.

Histologically it is composed of irregular masses of small cells containing darkly staining oval nuclei, which show peripheral palisading, and resembles basal cell carcinoma. Some of the epithelial masses contain keratin-filled cysts of varying size, while others remain solid and develop short branching processes (Fig. 15.4); at times structures resembling rudimentary hair papillae are present as well. The epithelial elements are accompanied by a stroma composed of fibrous tissue but without an inflammatory infiltrate.

When trichoepitheliomas are solitary they may have a histological appearance similar to those seen in epithelioma adenoides cysticum, but in other instances it may be impossible to separate them from basal cell carcinomata showing differentiation towards hair follicles. There is one variety of solitary tumour which should be recognised, namely the *desmoplastic trichoepithelioma*, as it may be misdiagnosed as a morphoeic basal cell carcinoma. It occurs on the face in all age groups and consists of small nests and strands of basiloid cells embedded in a dense fibrotic stroma. These strands show differentiation towards hair papillae, foci of keratin cyst formation and areas of calcification (Fig. 15.5).

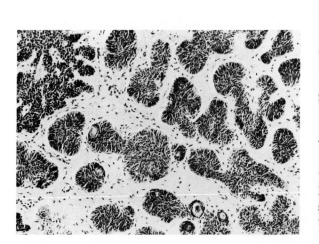
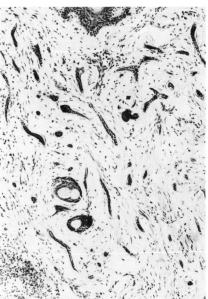

Fig. 15.4 (*left*) Trichoepithelioma (epithelioma adenoides cysticum). The tumour is composed of irregular masses of small, darkly staining cells similar to those of basal cell carcinoma, separated by a fibrous tissue stroma. Some of the masses contain tiny cysts of keratin while others remain solid and show short branching processes. There may be peripheral palisading of the cells.

Fig. 15.5 (*right*) Desmoplastic trichoepithelioma. Duct-like structures and thin strands of basal cells are embedded in loose, cellular, connective tissue. These strands of basal cells may show differentiation towards hair follicles. Keratin-filled cysts are usually seen in the upper third of the dermis.

Sebaceous gland tumours

These can vary from a simple hyperplasia of sebaceous glands seen in the elderly (Fig. 15.6) through all gradations to frank invasive and metastasising sebaceous carcinoma, seen especially in relation to the Meibomian glands of the eyelids.

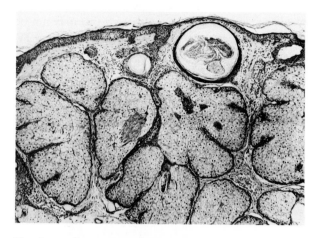

Fig. 15.6 Sebaceous hyperplasia (senile sebaceous naevus), showing marked hyperplasia of normal sebaceous glands around a central squamous-lined opening. It can be mistaken clinically for a basal cell carcinoma.

Benign sebaceous adenoma

These occur, but are rare. In structure they resemble sebaceous glands. The lobular pattern is not quite so regular and the periphery is composed of several layers of darkly staining, basal-cell-like elements, while the central lipid-filled cells are much smaller than normal sebaceous cells (Fig. 15.7). Great care must be taken, however, in attempting to diagnose sebaceous gland hyperplasia or adenoma when only a small biopsy specimen is available, especially from the face where the glands are normally large and numerous.

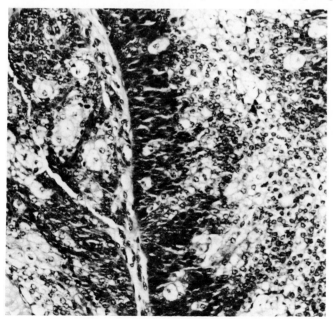

Fig. 15.7 Sebaceous adenoma. The edge of a lobule is composed of layers of darkly staining basiloid cells which merge with lipid-filled cells, similar to but often smaller than those of normal sebaceous gland.

Carcinoma of sebaceous gland

These malignant tumours of the sebaceous gland are rare, although sebaceous differentiation is seen not uncommonly in basal cell carcinoma. When malignant tumours do occur, the common site is in the sebaceous glands of the eyelids.

Histologically they are composed of lobules of large foamy cells, which have a high lipid content, and may resemble those of sebaceous glands (Fig. 15.8), although this may not be evident in the more poorly differentiated tumours. Frozen sections stained with Sudan IV will confirm the presence of lipid in these tumours. Characteristically they spread in a pagetoid fashion in the conjuctiva from one eyelid to the other.

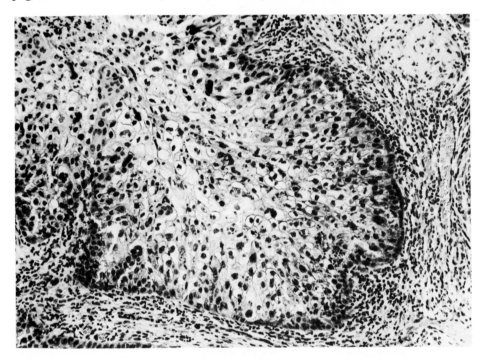

Fig. 15.8 Carcinoma of sebaceous gland. A lobule of tumour composed of pale foamy cells, which special stains show to contain lipid. There is considerable nuclear pleomorphism and hyperchromatism. The tumour illustrated is relatively well differentiated and shows a peripheral layer of darkly staining basal cells, which is not always present.

Apocrine gland tumours

Apocrine cystadenoma

This is a cystic lesion usually found in the skin around the eyes. The cysts are lined by a double layer of cells, an outer layer of myoepithelial cells and an inner layer consisting of high columnar cells which may show evidence of apocrine secretion (Fig. 15.9). Small papillary projections into the cyst cavity are sometimes present. A similar lesion, the hydrocystoma, lined by cuboidal cells is derived from eccrine glands.

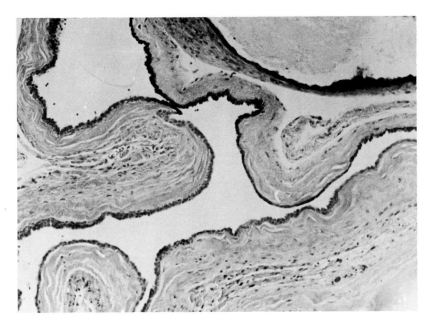

Fig. 15.9 Apocrine cystadenoma. The collapsed and folded cyst wall is seen lined by columnar cells with an outer layer of myoepithelial cells. The lining cells are often flattened by the contents of the cyst.

Syringocystadenoma papilliferum (syringadenoma papilliferum)

This tumour of possible apocrine or eccrine duct origin often occurs in a pre-existing organoid naevus and therefore is seen most commonly on the scalp and face, although it may be seen elsewhere as an independent lesion. Clinically it presents as a papillomatous lesion on the verrucous background of the organoid naevus, and, as the ductal epithelium is in direct contact with the surface, it often appears to be ulcerated.

Histologically it consists of numerous duct-like structures which have proliferated, arborised and communicated with the surface, giving the lesion its characteristic papillary appearance (Fig. 15.10). The double layer of epithelium lining the duct-like spaces and covering the papillary projections has a superficial layer of columnar cells, with eosinophilic cytoplasm and oval pale-staining nuclei, and a deeper layer of small cuboidal cells with darkly staining nuclei. There is a fibrous tissue stroma in which the striking feature is the very large number of plasma cells (Fig. 15.11).

Hidradenoma papilliferum

This benign adenoma occurs only in the vulva and perineum of adult women. Regarded as of apocrine origin,[3] its uniqueness of site is of interest.

It presents clinically initially as a circumscribed, mobile nodule in the deeper tissues, but it may eventually ulcerate on to the surface.

Histologically it is essentially a cystic lesion, surrounded by a pseudocapsule of condensed fibrous tissue, containing branching villous processes, multiple cysts and duct-like spaces. The lining of the cysts and the covering of the papillae are double layered, consisting of a

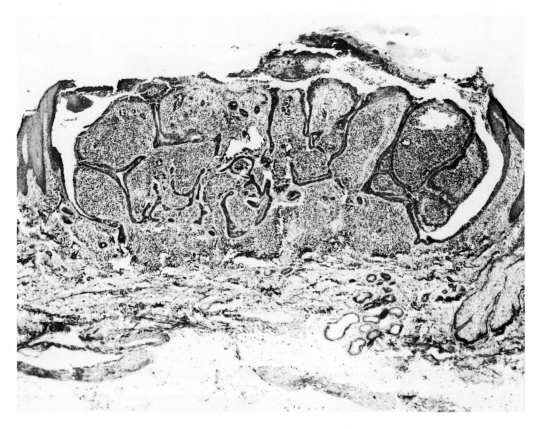

Fig. 15.10   Syringocystadenoma papilliferum. The papillary tumour is composed of duct-like structures arborising in a fibrous tissue stroma in which there are numerous plasma cells. This lesion occurred in an organoid naevus and the hyperplastic epidermis can be seen on the left.

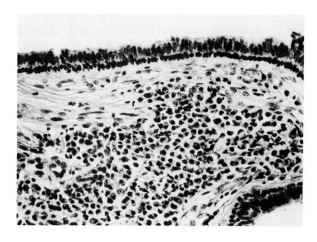

Fig. 15.11   Syringocystadenoma papilliferum, showing the lining of tall columnar cells, the outer layer of cuboidal cells and the numerous plasma cells in the stroma.

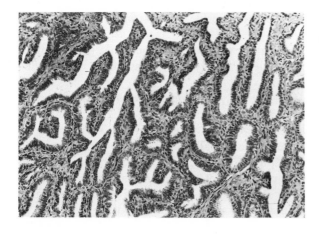

Fig. 15.12 Hidradenoma papilliferum. This lesion is composed of branching villous projections and cystic spaces, lined by a double layer of cells. The inner cells are usually columnar, but may show apocrine or sebaceous differentiation. The fibrous tissue stroma lacks the plasma cell infiltrate seen in the syringocystadenoma papilliferum.

superficial layer of columnar epithelial cells with eosinophilic cytoplasm containing PAS-positive diastase-resistant granules, and a deeper layer of myoepithelial cells. The epithelial cells show apocrine differentiation similar to that seen in the breast, and may also show sebaceous differentiation. There is a fine fibrous tissue stroma which lacks the inflammatory infiltrate seen in the syringocystadenoma papilliferum (Fig. 15.12).

Cylindroma

There is still some doubt about the exact origin of these tumours, but in view of the fact that they occur only in sites where apocrine glands are found and because of their association

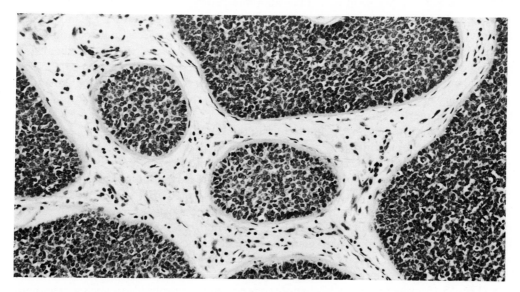

Fig. 15.13 Cylindroma. The varying-sized epithelial islands are embedded in a fibrous stroma and are composed of two cell types. The centrally placed cells have pale-staining cytoplasm with open vesicular nuclei, and these are surrounded by smaller cells with darker-staining oval nuclei. The islands are surrounded by a dense hyaline membrane. This hyaline material may also be seen between the cells.

with trichoepitheliomata they are classified with the apocrine tumours and are thought to be derived from their ducts.

They occur most often in the scalp, either singly or as multiple lesions when they are often referred to as 'turban tumours'. In their multiple form they may be associated with tricho-epitheliomata and inherited as a dominant trait.

Histologically they are composed of islands of darkly staining epithelial cells enclosed by a hyaline membrane and separated by a fine connective tissue stroma. The epithelial component consists of a central core of pale cells with open vesicular nuclei surrounded by smaller cells with darkly staining oval nuclei. These smaller cells tend to form a palisade where they abut on the hyaline membrane (Fig. 15.13). Between the epithelial cells, and occasionally within the cytoplasm of the pale cells, droplets of hyaline material may be seen. This material is strongly PAS-positive after diastase, as is the hyaline membrane. Small clefts and duct-like structures are frequent in some of the epithelial islands.

Apocrine adenocarcinoma

Apocrine adenocarcinomata have been described mainly on the areola of the nipple of the mammary gland or in the axilla. It is probable that these are mammary carcinomata occurring in the gland itself or its axillary tail.

Paget's diesase

This malignant infiltration of the epidermis from elsewhere is discussed under the heading of apocrine tumours because the majority of cases arise in connection with neoplasms of apocrine or modified apocrine glands. The commonest site is the areola of the nipple, where it is associated with carcinoma (often confined to the ducts) of the mammary gland. Extra-mammary Paget's diesase occurs mainly in the pubic and vulvar areas in association with adenocarcinoma of the apocrine glands in these sites. The disease is not necessarily always associated with neoplasia of apocrine glands. Cases have been recorded of Paget's disease on the abdominal wall, secondary to transitional cell carcinoma of the bladder, in the skin of the groin secondary to adenocarcinoma of the rectum, and on the vulva secondary to squamous carcinoma of the uterine cervix.

On histological examination the epidermis is thickened and infiltrated by large, pale-staining cells with clear cytoplasm (Paget cells). These cells, which may be single or in nests, may be found at any level in the epidermis, although they are most common in the mid zone. In the papillary dermis there is always a marked inflammatory reaction in which plasma cells and lymphocytes predominate (Fig. 15.14). When the Paget cells are derived from an underlying mucin-secreting adenocarcinoma they contain deposits of mucin which can be demonstrated by a mucicarmine or alcian blue stain. This can be a most useful diagnostic aid. In cases involving the mammary gland or other apocrine areas an intraduct carcinoma may be seen in the deeper parts of the sections. When the Paget cells are not derived from a mucus-secreting epithelium but are, for example, secondary to squamous carcinoma of the cervix (Fig. 15.15), mucin cannot be demonstrated in their cytoplasm. In such a case there will be considerable diagnostic difficulty in distinguishing the lesion from atypical melano-cytic hyperplasia or squamous carcinoma *in situ*. The use of a silver stain for melanin can usually resolve the question of a possible melanocytic lesion. In some instances Paget cells may have acquired melanin granules by passive transfer and then the only way to settle the

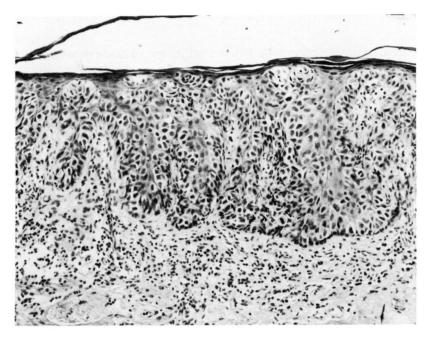

Fig. 15.14 Extramammary Paget's disease of the abdominal wall. The epidermis is infiltrated by large cells with hyperchromatic and pleomorphic nuclei. With special stains mucin can be demonstrated in the cytoplasm. There is an inflammatory infiltrate in the dermis consisting mainly of plasma cells and lymphocytes.

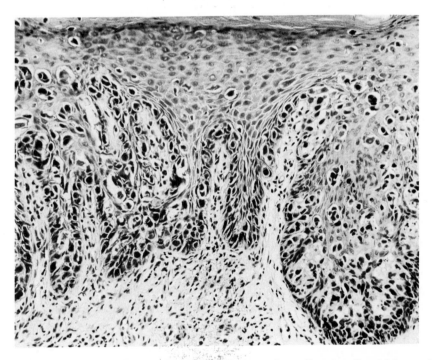

Fig. 15.15 Paget's disease of the vulva. The irregular malignant cells with hyperchromatic nuclei are infiltrating the normal epidermis. These cells did not contain mucin and the lesion was secondary to a carcinoma of cervix. (Reproduced by courtesy of the Editor, the *Journal of Obstetrics and Gynaecology of the British Commonwealth*).

diagnosis is to perform a DOPA reaction on fresh, unfixed tissue. The distinction from carcinoma *in situ* of Bowen's type may be more difficult. Paget cells frequently show mitosis, but the grossly abnormal mitoses of Bowen's disease are not encountered and there is no individual cell keratinisation.

Eccrine gland tumours

The classification of sweat gland tumours is extensive and confusing because there is no general agreement on terminology. 'Hidradenoma' is the most commonly used generic term for benign tumours of the sweat apparatus, but some tumours of probable apocrine origin such as hidradenoma papilliferum of the vulva also have this generic term. Some authors have used the names 'acrosyringoma' and 'syringoadenoma' to describe tumours of ductal origin, and spiradenoma for tumours of the secretory coil. These tumours, however, probably arise from the coiled segment of the duct connecting with the secretory coil. Others authors have used the adjectives 'superficial' and 'deep' for the same purpose, but it would seem to be more logical to try to classify these tumours according to the part of the sweat gland from which they are derived and towards which they differentiate. However, even this is not always possible either, as tumours are encountered which differentiate in various directions and seem to have elements of the acrosyringium as well as secretory elements.

One of the most useful diagnostic features of sweat duct tumours in general is their tendency to maintain a double layer of epithelium.

Syringoma

This benign hamartomatous lesion commonly affects the skin around the orbit, often in a multiple form, but it may occur in the axilla or, more rarely, in the pubic region. Although its distribution parallels that of the apocrine glands the finding that it contains succinic dehydrogenase and phosphorylases suggests that it may be of eccrine origin.

Histologically it consists of duct-like structures each lined by a double layer of epithelium and containing PAS-positive structureless material, embedded in a connective tissue stroma which merges imperceptibly into the surrounding dermis. In some instances the ducts are flattened and compressed into slit-like strands; in other places the epithelium forming the ducts is continued into a solid comma-like tail (Fig. 15.16). The inner lining cells may show squamous or sebaceous differentiation.

Hidroacanthoma simplex

This is a benign superficial lesion which clinically resembles a basal cell papilloma but has been shown to be of intraepidermal sweat duct origin.

Histologically, well-defined islands of glycogen-containing basiloid cells are seen in an acanthotic epidermis (Fig. 15.17). The tumour was one of the several lesions referred to in the past as an 'intraepidermal epithelioma of Borst Jadassohn', but its true origin can be demonstrated histochemically.

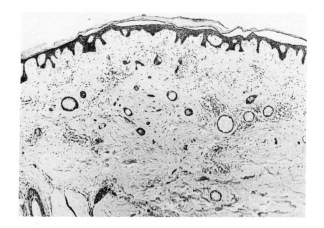

Fig. 15.16 Syringoma. Scattered throughout the dermis and embedded in a fibrous tissue stroma are duct-like structures lined by a double layer of epithelium. These structures are often comma shaped. They contain structure less material which is strongly PAS-positive.

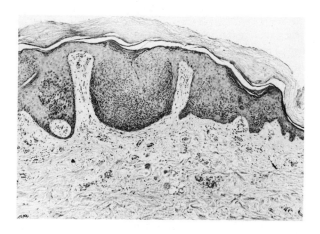

Fig. 15.17 Hidroacanthoma simplex. Sharply circumscribed whorls of basal cells can be seen within the epidermis.

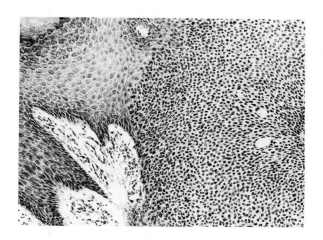

Fig. 15.18 Eccrine poroma. The tumour arises within the epidermis although it is sharply delineated from it, and grows down into the dermis. It is composed of small regular-shaped cells with dark oval nuclei, which lack any regular arrangement. Small lumina can be seen among the tumour cells. (Section by courtesy of Dr D.C. Carfrae, Stirling).

Eccrine poroma

This is a benign tumour of the acrosyringium, most commonly found on the palms and soles but which can occur elsewhere in the skin. The lesion consists of a mass of small, regular-sized cells with centrally placed oval nuclei, is superficial and arises within the epidermis although sharply demarcated from it. The tumour grows down into the dermis as an irregular mass. The cells resemble those of a basal cell carcinoma but do not stain as darkly, and the tumour lacks marginal palisading (Fig. 15.18). Small slit-like lumina lined by a PAS-positive membrane are found scattered throughout the cell mass, and granules of keratohyalin may be found in the cells adjacent to these spaces.

A malignant variant, the **porocarcinoma**, does occur but is rare.

Dermal duct tumour

This has an appearance similar to that of the eccrine poroma but occurs deeper in the dermis. It may have dilated ductal structures present in the islands of tumour cells.

Chondroid syringoma (tubular hidradenoma, mixed tumour of skin)

This tumour, which occurs mainly on the face, resembles the pleomorphic adenoma of salivary duct origin. Considered in the past to arise in ectopic salivary tissue, it was called a 'mixed tumour of skin'. It is now recognised as being of skin appendage origin and has been found elsewhere on the body, particularly on glabrous skin.

Histologically it consists of branching tubular structures and cystic spaces embedded in a varying amount of stroma which may have chondroid, myxoid or mucoid areas in it (Fig. 15.19). The tubular structures are lined by a double layer of epithelial cells, an inner basophilic cuboidal layer and an outer flatter layer. Sheets of the epithelial cells are also seen, and they occasionally show squamous differentiation. PAS-positive material is found in the lumen of some of the ducts and the stroma contains mucopolysaccharides.

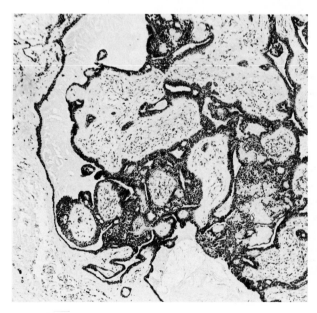

Fig. 15.19 Chondroid syringioma (tubular hidradenoma). The tumour is composed of branching duct-like structures containing PAS-positive material, and lined by a double layer of epithelium. In this instance they are embedded in a prominent fibrous tissue stroma, although it may be chondroid or myxoid.

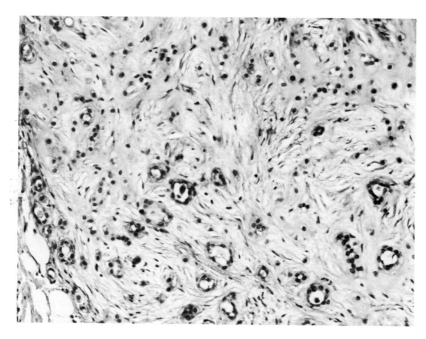

Fig. 15.20   Chondroid syringoma (tubular hidradenoma) 'variant'. There are small tubules lined by a single layer of cells which seem to merge with the cells of the surrounding chondroid matrix.

A variant of chondroid syringoma can occur in which there are small tubules lined only by a single layer of flat epithelial cells which seem to merge with the cells of the surrounding matrix (Fig. 15.20). Headington[4] postulated that this latter variety has an eccrine origin and that the more usual type is apocrine derived.

Spiradenoma (eccrine spiradenoma)

This tumour presents clinically as a deep-seated nodule which may give rise to spontaneous pain. It has been shown to differentiate towards both secretory and ductal epithelium, and may arise from the cells at the junction between the coiled duct and the secretory coil.

There is doubt regarding whether it is eccrine or apocrine in origin. Both spiradenomata and cylindromata have been seen in the same patient with multiple trichoepitheliomata, and tumours which appear to be a mixture of spiradenoma and cylindroma have also been described.

Histologically (Fig. 15.21) it consists of one or more well-defined cellular nodules, surrounded by a pseudocapsule of condensed fibrous tissue and divided by a variable amount of vascular and oedematous stroma. The cellular tissue consists of small basophilic cells of two types—one with a darkly staining nucleus and clear cytoplasm, and one with a larger paler-staining nucleus. On casual examination these two cell types appear to be mixed together except where they abut on to the stroma where the small dark cells palisade around the periphery. The stroma is often so oedematous that a false impression of cystic spaces is created. Careful examination of the cellular parts shows that there is an attempt to form duct-like spaces lined by the paler cells with the dark cells arranged peripherally. The lumina

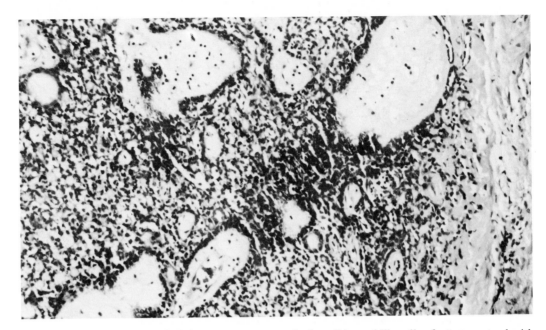

Fig. 15.21   Spiradenoma. Cellular tumour composed of small basophilic cells of two types and with a vascular and oedematous stroma. The cells appear to lack organisation but close examination shows that the larger paler cells are attempting to line duct-like spaces, and the smaller cells with darker nuclei are arranged peripherally and palisade around the oedematous stroma.

contain PAS-positive diastase-resistant material. As these lesions age, PAS-positive hyaline material is deposited in the stroma around the duct-like elements and between the cells. At this stage it may be difficult to separate these tumours from cylindromata, but there should be less difficulty if areas are present where the hyaline material has not been deposited. Sometimes these tumours are so cellular, with relatively frequent mitoses, that the possibility of low-grade malignancy should be considered. On occasion the stroma is so vascular that a misdiagnosis of angioma is made.

Clear cell hidradenoma (nodular hidradenoma, eccrine acrosyringoma, solid cystic hidradenoma, myoepithelioma)

The variety of names given to this tumour indicates that its origin has been in doubt, but it has now been shown to contain eccrine enzymes and, at the ultrastructural level, cells resembling those of the secretory coil of the eccrine gland.[2, 5] However, ductal elements are also present and the lesion should probably be regarded as an organoid tumour.

Histologically it has a lobular structure with a moderately well-defined capsule. It consists of solid sheets of cells within which there are a number of cystic spaces lined by a single layer of PAS-positive, diastase-resistant, cuboidal cells (Fig. 15.22). The solid areas are composed of two types of cells in varying proportions: one type is polygonal or fusiform with an open vesicular nucleus and clear cytoplasm containing glycogen; the other type is small with a more basophilic cytoplasm and a dense nucleus. Cells intermediate between these two types are often seen. Mitotic figures are not infrequent in the solid areas. Ductal elements may also

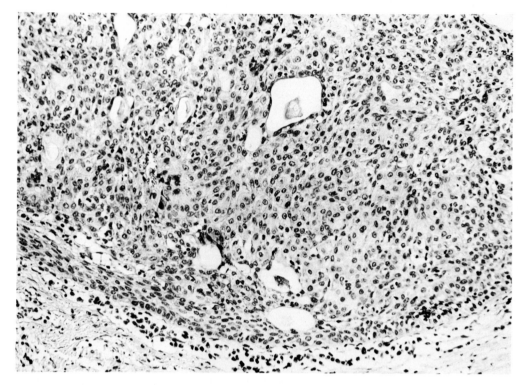

Fig. 15.22 Clear cell hidradenoma, showing a solid area of fusiform cells with open vesicular nuclei and clear glycogen-containing cytoplasm. Cystic spaces lined by PAS-positive cuboidal cells are present. Other areas in this tumour consisted of smaller, more basophilic cells, and ductal elements were also present.

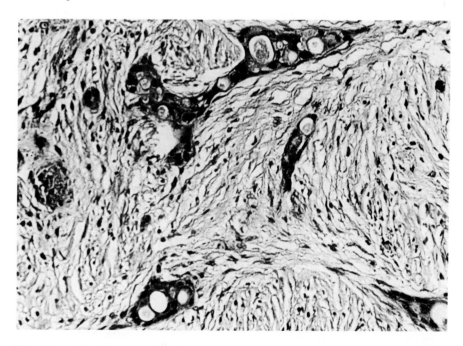

Fig. 15.23 Eccrine carcinoma. These tumours are often poorly differentiated and are mistaken for squamous carcinoma. However, in the more deeply infiltrating parts, poorly formed duct-like structures may be seen in a dense stroma as shown above. Each lumen contains PAS-positive material.

be present, and when the tumour connects with the surface its upper part resembles an eccrine poroma.

Eccrine carcinoma

These tumours are rare but various patterns have been described—*porocarcinoma* arising in the intraepidermal sweat duct, *clear cell carcinoma* thought to arise from clear cell hidradenoma, *mucinous carcinoma* in which islands of small dark basophilic cells are surrounded by lakes of mucin, and a poorly differentiated diffusely infiltrating tumour which can be mistaken for anaplastic squamous carcinoma. In this last tumour glandular spaces containing mucin can be found if carefully looked for (Fig. 15.23).

These malignant tumours have the capacity to metastasise to regional lymph nodes, as well as to the skin where they form nodules.

References

1. Ten Seldam REJ, Helwig EB. *Histological typing of Skin Tumours*. Geneva: World Health Organization, 1974: pp. 47–50.
2. Hashimoto K, Lever WF. *Appendage Tumors of the Skin*. Illinois: Springfield, Charles C Thomas, 1968.
3. Meeker JH, Neubecker RD, Helwig EB. Hidradenoma papilliferum. *Am J Clin Pathol* 1962; **37**: 182–95.
4. Headington JT. Mixed tumors of the skin: eccrine and apocrine types. *Arch Dermatol* 1961; **84**: 989–96.
5. O'Hara JM, Bensch KG. Fine structure of eccrine sweat gland adenoma, clear cell type. *J Invest Dermatol* 1967; **49**: 261–72.

16

Disorders of the Cutaneous Melanocyte

It is now well established that the epidermal melanocyte is of neuroectodermal origin and migrates during fetal life to its normal position in the basal layer of the epidermis. Here it is recognised on haematoxylin and eosin (H & E) sections as a relatively clear cell with marked cytoplasmic retraction artefact and a dark nucleus. The exact ratio of epidermal melanocytes to surrounding basal layer keratinocytes varies according to the body site, the past history of sun exposure and possibly the age of the patient.[1,2] As a rough rule of thumb, the ratio averages at around 1 melanocyte to 10 basal keratinocytes, but this can be higher on the face and lower on covered parts of the trunk. For accurate visualisation of melanocytes, a histochemical DOPA (dihydroxyphenylalanine) preparation is used. This utilises the DOPA oxidase and tyrosinase enzyme systems present in the melanocyte and forms a brown reaction product. Normally, however, a reasonable guide to melanocyte numbers can be gained by using an H & E or a Masson stain. The latter shows up the melanocyte particularly well.

The function of the epidermal melanocyte is to synthesise the pigment melanin protein and to distribute this pigment to surrounding keratinocytes. This is achieved first by synthesis of melanosomes or melanin granules in the melanocytes and then transfer of these granules via the melanocyte dendrites to the cytoplasm of the adjacent keratinocytes. The pigment granules then gather above the nucleus to protect the keratinocyte from ultraviolet damage. The cluster of one melanoctye and the surrounding keratinocytes which it supplies with pigment is termed the 'epidermal melanin unit'. The numbers of melanocytes are similar in matching sites in Caucasian and Negro skin but melanin is synthesised more rapidly in coloured skin and the size of individual melanin granules and packeting of these granules is different.[3]★

In normal human skin dermal melanocytes are very rarely seen, with the exception of the Mongolian spot found over the sacrum in some darker-skinned races. Dermal melanocytes are thought to have been arrested during their fetal migration from the neural crest towards the epidermis and are characterised by their bipolar and neural appearance. They frequently contain large, coarse melanin granules.

The range of benign lesions which may arise from epidermal or dermal melanocytes is shown in Table 16.1. It is generally believed that the epidermal melanocyte may transform into the naevus cell seen in the junctional, compound and intradermal naevi. Naevus cells vary in their morphology according to their position in the dermis. Thus, naevus cells high in the papillary dermis are relatively large and comparable in size with overlying melanocytes, while those in the deeper parts of the papillary dermis and high reticular dermis tend to be smaller and to be packeted in clumps of regular and uniformly sized cells. The deepest

★Thus although silver stain identifies melanin pigment it is not necessarily situated in a melanocyte.

Table 16.1   Types of pigmented naevi which arise from the dendritic melanocyte.

Name	Main histological features
Lentigo	Partial or complete replacement of stratum basale of epidermis by normal melanocytes
Junctional pigmented naevus	Focal proliferation of melanocytes with formation of clusters which project into the dermis—junctional change
Compound pigmented naevus	Junctional change in epidermis associated with nests of mature naevus cells in the dermis
Intradermal pigmented naevus	No junctional change in epidermis. Nests of mature naevus cells in dermis
Blue naevus	No constant epidermal changes. May range from normal epidermis to overlying junctional or compound naevi. In dermis bipolar spindle cells containing melanin granules

naevus cells frequently have a somewhat neural appearance and this morphological impression is confirmed on functional testing as some of these cells are cholinesterase positive. These different morphological appearances of naevus cells may be termed type A, type B and type C naevus cells respectively, and are thought to represent degrees of maturation as the cells 'drop off' the basal layer and move downwards through the dermis. Pigment production is rarely seen in the deeper cells of a naevus which has arisen from epidermal melanocytes, and the presence of fine cytoplasmic pigment in deeper cells together with a lack of orderly maturation are both important factors in identifying malignant change within a pre-existing naevus.

The frequency of malignant change within melanocytic naevi is a matter of some debate. At the present time it is generally agreed that malignant change within acquired melanocytic naevi is rare, as most young adults have 10–20 benign melanocytic naevi, the vast majority of which never become malignant.[4] The situation with the rarer congenital type of naevus is somewhat different, as a much higher incidence of malignant change within these lesions has been reported in the past.[5] Current views are that this problem has almost certainly been over-reported and that, although the risk of malignant melanoma developing within these giant congenital melanocytic naevi is greater than the risk of acquired naevi undergoing malignant change, it is not as big a problem as has been suggested. Prospective studies are currently in progress to confirm this, and also to establish whether or not smaller congenital naevi behave in a similar manner to the larger congenital lesions. This is obviously an important point to establish because while prophylactic removal of the giant naevi is rarely practical, smaller congenital naevi could be removed relatively easily.

Benign lesions arising from the epidermal melanocyte

Ephelis (freckle)

The ephelis, or freckle, is a functional rather than a morphological abnormality. Under ultraviolet stimulation some melanocytes produce larger amounts of melanin than others. This is visible clinically and presents histologically as an irregular increase in melanin granules in the basal layer keratinocytes. This functional anomaly is genetically determined.

Freckles disappear in the winter months or in the absence of ultraviolet stimulation. They are common in fair-skinned individuals and seen more frequently in the younger age groups.

Lentigo (Fig. 16.1)

This lesion is characterised clinically by the permanent present of a macular brown lesion on the skin surface. Although it may darken in the summer months, it does not disappear completely in the winter. It is commoner on older skin. The lesion is due to replacement of the basal layer melanocytes by melanocytes in a linear fashion. The melanocytes are of normal size and configuration, and mitotic figures are rare. There is no migration of melanocytes upwards through the epidermis or downwards into the papillary dermis.

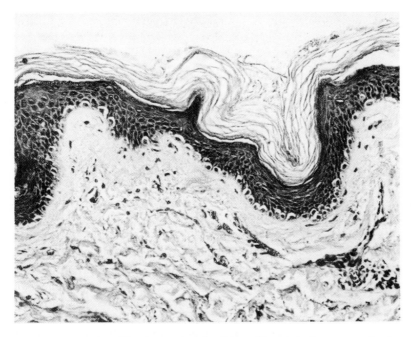

Fig. 16.1   Lentigo. The stratum basale of the epidermis is almost completely replaced by histologically normal melanocytes.

Junctional melanocytic naevus

This acquired lesion, which is usually flat and pale brown, is characterised by focal proliferation of groups or 'thèques' of melanocytes, all of which are still in contact with the basal layer of the epidermis (Fig. 16.2). These thèques, or packets of melanocytes, tend to gather at the deepest parts of the epidermal ridges in a regular fashion. The nuclei of the cells are similar in size to that of the surrounding keratinocytes and they tend to have abundant, sometimes rather vacuolated, cytoplasm. The nuclear/cytoplasmic ratio is thus frequently fairly low. These cells contain a fine dusting of melanin pigment and retain their ability to synthesise melanin, proved by a positive DOPA reaction.

Junctional melanocytic activity is most commonly seen at the dermo-epidermal junction on the epidermal surface but may also be seen in the hair follicles, particularly in congenital melanocytic naevi (see below).

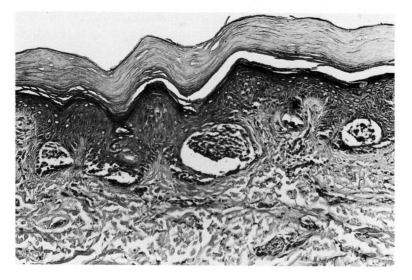

Fig. 16.2   Junctional naevus of sole. Note five 'thèques' or nests of melanocytes in contact with the basal layer.

It has been suggested that melanocytic naevi with so-called 'junctional activity' or large aggregates of naevus cells at the dermo-epidermal junction are the only naevi arising from epidermal melanocytes which have the potential for malignant change. It is clearly impossible to prove the accuracy of this statement and recently isolated case reports have suggested that on rare occasions malignant change may develop in the intradermal component of melanocytic naevi.[6,7,8] It is likely that the chances of malignant change are related to the frequency of cell division, and as evidence of active cell division within the deep dermal component of melanocytic naevi is rare, malignant change in these cells will also be an unusual event.

Compound naevus

These are mid to dark brown papular lesions. They are common in early adult life and numbers thereafter decrease with increasing age.

Lesions of this type are composed both of clusters of naevus cells which retain contact with the basal layer and also of naevus cells which are lying free in the underlying dermis (Fig. 16.3). The assumption is that a 'dropping off' or 'abtropfung'[9] of cells from the basal layer has occurred and that the intradermal cellular aggregates are older or more mature. Melanin pigment may be seen in the cells in the papillary dermis but is rare in the deeper parts of the lesion. Free melanin and melanin-laden macrophages are likewise unusual in benign non-irritated melanocytic naevi.

Both compound and junctional naevi may be stimulated to activity by incomplete excision or a shave biopsy. The resultant picture (Fig. 16.4) may be very similar to that of an early

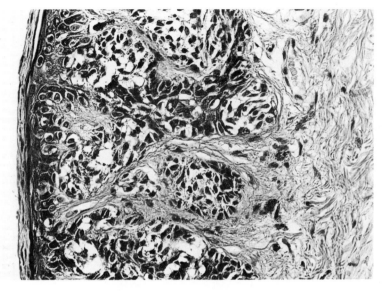

Fig. 16.4 Traumatically stimulated melanocytic naevus. This lesion had been incompletely excised 1 month previously. It has many features in common with the so-called dysplastic naevus.

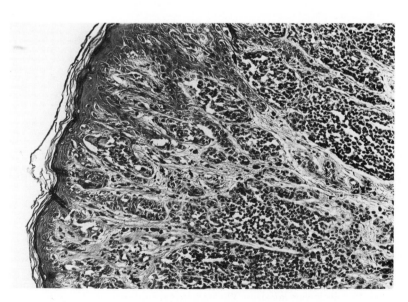

Fig. 16.3 Compound naevus. Note the obvious increase in naevus cells adjacent to the basal layer and also the presence of smaller possibly more mature naevus cells in deeper parts of the dermis.

invasive melanoma and give rise to considerable diagnostic confusion unless a clear history is sent with the lesion. The term 'pseudomelanoma'[10] has been suggested for such lesions but could obviously cause confusion. The alternative of 'traumatically stimulated naevus' is a safer and more accurate description.

Intradermal naevus

This lesion has no overlying abnormality of melanocytes, and no naevus cells in direct contact with cells of the basal layer of the epidermis. All the naevus cells lie free in the dermis and are generally packeted or clumped (Fig. 16.5). The deeper parts of these lesions may show a marked resemblance to neural cells (Fig. 16.6).

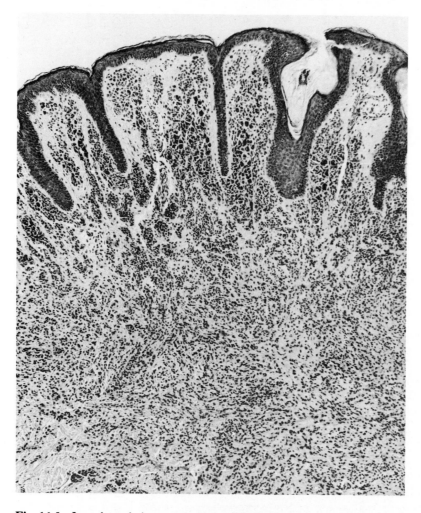

Fig. 16.5 Intradermal pigmented naevus. There is no junctional change in the epidermis. The dermis contains packets of mature naevus cells in varying sizes. The packeted arrangement of the naevus cells is more obvious towards the surface. The darker-staining cells visible within the packets are macrophages containing coarse melanin granules. Towards the bottom of the microphotograph the naevus cells become more diffuse and early fibrosis can be seen.

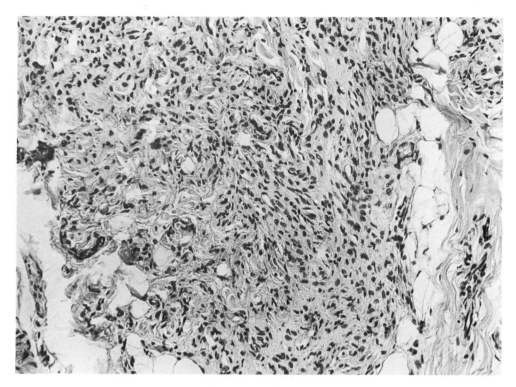

Fig. 16.6 Intradermal pigmented naevus. This microphotograph of the deeper portion of an intra-dermal pigmented naevus shows the naevus cells arranging themselves in a linear fashion with some palisading, an appearance reminiscent of that seen in neurolemmoma. (cf. Fig. 17.11; Chapter 17).

In general, it is considered that the deeper areas of both compound and intradermal naevi are relatively inert structures with very few mitotic figures to be seen. Occasionally, mel-anocytic naevus cells appear to cause obstruction to outflow of a pilosebaceous follicle, resulting in the rapid development of inflammation and progression to a granulomatous reaction (Fig. 16.7). If persistent, this can even result in bone formation in the depths of the naevus (Fig. 16.8). This sequence of events is a relatively common cause of sudden and dramatic growth of a previously inert naevus. Because of rapid expansion of the lesion, clinical concern over malignant change may have been aroused, but this is an entirely benign process. Clinical evidence of malignant change in association with a melanocytic naevus generally develops over a period of months rather than the days or weeks seen in the case of this obstructive process.

The end stage of the intradermal naevus is seen in the elderly as a *pedunculated skin tag*. Patients will frequently give a good history of having had a mole on the site for many years which has gradually lost all evidence of melanin pigmentation and matured into a loose pedunculated lesion composed of fibrous tissue stroma surrounded by normal epidermis.

The *fibrous papule of the nose* may also represent the end stage or part of a maturation process of melanocytic naevi. These lesions present on the face as raised, slightly pigmented nodules which are shown on biopsy to be composed of discrete islands of fibrous tissue underlying a normal epidermis with, on occasion, a slight increase in the normal melanocyte/

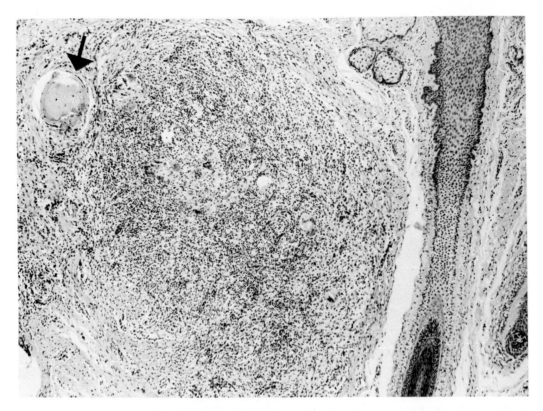

Fig. 16.7   Granuloma formation in benign pigmented naevus. This microphotograph shows a sub-acutely inflamed foreign body granuloma occurring in the depth of a fibrosed intradermal naevus which had clinically shown a recent and sudden increase in size. The small portion of bone (arrowed) indicates that a similar event, possibly on a smaller scale, has occurred in the past (see text and Fig. 16.8).

keratinocyte ratio. Many of these lesions contain cells which have a striking morphological resemblance to naevus cells.

Benign epithelioid or spindle cell melanocytic naevus[11] (Spitz tumour, juvenile melanoma)

These benign melanocytic naevi are lesions which may cause dermatopathologists considerable anxiety in the differentiation between a benign melanocytic naevus and an early malignant melanoma. Indeed, it is only in the last 30 years that they have been separated from malignant melanoma as a result of keen observation and clinicopathological correlation by the late Sophie Spitz.[12]

As one of their synonyms implies, these lesions are commoner in children, but may be seen in adults and even in elderly individuals. The classic lesion presents on the face of a child as a reddish-brown, tumid, raised lesion. Clinically these are easily identified. In older individuals the clinical appearance may be more like that of the commoner variety of compound naevi.

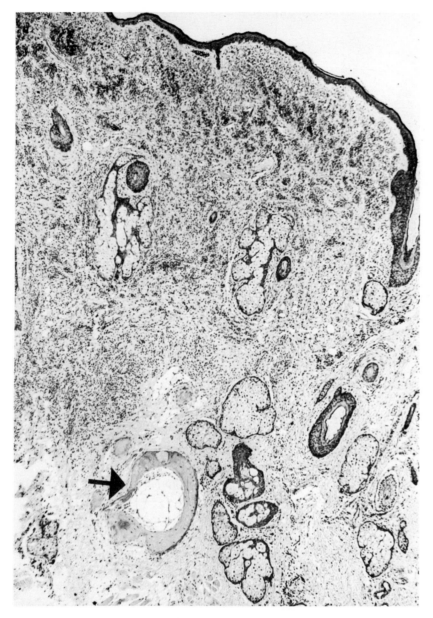

Fig. 16.8 Bone formation in benign pigmented naevus. A portion of cancellous bone (arrowed) containing bone marrow can be seen in the depth of this benign intradermal naevus.

Histologically these lesions appear to be a variant of compound naevi with the following additional and distinctive features (Figs. 16.9–16.11):

1. Obvious and at times gross oedema surrounding the individual cells.

2. Easily visible, large, dilated capillaries admixed with the melanocytic cells. This feature may explain the oedema.

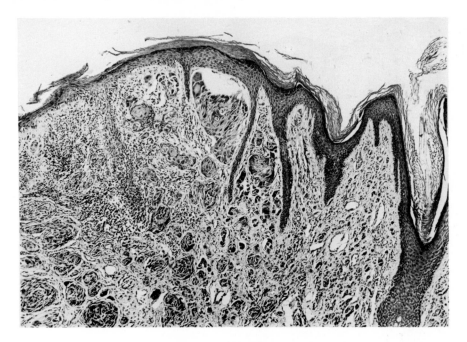

Fig. 16.9 Spitz naevus. Note the pseudoepitheliomatous hyperplasia overlying circumscribed nests of naevus cells.

3. The presence of large, pale, epithelioid or spindle cells, many of which contain hyperchromatic nuclei and have visible mitotic figures. Melanin pigment in these cells is often scanty.

4. The presence of small numbers of Langhans-type giant cells among the naevus cells.

5. The presence of a lymphocytic infiltrate admixed with the cells in the deeper parts of the lesion.

6. The presence in some cases of overlying pseudoepitheliomatous hyperplasia of the epidermis.

These lesions may at times have individual features strongly suggestive of a true malignancy and this is particularly apparent if one focuses rapidly on high-power examination of individual hyperchromatic cells. The pattern of the lesion at a lower power, and the presence of some degree of orderly maturation in the deeper parts of the lesion, should help to clarify the diagnosis, as will an accurate clinical history. There is no doubt, however, that differentiation between an atypical or unusual Spitz naevus and an early malignant melanoma is one of the most difficult tasks confronting a dermatopathologist. In the few cases in which a definitive diagnosis cannot be reached, adequate local excision and follow-up are essential.

The recent report of the presence of eosinophilic globules in Spitz naevi requires further confirmation as to its specificity. While the majority of Spitz lesions do appear to have these globules, they may also be seen in some melanomata and therefore cannot be regarded as a specific diagnostic feature.

Pigmented spindle cell naevus of Reed[13]

This lesion has many features suggesting that it is a variant of the classic Spitz naevus, but

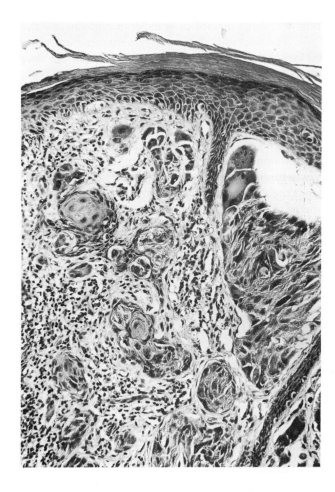

Fig. 16.10 Spitz naevus. Higher magnification view of 16.9 showing obvious oedema, dilated capillaries and giant cells.

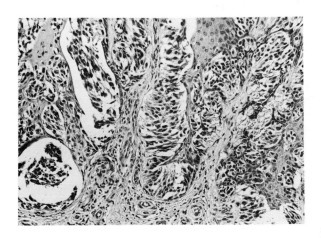

Fig. 16.11 Spitz naevus (spindle cell type). In the central portion of this microphotograph the melanocytes in the packets of junctional change are spindle shaped. This should not be mistaken for spindle cell melanocarcinoma. The section is from the margin of a benign spindle cell juvenile melanoma in a child.

is distinguished by the production of relatively large quantities of melanin pigment and the strikingly monomorphic spindle cell type. The naevus cells tend to remain localised in the papillary dermis and frequently elicit a lymphocytic host response. The picture can thus cause considerable confusion between an early malignant melanoma of the spindle cell type.

Halo naevus[14] (Fig. 16.12)

This lesion is easily identified clinically by the striking depigmented halo seen around a centrally placed melanocytic naevus. A local immunological response appears to have been mounted against melanocytes and naevus cells as the depigmentation is due to local destruction of melanocytes, and the central naevus shows infiltration with lymphocytes. The natural history of lesions is complete disappearance of the melanocytic naevus.

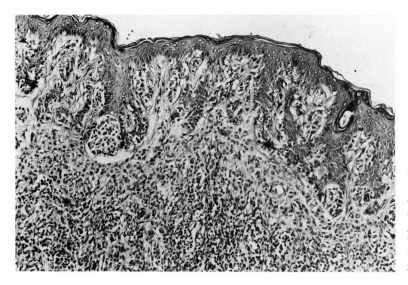

Fig. 16.12 Halo naevus. Note the naevus cells at the dermo-epidermal junction and a gross lymphocytic infiltrate in the underlying dermal component of the lesion.

Provided that a good clinical history is supplied with the specimen, this lesion should not present diagnostic difficulty. In the absence of this, a compound or intradermal melanocytic naevus with a dense lymphocytic infiltrate in and around the lesion and no other signs suggestive of malignant melanoma (upward migration of melanocytes through the epidermis, the presence of mitotic figures, the presence of cells with a high nuclear/cytoplasmic ratio) should indicate the diagnosis.

Lesions arising from dermal melanocytes

Mongolian spot

This is rarely biopsied as it is recognised clinically as a benign physiological variant. Under a normal epidermis large bipolar spindle cells are seen in association with large coarse clumps of melanin pigment, lying free in the dermis, in the naevus cells and also in macrophages.

Blue naevus

There are two distinct variants of this lesion. The commoner blue naevus has a histological appearance identical to that of the Mongolian spot with striking deposits of melanin in the papillary dermis within and around naevus cells which may be difficult to visualise because of the density of the melanin pigmentation. If this is the case, a melanin bleach will make accurate identification of individual cells very much easier (Fig. 16.13).

An extremely rare pair of blue naevus variants are the naevus of Ota, which is seen over the area of the face served by the trigeminal nerve, and the naevus of Ito, seen over the acromioclavicular area. These present as dusky, macular areas due to dermal melanin pigment.

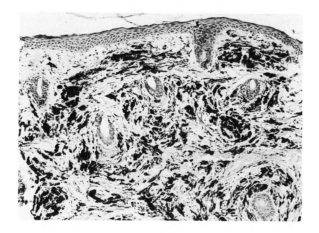

Fig. 16.13 Blue naevus. In the dermis are seen numerous elongated spindle cells containing melanin. The rounded dark-staining cells are melanin-laden macrophages. At this magnification the bipolar dendritic processes of the spindle cells are not evident. They are seen more clearly in silver stained preparations from lesions containing only a few spindle cells.

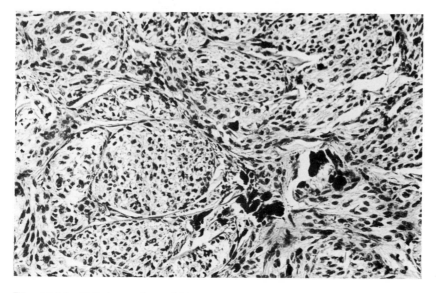

Fig. 16.14 Cellular variant of blue naevus. The tumour is composed of well-defined bundles of spindle cell which, because they run in all directions, are cut in different planes. The black masses towards the centre of the picture are aggregations of melanin-laden macrophages contained in the stroma.

The rarer *cellular blue naevus* is said to be found more commonly on certain body sites such as the wrists and buttocks. These lesions are frequently raised pink nodules with little obvious melanin pigment. Histologically they are composed of bundles of naevus cells which interlace and are thus seen cut at different planes in the dermis. Melanin pigment may be very scanty and present only in macrophages or lying free in the dermis (Fig. 16.14). A Fontana stain will help to identify small quantities of melanin in difficult cases. Mitotic figures may be present in the naevus cells but are regular and normal.

The differentiation of these relatively rare tumours from other spindle cell tumours of the dermis may at times be difficult (Chapter 17). In cases of doubt, ultrastructural examination may reveal the classic large melanosomes seen in blue naevi. Often, however, a specimen has not been taken specifically for ultrastructural processing and the degree of preservation in the material available may be inadequate to allow accurate identification of these melanosomes.

Although malignant change in cellular blue naevi has been reported, it is extremely rare. Atypical mitoses and areas of tumour necrosis are features which should alert the observer to this possibility.

Occasionally some increase in epidermal melanocytes is seen overlying a blue naevus. This implies activity on the part of both dermal and epidermal melanocytes or naevus cells and is called a *combined naevus*. It has no sinister or adverse prognostic significance.

Congenital naevi

The majority of congenital naevi are frequently hamartomatous with melanocytic cells comprising only a part of the picture. Excessive and malformed skin appendages may be present, and the lesions contain naevus cells of both epidermal and dermal origin. Thus areas similar to a blue naevus are seen underlying junctional activity at the basal layer of the epidermis. Melanocytic activity is frequently seen extending down the root sheath of the pilosebaceous follicle, and the lesion may extend well into the subcutaneous fat (Fig. 16.15). The impression is one of irregularity and disorder but high-power examination reveals relatively few mitotic figures in the naevus cells.

Although it seems clear that congenital melanocytic naevi have a higher incidence of malignant transformation than acquired naevi, the true incidence is not yet established.

Malignant melanoma

There is good evidence from certain parts of the world, such as Scandinavia and Queensland, Australia, that the incidence of cutaneous melanoma is rising.[15] This being so, it is likely that dermatopathologists will see an increasing number of these important lesions. For many years it has been recognised that the lentigo maligna melanoma (Hutchinson's malignant freckle, precancerous melanosis of Dubreuilh) is a distinct entity on the grounds of age at presentation, sites of involvement and response to therapy.[16] In the past decade the other primary cutaneous melanomata have been subdivided on clinicopathological criteria into three main groups—the superficial spreading, nodular, and acral lentiginous (palmoplantar mucosal) varieties.[17] While these variants can usually be recognised with little difficulty, it is not yet clear whether such identification has any prognostic significance for the individual patient. It may well be that these three subtypes are all part of a spectrum of disease. At the present time, however, it is common practice to try to assign primary cutaneous malignant melanoma to one of these subsets, and it may be that such classification will in time throw

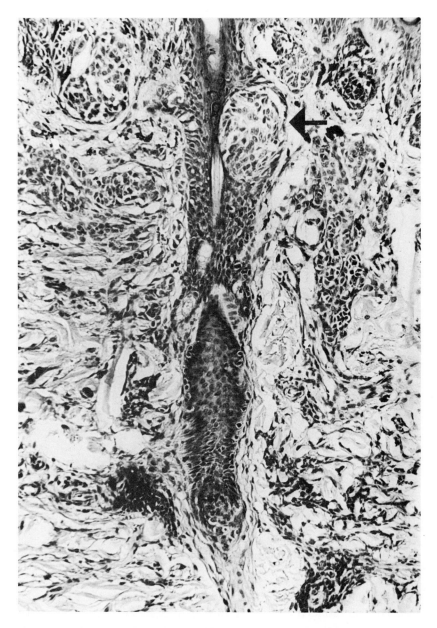

Fig. 16.15 Congenital melanocytic naevus. Note the melanocytic activity deep in a pilosebaceous follicle.

light on the aetiological factors at work in this disease. The evidence incriminating excessive exposure to sunlight as a major aetiological factor is accumulating steadily, but only in the case of lentigo maligna melanoma does this appear to be a direct cumulative effect of total lifetime sun exposure. In the case of the other varieties, short sharp intensive exposure and ultraviolet-induced burns appear to be more important. The role of other factors such as hormones, diet, and ingestion of photosensitising drugs is not yet established.

Lentigo maligna and lentigo maligna melanoma

The preinvasive phase of this lesion, *lentigo maligna*, is found commonly on the cheeks of elderly people who have spent considerable periods in the sun or in an outdoor occupation. The lesions present as dull brown macular areas which, over a period of years, advance laterally across the face. This lateral growth is frequently accompanied by some central regression and development of pallor and scar tissue.

Histologically the lesion is recognised as a replacement of the basal layer keratinocytes by large atypical melanocytes, usually spindle shaped. The overlying epidermis is thin and atrophic and the underlying dermis shows gross and obvious actinic damage (Fig. 16.16). A

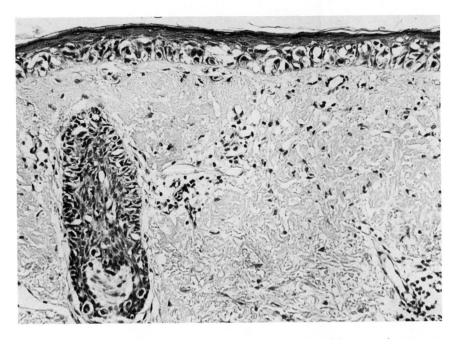

Fig. 16.16 Lentigo maligna. The stratum basale is replaced by a continuous row of pleomorphic melanocytes with irregular hyperchromatic nuclei. In some areas these aberrant melanocytes are seen at a higher level in the epidermis than the stratum basale. The epithelium of the pilosebaceous follicle to the left of the picture also contains numerous aberrant melanocytes. The dermal collagen shows a marked degree of solar elastosis.

considerable degree of vacuolation occurs in the atypical melanocytes during processing, giving rise to a very characteristic 'honeycomb' appearance in the basal layer of the epidermis. This striking change can extend for a considerable distance down the epithelial lining of pilosebaceous follicles. Lentigo maligna is usually a lesion which covers a considerable area of the epidermis and the typical changes are frequently seen extending throughout the entire excised specimen. It is very common for the limits of excision of the specimen to show changes of lentigo maligna but despite this, local recurrence is relatively unusual due, first, to the fact that this is a slowly evolving lesion and, secondly, to the fact that these lesions commonly affect patients in the seventh decade or later, who tend to die of unrelated disease before the lesion has regrown.

In an undetermined proportion of these lesions the *in situ* malignant change of *lentigo*

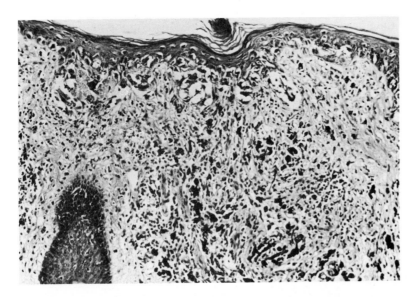

Fig. 16.17 Lentigo maligna melanoma. Note the replacement of basal layer keratinocytes by large atypical melanocytes and, in addition, invasion of lymphocytes into the underlying dermis which shows gross actinic damage.

maligna progresses to the invasive *lentigo maligna melanoma* (Fig. 16.17). This usually occurs after a lesion has been present for years or even decades, and clinically is characterised by the development of areas of hyperkeratosis or frank nodule formation within the lesion. The early histological changes show extension of isolated atypical melanocytes into the dermis. This development is frequently accompanied by the presence of a striking lymphoid cell infiltrate which may mask individual neoplastic melanocytes and make them difficult to identify. The presence of such an infiltrate under an area of apparently non-invasive lentigo maligna should alert the observer to cut in on the block and search carefully for individual invasive malignant melanocytes. In the later stages of lentigo maligna melanoma the presence of invasive melanocytes is easily seen. The overlying epidermis frequently becomes acanthotic relative to the surrounding thin epidermis and a degree of pseudoepitheliomatous hyperplasia may be seen. The invasive malignant melanocytes are large and hyperchromatic, frequently spindle shaped, and exhibit a variety of bizarre mitotic figures.

Even when lentigo maligna melanoma is obviously invading well into the dermis, the presence of neoplastic cells in lymphatic vessels and subsequent metastases are relatively rare events. This may be related to the gross actinic damage seen in the dermis around these lesions.

Superficial spreading malignant melanoma

This lesion accounts for over 50 per cent of all cutaneous malignant melanomata in reported series from Europe and North America.[18] They occur commonly on the female leg and the male trunk, frequently on individuals two to three decades younger than those presenting with lentigo maligna melanoma. The preinvasive or *in situ* phase of growth of these lesions is identified as an area of epidermis in which large numbers of atypical melanocytes are seen clustered together at the dermo-epidermal junction. Overlying these areas individual atypical melanocytes are seen in the upper layers of the epidermis. A scanty lymphoid infiltrate may be seen in the papillary dermis, but no invasive melanocytic cells. Such lesions are sometimes termed 'atypical melanocytic hyperplasia' or 'Clark level I malignant melanoma'. The use of the latter term is discouraged outside research studies and is not recommended for routine reporting because inappropriately wide excision of the lesion might result. We have no evidence as to how many of these lesions would progress to frank invasive superficial spreading melanoma if left *in sutu*.

The invasive phase of superficial spreading melanoma is recognised clinically by an

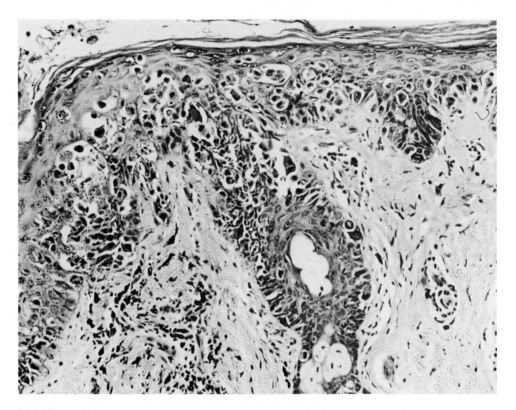

Fig. 16.18   Superficial spreading melanoma. Note the Pagetoid invasion of the epidermis by large atypical melanocytes.

irregular brownish-black lesion with marked pigmentary variation. The lateral margin of the lesion frequently has an irregular scalloped edge, and areas of dark melanin pigmentation alternating with reddish inflammatory zones within the lesion are common. Frank ulceration is usually a late event but microscopic evidence of ulceration may be seen in lesions excised at a relatively early stage of growth. Histologically the lesion commonly shows an area of thickened and acanthotic epidermis with large atypical melanoctytes scattered through it in a manner strongly resembling extramammary Paget's disease (Figs. 16.18 and 16.19). If there is genuine difficulty in differentiating between these two lesions, a PAS stain before and after diastase will clearly identify the latter condition. Invasion of neoplastic melanocytes into the dermis is generally seen in the centre of the lesion, with the Pagetoid change

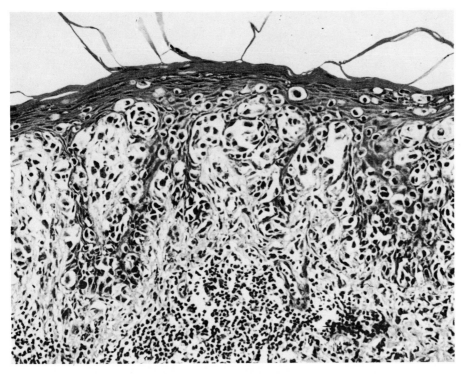

Fig. 16.19 Superficial spreading melanoma. Note the nests of atypical melanocytes invading the epidermis and also extending into the underlying dermis. There is a desultory lymphocytic infiltrate underlying the lesion.

persisting in the epidermis for several millimetres around this area. In addition to this Pagetoid pattern, superficial spreading melanomata may show significant epidermal hyperplasia associated with aggregates of neoplastic spindle cell melanocytes around the dermo-epidermal junction. This pattern is frequently seen in lesions of the lower leg and may coexist with the Pagetoid pattern within any one lesion.[19] Melanin pigment is easily seen within melanoma cells and lying either free in the dermis or in macrophages. Important features of prognostic significance include the presence of neoplastic cells in vascular channels, and the presence of streaks of melanin pigment in the mid dermis surrounded by granulation or scar tissue. This latter observation suggests a degree of spontaneous regression, and in thin lesions (see below) may be associated with a relatively poorer prognosis.[20] As with the lentigo maligna melanomata, a lymphoid cell infiltrate is seen in some cases admixed with the invasive tumour cells. If the lesion is ulcerated, a more mixed infiltrate including plasma cells may be present.

Nodular malignant melanoma

Nodular malignant melanoma is commoner in younger individuals and frequently occurs on the non-exposed skin of the trunk. These lesions appear to develop an invasive capacity at a very early stage in their evolution so that any trace of *in situ* growth confined to the epidermis has been obliterated by the time the lesion is submitted for pathological study.

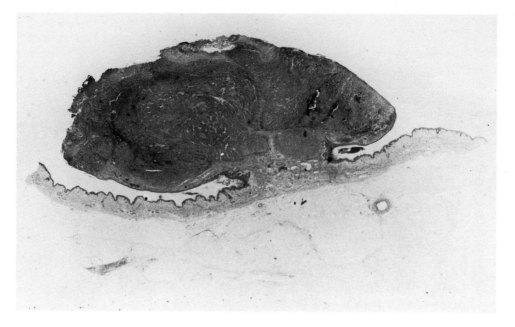

Fig. 16.20 Polypoid melanoma. This lesion is obviously a pedunculated one with remarkably normal epidermis on either side of the stalk.

Clinically these lesions are raised nodules, and frequently melanin pigment is scanty or absent. Ulceration occurs rapidly and clinical confusion with vascular lesions is common.

Histologically the lesions consist of discrete nodules of invasive neoplastic melanocytes invading both upwards through the epidermis and downwards into the dermis. Adjacent to this area the epidermis appears remarkably normal with no *in situ* change.

A variant of the nodular melanoma is the polypoid variety where a great deal of growth takes place above the level of the surrounding normal epidermis (Fig. 16.20). Ulceration is common, and there is some evidence to suggest that they have an even poorer prognosis than other nodular lesions.

Acral lentiginous melanoma[21, 22]

These lesions are found on the thick epidermis of the palms and soles, and the majority are on the foot. Approximately 50 per cent of all primary melanomata arising on the foot are of this histogenetic variety, as both superficial spreading and nodular melanomata are also seen on the soles. Clinically the lesion may appear relatively benign and present as a flat macular pigmented lesion. The more rapidly growing raised lesions are not infrequently misdiagnosed as plantar warts and treated inappropriately for some time before referral for definitive therapy.

Histologically the lesions show striking replacement of the basal layer keratinocytes by large spindle-shaped malignant melanocytes, with proliferation of these neoplastic cells both upwards through the epidermis and downwards into the dermis (Fig. 16.21). A striking lymphocytic infiltrate may be present around these cells, and in early non-ulcerated lesions some acanthosis may be present.

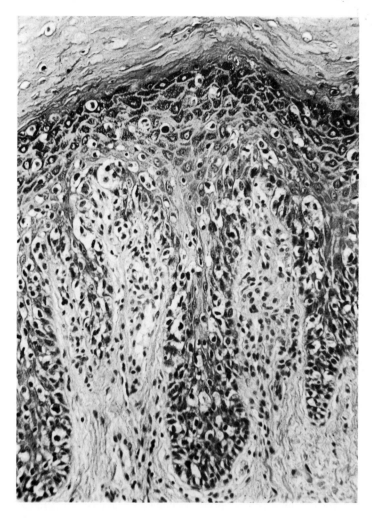

Fig. 16.21 Acral lentiginous melanoma. Note the upward migration of atypical melanocytes through the epidermis and smaller numbers of neoplastic cells invading the dermis.

Subungual melanoma[23]

These lesions are often misdiagnosed as 'ingrowing toenail' or warts, and delays in referral for appropriate surgery may account in part for their particularly poor prognosis. Histogenetic typing may be difficult because of topographical considerations, but the majority of lesions fall into either the nodular or the acral lentiginous type.

Minimal deviation melanoma

This term was coined by Reed to describe melanomata arising in association with melanocytic naevi in which evidence of malignant transformation was subtle and not instantly recognisable.[13] Features which might suggest such a diagnosis include a lack of maturation of individual cells in the deeper parts of an apparently benign naevus, the presence of mitotic figures and aberrant mitoses in these cells, and fine 'dusty' melanin pigment in cells deep in the dermis.

Malignant melanoma of unclassified histogenetic type

This term is used to describe a lesion which does not fit easily into any of the four major currently recognised 'subsets'—lentigo maligna melanoma, superficial spreading melanoma, nodular melanoma and acral melanoma. The incidence of this type will vary according to the pathologist's experience and enthusiasm for classification but is commonly around 5–10 per cent in large reported series. Such lesions may have features in common with both lentigo maligna melanoma and superficial spreading lesions, or may show an invasive nodule with areas of *in situ* adjacent intraepidermal activity which is not easily classified.

Desmoplastic melanoma[24]

A few cases of this rare variant have been described. The lesion is composed of spindle cells and appears to elicit a very striking and intense stromal reaction. Prognosis is poor. Some of these lesions appear to acquire the quality of neurotropism.[25]

Features of prognostic significance (Table 16.2)

From the many studies in the past decade of pathological features of prognostic value for the individual patient, it has now clearly emerged that the single most important prognostic feature is the thickness of the tumour.[26,27,28] This was established by the late Alexander Breslow, and the Breslow thickness measurement is one which all surgeons involved in melanoma surgery should request from their pathologists. The measurement is obtained by using an ocular micrometer to measure in millimetres the distance between the granular layer of the epidermis and the deepest easily identified tumour cell in the underlying dermis (Fig. 16.22). A direct inverse linear correlation exists between five-year survival and Breslow

Table 16.2   Features of possible prognostic significance in primary cutaneous malignant melanoma.

Tumour thickness	Over-rides all other factors
Clark level of invasion	Valuable but less significant than tumour thickness
Vascular invasion	Valuable
High mitotic rate and abnormal mitoses	Probably of supplementary value to thickness
Ulceration	Indicates aggressive destructive cell type. Probably indicates poor prognosis
Clear evidence of regression	Conflicting reports. May indicate a poorer short-term prognosis in thin tumours
Lymphocytic infiltrate	Conflicting results. Obvious lymphocytic response to deeper invasive tumour cells may be a good prognostic sign
Cell type	No clear difference between spindle, epithelioid or mixed cell type. 'Intralesional transformation' may be a poor prognostic sign
Degree of melanisation	No obvious significance
Pre-existing naevus	Possibly a good prognostic feature

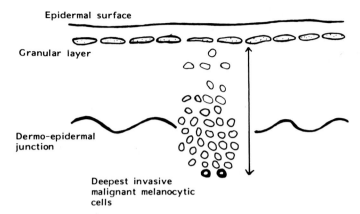

Fig. 16.22 Diagrammatic representation of measurement of melanoma thickness by the Breslow technique.

thickness so that the measurement can be used to divide lesions into those with a relatively good prognosis (1.5 mm or less in thickness) and intermediate and poor prognosis lesions (1.5–3 mm and >3 mm respectively).

If this measurement is to be obtained accurately, it clearly is essential that blocks be taken from what appears to be the most deeply invasive part of the tumour. This is an important point to consider in reports of retrospective surveys of material.

Overlying ulceration makes accurate tumour thickness measurement slightly more difficult to obtain and there is some evidence that the presence of tumour regression

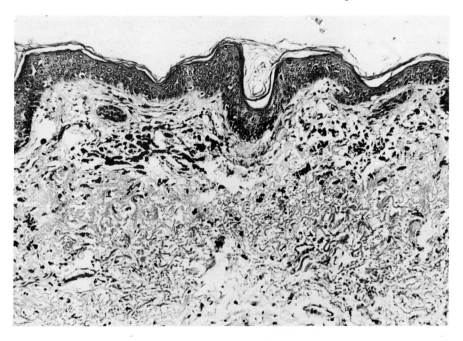

Fig. 16.23 Evidence of regression adjacent to a primary melanoma. Note the gross melanin streaking in the papillary dermis.

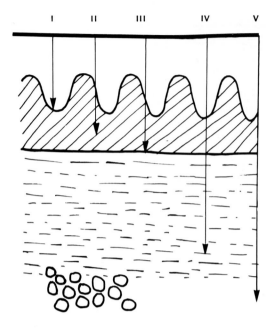

Fig. 16.24   Clark levels of invasion: I, intraepidermal only; II, papillary dermis; III, interface between papillary and reticular dermis; IV, reticular dermis; V, subcutaneous fat.

may result in a falsely thin measurement and a relatively poor prognosis for the individual patient. Regression is generally recognised by the presence of streaks of coarse melanin pigment within the dermis, and collagen changes resembling granulation or even scar tissue (Fig. 16.23).

Measurement of Clark levels of invasion (Fig. 16.24) is also a useful guide to prognosis, but correlation between pathologists is poorer than for Breslow thickness measurements. The Clark levels used in Europe and North America are:

Level I   Intraepidermal (non-invasive, *in situ*)
Level II   Neoplastic cells in the papillary dermis
Level III   Neoplastic cells filling and distorting the papillary dermis and abutting on the reticular dermis
Level IV   Neoplastic cells invading into the reticular dermis
Level V   Invasion of cells beneath the reticular dermis into the subcutaneous fat

A connective tissue stain such as Masson trichrome will facilitate identification of the papillary and reticular dermis. This differentiation can also be made with ease using polarised light.

The presence of neoplastic cells in vascular channels is generally regarded as a poor prognostic sign, and a search should be made for this feature (Fig. 16.25). Unlike ocular melanomata, there is no clear evidence that the cell type comprising the bulk of the tumour affects prognosis, although it has been suggested recently that 'intralesional transformation' or the development within a tumour of a morphologically distinct clone of cells is a poor prognostic sign.[29] Quantity of melanin pigment present does not appear to affect prognosis. Ulceration is generally regarded as a poor prognostic sign and its presence should be included in the report.[30] In many early lesions a lymphoid infiltrate is present but there is no clear evidence that this is a useful prognostic guide. Counting of mitoses is a time-honoured and time-consuming exercise, and in general a high mitotic rate and the presence of abnormal

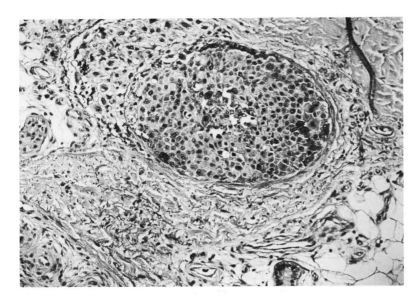

Fig. 16.25 Cluster of melanoma cells within a vascular channel deep to a primary lesion.

mitoses are indicative of a poor prognosis. Schmoekel has suggested that the combination of Breslow thickness measurement and mitotic rate together give a more accurate prognostic index for the individual patient than thickness measurement alone.[31]

Differential diagnosis of malignant melanoma

For the pathologist there are two main problems. The first is differentiating between a benign but apparently active melanocytic naevus and early primary cutaneous malignant melanoma. The second is when faced with an obviously malignant anaplastic tumour to establish whether or not the tumour is melanocytic in origin.

Differentiation between active melanocytic naevi, including Spitz naevi and early invasive melanoma, depends on a variety of features listed in Table 16.3. No one feature can be regarded as the definitive arbiter between benignity and malignancy, but features which should alert the pathologist and prompt careful inspection of multiple sections include upward migration of melanocytes through the epidermis, the presence of a lymphoid infiltrate around melanocytic cells in the dermis and the presence of mitotic figures within these melanocytic cells. Deciding that an anaplastic tumour is melanocytic in origin is frequently equally difficult. Any evidence of origin from basal layer melanocytes is of great value but frequently the lesion is ulcerated, and, as the lesion may be a secondary deposit rather than a primary tumour, this evidence is not always present. The presence of pigment presumed to be melanin is not a reliable guide, as other tumours may trap melanin granules in their framework. If fresh or frozen material is available a positive DOPA reaction is a most useful guide, but frequently it is necessary to process residual tissue for ultrastructural examination for melanosomes. The preservation of such samples is very variable and a definitive answer is not always possible.

Recent experimental developments in the use of immunocytochemical techniques to identify cells of melanocytic origin may in time prove a valuable aid to the diagnostic

Table 16.3 Features of value in differentiating between a benign melanocytic lesion and invasive malignant melanoma.

	Benign melanocytic naevus	Malignant melanoma
Upward migration of melanocytes through epidermis	Unusual	Common
Pattern of melanocytic activity within the basal layer of the epidermis	Concentrated in deeper parts of epidermal pegs	Tends to replace basal keratinocytes at all levels
Melanocytic cells in dermis	Evidence of maturation and neuroid features in deeper cells. Very few if any mitotic figures. Very little intracellular melanin	No obvious maturation. Mitoses often present. Fine melanin dusting in deeper cells
Dermal lymphoid infiltrate	Unusual except in Spitz naevi	Common in primary tumours
Symmetry of lateral margins of lesion	Usually symmetrical	Frequently asymmetrical

pathologist. Although many of these methods utilising monoclonal antibodies with selectivity but not total specificity for melanoma originally required fresh-frozen tissue, there are now three approaches which give positive results on formalin-fixed paraffin-processed material. These are the use of S–100 protein,[32] neurone-specific enolase[33] and the NKI/C–3 antibody.[34,35] While each of these techniques yields a small percentage of false positives, they could, if used together as 'melanoma antibody battery', help reduce the number of undiagnosed poorly differentiated tumours.

Epidermotropically metastatic melanoma[36]

In a small proportion of patients with metastatic melanoma the tumour cells appear to 'home in' on the dermo-epidermal junction area. Differentiating these lesions from multiple primary melanoma may be difficult. The shape of the lesion (Fig. 16.26) may help and also the absence of any definitive evidence of basal layer origin in the secondary lesion (Fig. 16.27).

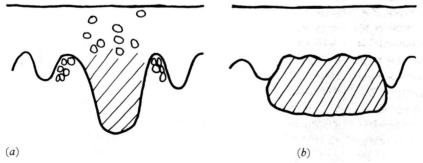

(a)   (b)

Fig. 16.26 Pattern of involvement of (a) a primary cutaneous melanoma compared with (b) an epidermotropically metastatic lesion.

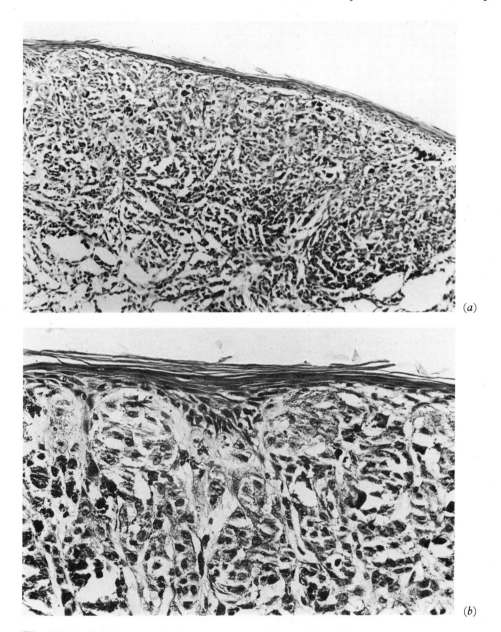

Fig. 16.27   Epidermotropically metastatic melanoma. (*b*) showing areas simulating 'junctional' activity adjacent to the basal layer.

Atypical melanocytic naevi and melanoma (dysplastic naevi, BK mole Syndrome, familial atypical mole–malignant melanoma syndrome)

Currently (1983) there is considerable interest in a syndrome which appears to exist both in familial and in sporadic forms consisting of multiple large melanocytic naevi and the develop-

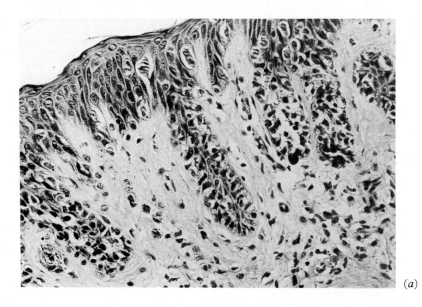

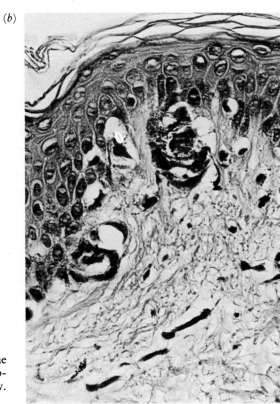

Fig. 16.28 Dysplastic naevus. (*a*) Note the large melanocytes and evidence of dermal papillary fibrosis. (*b*) Higher magnification view. Note the large, atypical melanocytes.

ment of multiple primary malignant melanomata. Naevi from these patients show increased numbers of atypical melanocytes in the basal layer, occasional suprabasilar melanocytes, a mild lymphocytic infiltrate in the papillary dermis, and in some cases thickening and coarsening of papillary dermis collagen[37, 38, 39] (Fig. 16.28).

In time the true incidence of this syndrome should be established. Once these patients are identified, careful and intensive clinical follow-up is essential to detect and excise early malignant melanoma.

The pathologist's report on a primary malignant melanoma[40]

The quantity of detail offered in such a report will clearly vary with the enthusiasm of the pathologist and the interest of the clinician. An absolute minimum is confirmation of the diagnosis and a statement as to the completeness or otherwise of excision (Fig. 16.29). The majority of surgeons would also nowadays welcome a measurement of tumour thickness. Other features are of interest but of doubtful practical value in managing the individual patient. Very extensive and detailed reports are of course required for prospective collaborative studies relating pathological features to prognosis and for therapeutic trials.

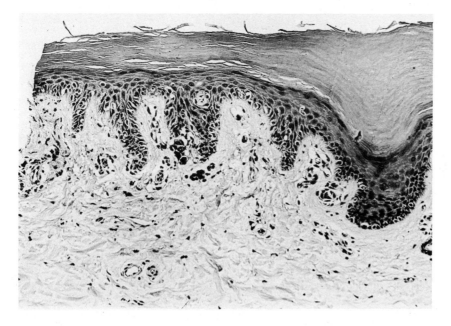

Fig. 16.29   Melanocarcinoma—excision margin. This section is from an excision margin through clinically normal skin of an apparently adequate excision of an early melanocarcinoma. It shows an increased number of melanocytes, with irregular hyperchromatic nuclei. Small areas of junctional activity can also be seen. Further excision of a 10-cm disc of skin revealed similar changes in the melanocyte population at the excision margins. Melanocarcinoma recurred 9 months later at the junction of the 'normal' skin and the graft used to repair the defect.

References

1. Szabo G. The number of melanocytes in human epidermis. *Br Med J* 1954; **1**: 1016–17.
2. Gilchrest BA, Blog FB, Szabo G. Effects of ageing and chronic sun exposure on melanocytes in human skin. *J Invest Dermatol* 1979; **73**: 141–3.
3. Toda K, Pathak MA, Parrish JA, Fitzpatrick TB. Alteration of racial differences in melanosome distribution in human epidermis after exposure to ultraviolet light. *Nature; New Biol* 1972; **236**: 143–5.
4. Stegmaier OC, Becker SW. Incidence of melanocytic naevi in young adults. *J Invest Dermatol* 1960; **34**: 125–9.
5. Kaplan EN. The risk of malignancy in large congenital naevi. *Plast Reconstr Surg* 1974; **53**: 421–4.
6. Okun MR, Bauman L. Malignant melanoma arising from an intradermal naevus. *Arch Dermatol* 1965; **92**: 69–72.
7. Okun MR, Di Mattia A, Thompson J, Pearson SH. Malignant melanoma developing from intradermal naevi. *Arch Dermatol* 1974; **110**: 599–601.
8. Benisch B, Peison B, Kannerstein M, Spivack J. Malignant melanoma originating from intradermal naevi. A clinicopathologic entity. *Arch Dermatol* 1980; **116**: 696–8.
9. Unna PG. Zu epithelalen abkemft der Naevuszellen. *Virchows Arch Pathol Anat* 1896; **143**: 224–42.
10. Kornberg R, Ackerman AB. 'Pseudomelanoma': recurrent melanocytic naevi following partial surgical removal. *Arch Dermatol* 1975; **111**: 1588–90.
11. Weedon D, Little JH. Spindle and epithelioid cell naevi in children and adults. *Cancer* 1977; **40**: 217–25.
12. Spitz S. Melanomas in childhood. *Am J Pathol* 1948; **24**: 591–609.
13. Reed RJ, Ichinose H, Clark WH, Mihm MC. Common and uncommon melanocytic naevi and borderline melanomas. *Semin Oncol* 1975; **2**: 119–47.
14. Frank SB, Cohen HJ. The halo naevus. *Arch Dermatol* 1964; **89**: 367–73.
15. Magnus K. Habits of sun exposure and risk of melanoma. *Cancer* 1981; **48**: 2329–35.
16. McGovern VJ, Shaw HM, Milton GW, Farago GA. Is malignant melanoma arising in Hutchinson's freckle a separate entity? *Histopathology* 1980; **4**: 235–42.
17. Clark WH, From L, Bernardino EA *et al*. The histogenesis and biological behavior or primary human malignant melanoma of the skin. *Cancer Res* 1969; **29**: 705–27.
18. Clark WH, Ainsworth AM, Bernardino EA *et al*. The developmental biology of primary human malignant melanomas. *Semin Oncol* 1975; **2**: 83–103.
19. Kühnl-Pedzoldt C. Superficial spreading melanoma: histological findings and problems of differentiation. *Arch Dermatol Forsch* 1974; **250**: 309–21.
20. Gromet MA, Epstein WL, Blois MS. The regressing thin malignant melanoma. A distinctive lesion with metastatic potential. *Cancer* 1978; **42**: 2282–92.
21. Krementz ET, Reed RJ, Coleman WP, Sutherland CM, Carter RD, Campbell M. Acral lentiginous melanoma. *Ann Surg* 1982; **195**: 632–45.
22. Feibleman CE, Stoll H, Maize JC. Melanomas of the palm, sole and nail bed. *Cancer* 1980; **46**: 2492–2504.
23. Patterson RH, Helwig EB. Subungual malignant melanoma. A clinico-pathologic study. *Cancer* 1980; **46**: 2074–87.
24. Conley J, Lattes R, Orr W. Desmoplastic malignant melanoma (a rare variant of spindle cell melanoma). *Cancer* 1971; **28**: 914–36.
25. Reed RJ, Leonard DD. Neurotropic melanoma. A variant of desmoplastic melanoma. *Am J Surg Pathol* 1979; **3**: 301–11.
26. Breslow A. Problems in the measurement of tumor thickness and level of invasion in cutaneous melanoma. *Hum Pathol* 1977; **8**: 1–2.
27. Balch CM, Murad TM, Soong S *et al*. A multifactorial analysis of melanoma. I. Prognostic histopathological features comparing Clark's and Breslow's staging methods. *Ann Surg* 1978; **188**: 732–42.
28. Prade M, Sancho-Garnier H, Cesarini JP, Cochran A. Difficulties encountered in the application of Clark classification and the Breslow thickness in cutaneous malignant melanoma. *Int J Cancer* 1980; **26**: 159–63.

29. Clemente C, Cascinelli N, Rilke F. Monomorphic cellular proliferation of malignant melanomas of the skin as a prognostic morphologic parameter. *Hum Pathol* 1981; **11**: 299–300.

30. Balch CM, Wilkerson JA, Murad TM, Soong SJ, Ingalls AL, Maddox WA. The prognostic significance of ulceration of cutaneous melanoma. *Cancer* 1980; **45**: 3012–17.

31. Schmoekel C, Braun-Falco O. The prognostic index in malignant melanoma. *Arch Dermatol* 1978; **114**: 871–3.

32. Cochran AJ, Wen E-R, Herschman HR, Gaynor RB. Detection of S-100 protein as an aid to the identification of melanocytic tumors. *Int J Cancer* 1982; **30**: 295–7.

33. Hageman Ph, Vennegoor C, van der Valk M, Landegent J, Jonker A, van der Mispel L. Reactions of monoclonal antibodies against human melanoma with different tissues and cell lines. In: Peeters H, ed. *Protides of the Biological Fluids*, vol. 89. Oxford: Pergamon Press, 1982; pp. 889–92.

34. Dhillon AP, Rode J. Patterns of staining for neurone specific enolase in benign and malignant melanocytic lesions of the skin. *Diagn Histopathol* 1982; **5**: 169–74.

35. MacKie RM, Campbell I, Turbitt ML. The use of the monoclonal antibody NKI C3 in the diagnosis of melanocytic lesions. *J Clin Pathol* in press.

36. Kornberg R, Harris M, Ackerman B. Epidermotropically metastatic malignant melanoma. *Arch Dermatol* 1978; **114**: 67–9.

37. Clark WH, Reimer RR, Greene M, Ainsworth AM, Mastrangelo MJ. The BK mole syndrome. *Arch Dermatol* 1978; **114**: 732–8.

38. Lynch HT, Fusaro RM, Pester J, Lynch JF. Familiar atypical multiple mole melanoma (FAMMM) syndrome: genetic heterogeneity and malignant melanoma. *Br J Cancer* 1980; **42**: 58–70.

39. Elder DE, Goldman LI, Goldman SC, Greene MV, Clark WH Jr. The dysplastic naevus syndrome. A phenotypic association of cutaneous melanoma. *Cancer* 1980; **46**: 1787–92.

40. McGovern VJ, Mihm MC, Bailly C *et al.* Classification of melanoma and its histological reporting. *Cancer* 1973; **32**: 1446–57.

17
Tumours of the Dermis

The mesenchymal lesions described in this chapter have been selected to include only those most likely to present initially to the dermatologist. Those sarcomata such as fibrosarcoma, liposarcoma and malignant fibrous histiocytoma which usually arise in deeper tissues and only involve the dermis at a late stage are not discussed.[1]

Tumour-like lesions of fibrous and elastic tissue

The term 'connective tissue naevus' embraces a group of rather uncommon, congenital, localised abnormalities of either the dermal collagen or elastic tissue. The changes vary from the overgrowth of collagen, as in the shagreen patches of tuberous sclerosis (p. 72), to the naevus elasticus with, paradoxically, its absence of elastic fibres and the juvenile elastoma with its localised increase.

Benign tumours of the skin producing collagen (*fibromas*) are probably rare. They are difficult to define and to distinguish from the end results of irritation or inflammation, while the so-called dermatofibroma is thought to be of histiocytic origin (see below).

Skin tag (so-called soft fibroma, fibroepithelial polyp)

These lesions consist of a vascularised core of loosely arranged collagen fibres covered by epidermis. In the neck and axillae they usually form small delicate filiform projections with overlying hyperplastic epithelium, while on the trunk and thighs a larger, pendulous, bag-like structure often containing fat is seen. Sometimes the formation of a skin tag is clearly related to chronic irritation.

Hypertrophic scars and keloids

Keloids sometimes develop following skin trauma such as surgery, ear-piercing, burns or tattooing or as a result of acne. They may merit excision, for, in contrast to hypertrophic scars, they are often painful, may extend beyond the original site of skin damage and do not disappear spontaneously. It would be helpful to the clinician if the pathologist could distinguish between the two conditions at an early stage, but this may be difficult or impossible because initially both consist of fibroblasts and collagen arranged in whorls and nodules and accompanied by abundant new capillaries. In hypertrophic scars the cellularity gradually decreases and eventually the collagen fibres lie parallel to the surface as in a normal scar. In true keloids, however, very thick, hyalinised eosinophilic strands of collagen remain ran-

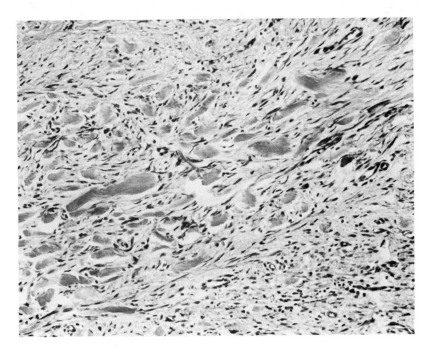

Fig. 17.1 Keloid. Strands of dense hyaline collagen are intermingled with plump spindle-shaped fibroblasts.

domly arranged and are associated with plump triangular fibroblasts similar to those seen following irradiation (Fig. 17.1).

Palmar fibromatosis (Dupuytren's contracture), plantar fibromatosis and knucklepads[2, 3]

In each of these self-limiting benign conditions, nodules which arise in fascia and sometimes extend into the dermis and adjacent fat may be sufficiently cellular to be mistaken for fibrosarcoma. Initially in all of these sites the normal fascia is expanded by, and imperceptibly merges with, highly cellular fasciculated fibroblastic foci which may contain numerous but normal mitoses. Some of these cells have been identified as myofibroblasts on electron microscopy. With time the nodules in palmar fibromatosis become less cellular and more collagenous, the proximal fascia stands out as a cord under the skin and the classic Dupuytren's contracture of the affected finger develops. The other hand is subsequently affected in about half the patients. There is more likely to be clinical concern over the less familiar, larger, tender and sometimes rapidly growing nodules in the plantar fascia (Fig. 17.2). These are not usually heavily collagenised and clinically there is seldom contracture of the toes. Brisk 'recurrence' as a result of field change may follow incomplete removal of the fascia. However, the presence of similar lesions in the other foot or in the palm or over the knuckles may be reassuring clinical evidence that the lesion is part of the Dupuytren diathesis.

Small, sessile, intradermal nodules of fibromatosis on the extensor surfaces of the fingers or toes of infants and children under 2 years old have a very high recurrence rate though an

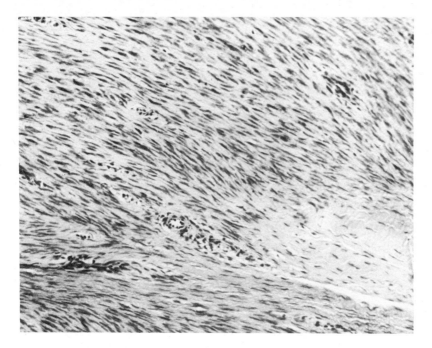

Fig. 17.2 Plantar fibromatosis. Delicate, elongated spindle cells with some mitoses but little pleomorphism gradually merge with the normal poorly cellular collagenous plantar fascia (lower right).

occasional one regresses spontaneously (infantile dermal fibromatosis, recurring digital fibrous tumours of childhood.[3b]) The fibroblasts contain, near to the nucleus, intracytoplasmic inclusion bodies which stain deep red with Masson's trichrome stain.

Another type of recurring fibromatosis found especially in the hands and feet of children and adolescents contains foci of calcification or chondroid differentiation; sometimes the surrounding fibroblasts are palisaded. The lesion may extend to involve fat, muscle and perineural tissue (so-called juvenile aponeurotic fibroma).[4] Musculoaponeurotic fibromatosis, as its name implies, arises in deeper tissue and is a more aggressive lesion.

Fasciitis (pseudosarcomatous or nodular fasciitis)[5]

This benign reactive lesion is important because it may readily be mistaken for a malignant tumour such as a fibro- or liposarcoma. Fasciitis may develop at any age and any site but the peak incidence is between 20 and 40 years, and the forearm is most often involved. Characteristically a tender subcutaneous nodule, seldom more than 2 cm in diameter, develops over a few weeks. Microscopically the lesion consists of spindle-shaped or triangular fibroblasts often haphazardly arranged in feathery, tissue-culture-like pattern in a loosely textured focally myxoid stroma (Fig. 17.3a). Foci of lymphocytes especially at the margins, scattered macrophages and mast cells and sometimes occasional multinucleated cells are seen. Capillary proliferation is prominent and may extend with the fibroblasts into surrounding fat, giving the lesion a saw-toothed margin or circumscribing fatty lobules (Fig. 17.3b). Occasionally small foci of osteoid, cartilage or ganglion-like cells form. Sometimes the fibroblasts are more closely packed in interconnecting bundles and the nodule is pseudoencapsulated.

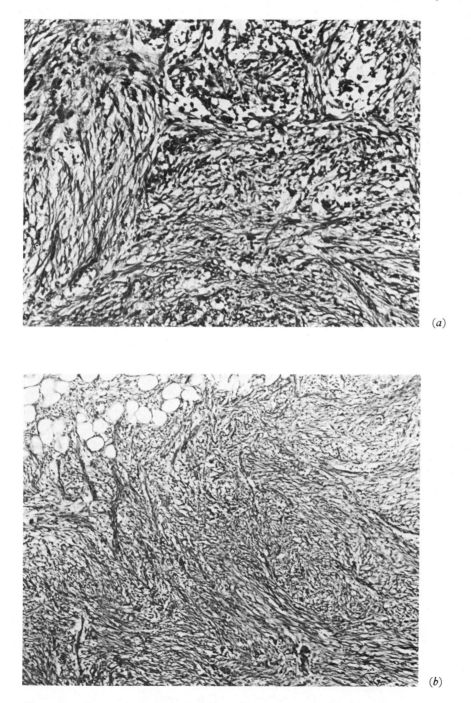

(a)

(b)

Fig. 17.3 Fasciitis. (*a*) Spindle-shaped fibroblasts are haphazardly arranged. There is a focus of myxoid change with some inflammatory cell infiltrate (upper right). (*b*) The feathery pattern of the fibroblasts is well seen. At the upper left corner the proliferating fibroblasts are extending into a fatty lobule and outgrowing capillaries are prominent, giving the lesion the suggestion of a 'saw-tooth' edge.

The cellularity, the mitotic activity (which may be as high as 1/high power field) and the infiltrative margins may suggest malignancy but follow-up shows that the lesion is unquestionably benign and some have regressed following incomplete excision. Recurrence is sufficiently unusual to warrant a review of the diagnosis.[6]

Focal mucinosis (cutaneous myxoma)

A single flesh-coloured and sometimes fluctuant nodule about 1 cm in diameter may be found on the face, trunk or limbs.[7] On microscopy the dermis is rich in mucopolysaccharides and there is a slight increase in plump fibroblasts. Similar nodules occur around the base of the nail, principally in the fingers, and at first have a similar microscopic appearance though later clefts may form and coalesce to give a mucin-filled cavity.

Tumours and tumour-like lesions perhaps of histiocytic origin

Dermatofibroma (nodular subepidermal fibrosis, histiocytoma cutis, benign or cutaneous fibrous histiocytoma, sclerosing haemangioma)

This is usually now regarded as a true neoplasm rather than as a reaction to some form of trauma such as an insect bite. The variety of names reflects the change in the predominant histological component as the lesion ages.

Dermatofibroma is found chiefly on the limbs, usually in adults, and presents as a firm, non-encapsulated nodule which is often reddish-brown clinically and yellow or tan on section. Occasionally, if the lesion contains telangiectatic blood vessels and there is much haemorrhage, it may appear black and be mistaken clinically for a melanoma.

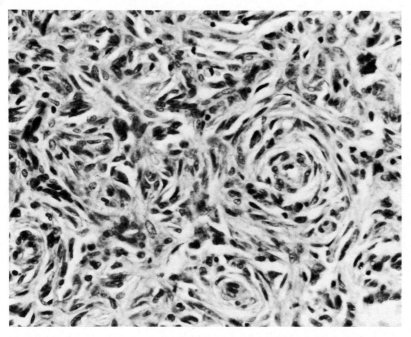

Fig. 17.4 Dermatofibroma. Capillaries are numerous and are surrounded by fibroblasts, collagen fibres and histiocytes. An occasional pale-staining foamy cell (xanthoma cell) is seen.

Histologically, dermatofibroma consists of a lenticular lesion in the mid dermis which merges imperceptibly with the adjacent dermal collagen. It is often separated from the epidermis by a band of collagen and there may be a collar of lymphocytes around its margin. The lesion is formed of histiocytes, fibroblasts with collagen fibres and a fine vascular meshwork (Fig. 17.4). In the early stages histiocytes predominate, and single or clusters of foamy cells with Touton-type giant cells are seen. Lipid is often in very fine droplets and its amount is likely to be underestimated unless frozen sections on fresh tissue are stained for fat. Haemosiderin-containing macrophages are often plentiful (Fig. 17.5) but may be absent. Spindle-shaped fibroblasts are scanty and the collagen is in fine strands forming a delicate meshwork.

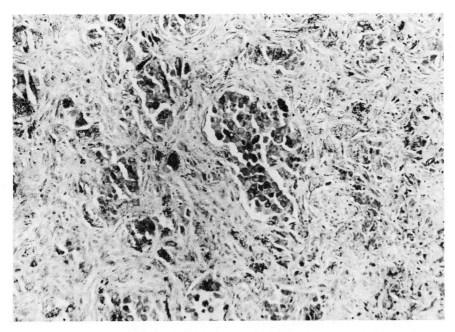

Fig. 17.5 Dermatofibroma. A number of histiocytes containing granules of haemosiderin are embedded in a fibrovascular stroma. Granules of haemosiderin can also be seen lying free.

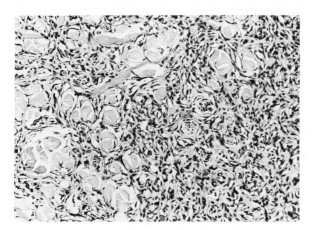

Fig. 17.6 Dermatofibroma. On the left, at the edge of the lesion, the normal collagen bundles of the dermis have been enveloped by curved fibroblasts and fibres. This appearance should not be mistaken for malignant infiltration.

As the lesion ages, the histiocytic component diminishes and the fibroblastic elements and collagen increase. If focal haemorrhages occur they provoke repair by the formation of vascular fibrous tissue and increase the amount of haemosiderin. At the lateral margins fibroblasts curve round and envelop the preformed collagen bundles of the dermis, simulating malignant infiltration (Fig. 17.6) while they may also extend on the deep surface into the fibrous septa of the subcutaneous fat. The increasing collagen usually forms intertwining, anastomosing bands rather than the storiform pattern characteristic of dermatofibrosarcoma protuberans (Fig. 17.7). Changes in the overlying epithelium occur in about half the dermatofibromata. These range from a simple acanthosis often with an increase in melanocytes, through a lesion indistinguishable from a basal cell papilloma to foci of pseudoepitheliomatous hyperplasia.

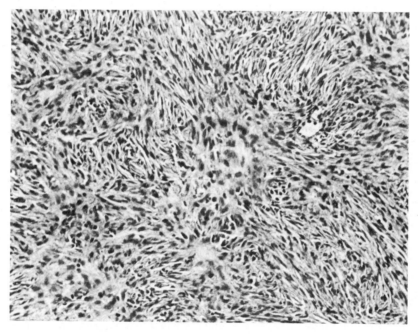

Fig. 17.7 Dermatofibrosarcoma protuberans. The plump spindle cells of the tumour radiate from a fibrous centre like spokes of a wheel, producing short bundles of cells and fibres—the so-called storiform pattern.

Dermatofibrosarcoma protuberans[8]

This tumour may start as a slowly growing, firm, indurated plaque in the dermis and then grow more rapidly to form several protuberant nodules. As there is often microscopic extension of tumour beyond the visible nodules there is a high risk of recurrence unless the lesion is widely excised. Metastases are extremely rare.

Microscopically the dermatofibrosarcoma consists of rather uniform plump spindle cells with infrequent mitotic figures. The centre of the tumour is cellular with little collagen but towards the margin the cellularity decreases and collagen increases to blend with the normal dermis. The spindle cells characteristically radiate from a fibrous centre to form a cartwheel or storiform pattern (Fig. 17.7). This storiform pattern is not usually a prominent feature in dermatofibroma, while in dermatofibrosarcoma haemosiderin, lipid-containing histiocytes and inflammatory cells are confined to areas of necrosis and the overlying epidermis is usually atrophic rather than hypertrophic. Myxoid foci may be striking, especially in recurrent tumours.

Atypical fibroxanthoma[9]

This lesion of uncertain origin has an alarming histological appearance which belies its behaviour. Most atypical fibroxanthomata are cured by local excision; only a few recur. Metastases, though occasionally reported, are very rare. The lesion presents as a firm solitary nodule or ulcer, chiefly on the sun-damaged skin of the face or neck of elderly patients. It may also develop at the site of previous irradiation or in younger patients in apparently normal skin of trunk or limbs. The commoner clinical diagnoses are of basal cell or squamous carcinoma or pyogenic granuloma. Microscopically atypical fibroxanthoma forms a fairly well circumscribed but unencapsulated expanding nodule surrounded by a collar of bowed pilosebaceous follicles and sometimes also by a zone of chronic inflammatory cells (Fig. 17.8a). Bizarre tumour cells with multipolar mitoses are mixed with spindle-shaped cells like fibroblasts and a random scattering of polyhedral histiocytic cells sometimes containing lipid (Fig. 17.8b), appearances similar to those of malignant fibrous histiocytoma. This

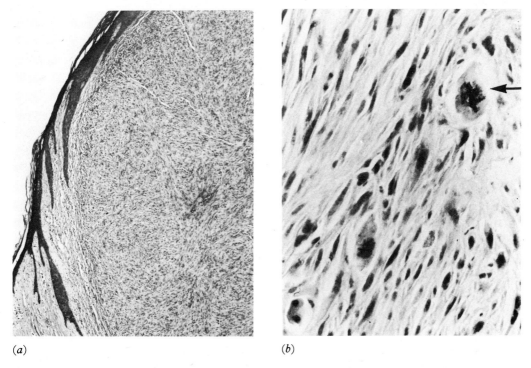

(a) (b)

Fig. 17.8 Atypical fibroxanthoma. This lesion arose on the chin of an elderly man who had received x-irradiation many years previously for sycosis barbae. (a) A well-circumscribed cellular nodule with some surrounding chronic inflammatory cell infiltrate has bowed the pilosebaceous units. (b) Histiocyte-like cells with prominent nucleoli are interspersed with bizarre giant cells. A multipolar mitotic figure is arrowed.

highly cellular nodule is often confined to the dermis; deep extension or widespread necrosis casts doubt on the diagnosis.

Tumours and tumour-like lesions of peripheral nerves[10]

Traumatic neuroma (amputation neuroma)

This may present as a tender, painful palpable nodule in the proximal end of a divided peripheral nerve. It is not a true tumour but results from reactive proliferation of Schwann cells and mesodermal elements which sprout from the cut end of the nerve. If the growing nerve fibres fail to make contact with the distal stump a tangled mass of sheathed axis cylinders embedded in collagenous scar tissue forms (Fig. 17.9).

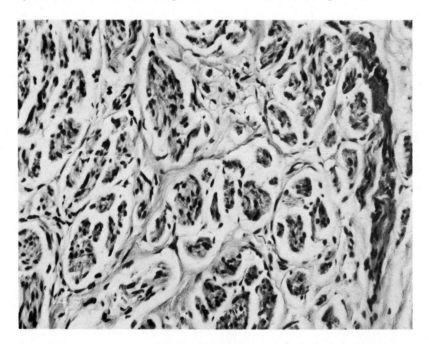

Fig. 17.9   Traumatic neuroma. Proliferated bundles of unorientated Schwann cells are surrounded by collagen strands. The accompanying nerve fibres are not identifiable in haematoxylin and eosin stained sections.

Digital neuroma (Morton's neuroma)

Digital neuroma is a localised painful swelling of a plantar nerve in the region of the metatarsal heads, often in the third cleft. There is marked concentric endo- and peri-neurial fibrosis with thickening and hyalinisation of endoneurial blood vessels. The frequent presence of fibrin and fat necrosis in the surrounding tissue suggests that the lesion is a reaction to repeated mild trauma.

Neurofibroma

Neurofibroma in the skin may occur as solitary or multiple soft pedunculated nodules sometimes with café au lait pigmentation of the overlying epidermis. Multiple nodules may be one of the manifestations of familial neurofibromatosis (von Recklinghausen's disease) which may also involve the dermis more diffusely, giving rise to thickened loose folds of redundant heavily pigmented skin.

Histologically the lesion is characterised by a diffuse proliferation of thickened cords of

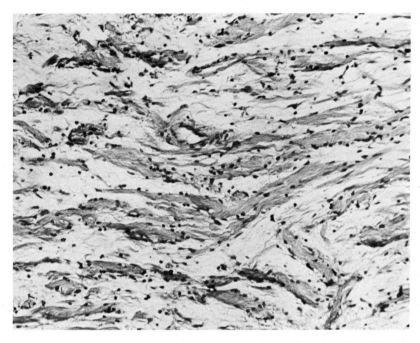

Fig. 17.10   Neurofibroma. Within a pale myxomatous stroma there are thickened cords of Schwann cells.

Schwann cells in a myxomatous stroma rich in mucopolysaccharides (Fig. 17.10) and containing scattered mast cells, fibroblasts and histiocytes. Streaming strands of wire-like reticulin may be seen, and neurites are diffusely scattered through the lesion. Occasionally poor facsimiles of Wagner–Meissner tactile corpuscles may be recognised.

Oedema and proliferation of Schwann cells within the perineurium give rise to thickening and tortuosity of nerves (plexiform neurofibroma) which is considered diagnostic of neuro-fibromatosis.

Neurofibrosarcoma (malignant Schwannoma)

Neurofibrosarcoma is diagnosed histologically on the basis of mitotic activity. It has been calculated to arise in about 4 per cent of patients over the age of 21 with neurofibromatosis,[11] and almost always affects large nerve trunks so that primary skin involvement is rare.

Schwannoma

Schwannoma—another form of benign peripheral nerve tumour—does not undergo malignant change and is rare in the skin. It forms an encapsulated tumour within the epineurial sheath so that, in contrast to the neurofibroma, the nerve fibres are spread out over its surface rather than incorporated in its substance. Histologically it consists of a mixture of compact

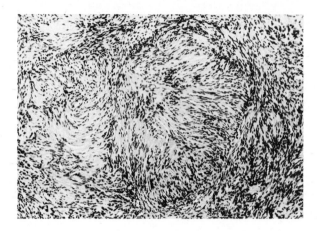

Fig. 17.11 Schwannoma. There is palisading of Schwann cell nuclei and the formation of an organoid structure (Verocay body).

masses of Schwann cells in fasciculi and cords along with loosely textured tissue rich in mucopolysaccharides. Characteristically, in some areas the Schwann cell nuclei are palisaded (Fig. 17.11) or assume an organoid appearance (Verocay body). Blood vessels are often filled with thrombus and surrounded by collars of hyalinised fibrous tissue. Mast cells are plentiful. In the absence of mitotic activity large, hyperchromatic and sometimes vacuolated Schwann cell nuclei should not be interpreted as evidence of malignancy. They are probably a degenerative phenomenon (ancient Schwannoma).

Tumours of smooth muscle

Benign smooth muscle tumours

Benign smooth muscle tumours are not particularly common in the skin and arise mainly from the arrectores pilorum muscles (leiomyoma; Fig. 17.12) and also from the media of the superficial veins (angioleiomyoma or vascular leiomyoma; Fig. 17.13). Those arising from the arrectores pilorum are usually multiple, small, tender and occasionally painful nodules arranged in lines or groups, often on the extensor surfaces of the limbs. Those arising from vein walls are more common in the subcutaneous tissue of the lower limbs, especially in women. They reach a larger size than the multiple lesions and are often extremely painful.

Both types of leiomyoma are composed of interlacing bundles of spindle cells with varying amounts of collagen between the bundles. In addition, the angioleiomyoma contains numerous thick-walled veins (Fig. 17.13). Helpful points in the sometimes difficult microscopic differentiation between smooth muscle and fibrous tissue tumours are that smooth muscle bundles are less curved, the cell nuclei longer and with blunt rather than pointed ends (see Fig. 17.12) while on cross-section the cytoplasm is faintly vacuolated. Further assistance in differentiation may be gained by using Van Gieson's stain or one of the

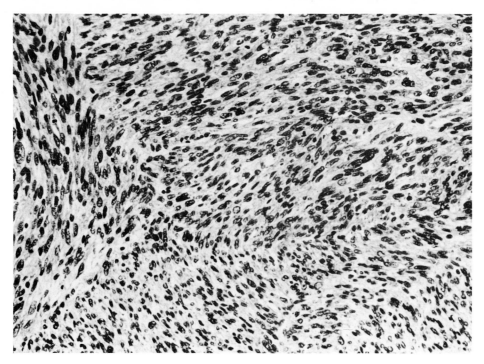

Fig. 17.12 Leiomyoma. The tumour is composed of long bundles of smooth muscle cells with elongated, blunt-ended nuclei. In this example there are a few collagen fibres.

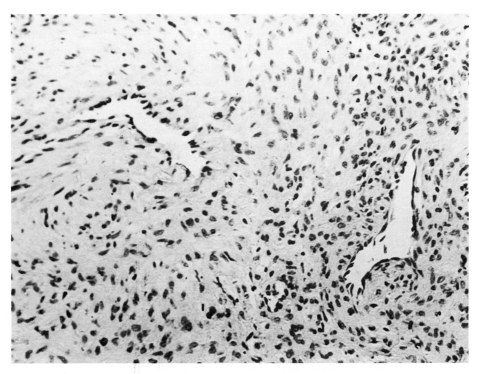

Fig. 17.13 Angioleiomyoma. Small veins are associated with bundles of smooth muscle. The tumour contains more collagen and is less cellular than that illustrated in Fig. 17.12.

modifications of Mallory's trichrome stain. Diagnostic intracytoplasmic myofibrils are most reliably demonstrated by electron microscopy though they may sometimes be recognised on light microscopy, especially using the phosphotungstic acid–haematoxylin stain. Nuclear palisading is occasionally found in leiomyomata as well as in Schwannomata.

Leiomyosarcoma[12]

The differentiation between leiomyoma and leiomyosarcoma may be difficult, and mitotic activity seems a more helpful guide than nuclear pleomorphism, for occasional large or multilobed nuclei may be seen in leiomyomata. Benign smooth muscle tumours seldom contain more than one mitotic figure per 50 high power fields (HPF) while there are usually more than 10/50 HPF in leiomyosarcomata.[13] Very occasionally an apparently benign tumour metastasises.

Leiomyosarcoma is rare in the skin. The prognosis depends more on site than on the microscopic appearances. Cutaneous tumours have an infiltrative pattern but, while they frequently recur, they are very unlikely to metastasise. In contrast, about a third of the more circumscribed, nodular and compressive subcutaneous leiomyosarcomata give rise to lung secondaries.[12]

Tumours and tumour-like lesions of blood and lymphatic vessels

While the term 'haemangioma' is used in this chapter many pathologists prefer to regard these lesions as vascular malformations or hamartomata (see p. 53 for definition) rather than as true tumours. Although the haemangiomata are divided for convenience into telangiectatic, superficial and deep lesions, in practice many are mixed having both a superficial capillary and a deeper cavernous component. The distinction between blood and lymphatic vessels is not always easy. Blood vessels may contain only eosinophilic fluid and some red blood cells may be found within lymphatic vessels; assessment must be made on the appearance of the whole lesion. The detection of factor-VIII-associated protein by the immunoperoxidase technique is a good marker for normal, hyperplastic and well-differentiated endothelial cells.

Flat haemangioma (portwine stain, naevus flammeus, naevus telangiectaticus)

The flat haemangioma is present at birth and usually involves the skin of the face, neck or thorax or, less frequently, of the limbs. The haemangioma grows slowly, in proportion to the patient, and does not regress. Occasionally it is associated with angiomatous malformations of the choroid and meninges or with varicosities and gigantism of a limb. Microscopically the lesion consists of large, dilated, thin-walled vessels lying haphazardly throughout the dermis (Fig. 17.14), and sometimes spreading more deeply in the subcutaneous tissue. These appearances probably represent permanent dilatation of pre-existing vessels rather than vascular proliferation.

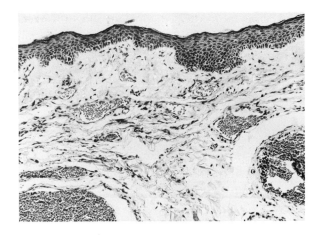

Fig. 17.14 Flat haemangioma (port-wine stain). Large, irregular, dilated capillaries lined by rather flattened endothelium are scattered through the dermis.

Immature haemangioma (capillary haemangioma, strawberry naevus, naevus vasculosus)

The immature haemangioma appears within the first two weeks of life and grows rapidly for a few months. It is a solitary, often lobular, raised tumour which becomes crimson and tense when the infant cries. It is composed of sharply circumscribed nodules of capillaries. Often

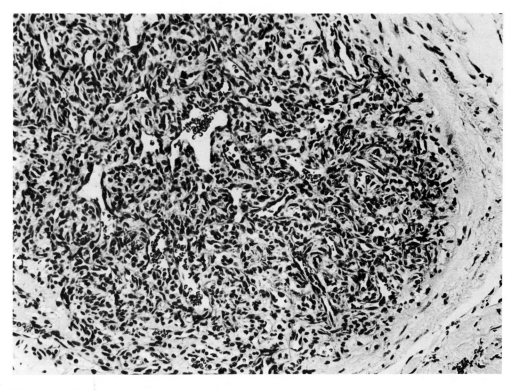

Fig. 17.15 Immature haemangioma (strawberry naevus). This shows a sharply circumscribed nodule of proliferated capillary vessels. In the centre there are a few patent vessels containing red cells but in many the lumen is obliterated by swollen endothelial cells.

in the early stages the endothelium is so swollen that blood-filled lumina are not apparent, the cells forming solid cords and masses (Fig. 17.15). Mitoses may be frequent and the lesion at this stage is sometimes called a benign haemangioendothelioma. As it matures, the endothelial cells shrink and the lumina become patent. Eventually spontaneous involution with fibrosis begins in the centre of the lesion, which gradually becomes flaccid, wrinkled and bluish and after some years may disappear completely.

Mature haemangioma (cavernous angioma)

The mature haemangioma appears as a deeper seated, purplish nodular mass and causes serious cosmetic problems. The overlying skin may be normal or the site of a capillary

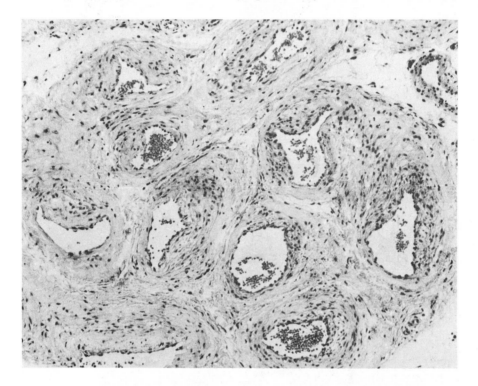

Fig. 17.16   Mature haemangioma (cavernous haemangioma). Numerous thick-walled vessels, lined by plump endothelium and containing red cells, are embedded in a fibrous stroma.

haemangioma. Histologically, cavernous angioma is composed of vascular spaces, probably of venous origin, lined by a single layer of endothelial cells and surrounded by a fibrous wall which may be thickened by adventitial cell proliferation (Fig. 17.16). Multiple cavernous haemangiomata often with radiological evidence of calcification may be seen in patients with multiple enchondromatosis (Maffucci's syndrome).

Pyogenic granuloma (granuloma pyogenicum, lobular capillary haemangioma)

This lesion is a rapidly growing, painless, red, bleeding, pedunculated nodule usually found on the oral mucosa, face or fingers. Whether these lesions represent an exuberant overgrowth

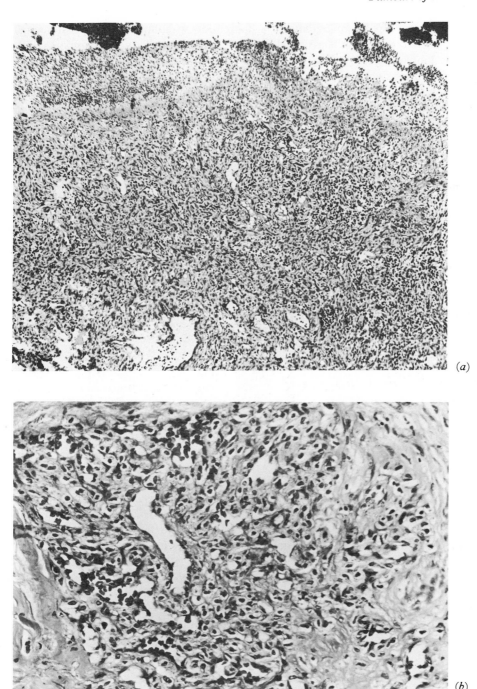

(a)

(b)

Fig. 17.17 Pyogenic granuloma. (*a*) The epidermis has ulcerated and is replaced by an area of serous crusting and fibrinoid necrosis. Beneath this, numerous capillaries are embedded in an oedematous fibrous stroma containing scattered inflammatory cells. (*b*) In the depths of the lesion a compact capillary lobule is seen surrounded by fibrous tissue devoid of any inflammatory infiltrate.

of a pre-existing capillary haemangioma is a matter for speculation. Some histological evidence suggests that the lesion is essentially a pedunculated capillary haemangioma with a characteristic lobular pattern[14] (Fig. 17.17). This is most easily recognised in its deeper part where the picture is not complicated by the oedema and inflammation associated with chronic irritation or actual ulceration of the overlying squamous epithelium. Rapid growth, a tendency to local recurrence, sometimes as multiple satellites or deep-seated nodules, and the presence histologically of mitotic activity should not be interpreted as evidence of malignancy.

Angiokeratoma

The variant of angioma which is associated with hyperkeratosis of the overlying epidermis is known as angiokeratoma (Fig. 17.18). Two clinical varieties of this lesion are recognised. They have similar appearances, consisting of dilatation and engorgement of the capillaries in the dermal papillae and a reactive acanthosis and hyperkeratosis of the epidermis. The

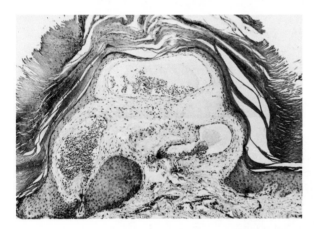

Fig. 17.18 Angiokeratoma (Mibelli type). There is dense laminated hyperkeratosis and some parakeratosis of the epidermis overlying several greatly dilated capillaries in the papillary dermis. The diffuse type (Fabry) shows a similar appearance in haematoxylin and eosin stained sections.

localised (Mibelli) type of angiokeratoma occurs on the fingers, toes and the scrotum (Fordyce) as localised patches and has no systemic component. A *diffuse* (Fabry) type, which is inherited as a sex-linked recessive, occurs over a wider area of the body and is the cutaneous manifestation of a systemic disorder in which di- and triglycosylceramides are deposited in the smooth muscle coats of the arterioles of the kidneys, heart and skin as a result of deficiency of the enzymes alpha- or beta-galactosidase. If the condition is suspected, electron microscopy or frozen sections stained with Sudan black or Nile Blue Sulphate will reveal the lipid droplets in the media of the cutaneous arterioles. The renal and cardiac complications of this vascular deposition are more important than the skin lesions.

Glomangioma

The glomangioma is not a true vascular tumour. It is derived from the neuromyoarterial glomus which is part of the arteriovenous shunt mechanism. The normal glomus has a temperature-regulating function and consists of a neuromuscular vascular channel (Fig. 17.19), known as the Sucquet–Hoyer canal, which runs between small arterioles and venules. Neoplastic proliferation of this structure therefore involves varying proportions of vascular, muscular and neural elements.

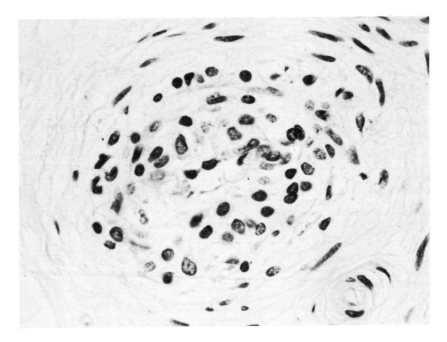

Fig. 17.19 Normal glomus (Sucquet–Hoyer canal). This typical glomus from a finger consists of a central vascular channel surrounded by a thick layer of epithelial-looking neuromuscular glomus cells.

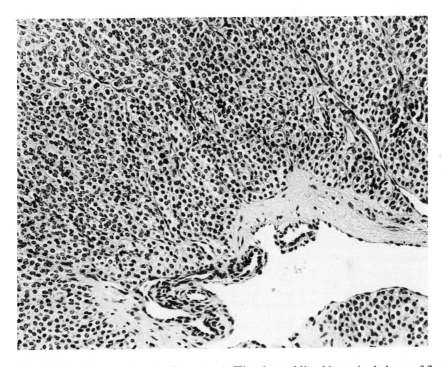

Fig. 17.20 Glomangioma (solitary type). The channel lined by a single layer of flattened epithelium is the lumen of a Sucquet–Hoyer canal. It is surrounded by a mass of spherical cells with sharply defined cell borders and central oval or round vesicular nuclei (glomus cells).

Clinically there are two types of glomus tumour. The solitary type, which may occur anywhere in the skin or occasionally in deeper soft tissues, is found most often on the fingers especially under the nails. It gives rise to spontaneous paroxysms of pain and may be misdiagnosed as an eccrine spiradenoma. A small pinkish nodule may be seen in the nailbed or fingertip, sometimes eroding the terminal phalanx, but often no lesion is visible to the naked eye and the diagnosis depends on microscopic examination of the excised painful area of skin. Multiple glomangiomata are less common; they present clinically as more obvious raised vascular lesions, often on the limbs, and are rarely painful.

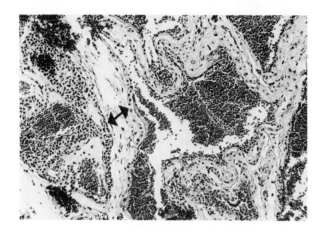

Fig. 17.21 Glomangioma (multiple type). This lesion bears a superficial resemblance to a mature (cavernous) haemangioma but the walls of the vascular channels are surrounded by one or two layers of typical glomus cells (arrowed).

Microscopically the solitary lesion consists of a sharply circumscribed mass of cells with pale faintly eosinophilic cytoplasm, sharply defined cell borders and a round central vesicular nucleus (Fig. 17.20). The pericellular reticulin pattern contrasts with the 'epithelial' appearance of the cells. Non-medullated nerve fibres may be demonstrated within the tumour, while the perivascular arrangement of the glomus cells around ovoid and slit-like endothelium-lined channels is usually best seen at the margins of the lesion. The histology of the multiple glomangioma closely resembles that of a cavernous haemangioma where the vessels are surrounded by one or several layers of glomus cells (Fig. 17.21) which may be so sparse as to be missed on a cursory examination.

Haemangiopericytoma

Haemangiopericytoma is a rare tumour derived from the pericytes of Zimmermann. It usually presents as a single, painless, well-circumscribed nodular mass, which is much more often situated in deep than in subcutaneous tissue.[15]

Histologically, haemangiopericytoma is composed of sinusoidal spaces and capillaries lined by flattened endothelium and surrounded by tightly packed, haphazardly arranged oval and spindle cells. Reticulin stains show that, in addition to a pericellular meshwork, a cuff of reticulin separates the tumour cells from the endothelium-lined spaces. This is helpful in differentiating the tumour from a haemangioendothelioma (see below). The lack of fasciculated pattern of the spindle cells in true haemangiopericytoma aids in its differential diagnosis from a number of tumours such as those of synovial, smooth muscle or neural origin which sometimes contain areas with a richly vascular pericytomatous pattern.

In about 20 per cent of tumours increased cellularity, a high mitotic rate, necrosis, haemorrhage and especially local recurrence are associated with metastatic spread.

Infantile or congenital haemangiopericytoma is a benign condition in spite of foci of necrosis and a worrying mitotic rate.

Haemangioendothelioma

The term 'haemangioendothelioma' is applied by some authors to any vascular lesion such as an immature (capillary) haemangioma in which vascular endothelium has proliferated to form solid cords or new capillaries. While this may be correct from an etymological point of view, by common usage the term is more often applied to a highly malignant tumour of vascular endothelium—perhaps, to avoid confusion, best called an angiosarcoma.

Angiosarcoma (malignant haemangioendothelioma, angioplastic reticulosarcoma)[16, 17, 18]

Apart from a few examples arising in irradiated skin, cutaneous angiosarcoma is almost exclusively a tumour of the face or scalp in patients between 60 and 80 years old. The tumour appears as one or more purplish plaques or nodules which usually grow slowly and bleed easily, sometimes forming apparent 'blood blisters' (Fig. 17.22a). Angiosarcoma tends to spread extensively both superficially and in depth, recurs persistently and in many patients metastasises to cervical lymph nodes and lungs. Sometimes lymph node involvement is evident when the patient first presents.

Microscopically the tumour involves the dermis and may spread to subcutaneous tissues. The most distinctive pattern is of an intricate network of dilated channels lined by atypical endothelial cells (Fig. 17.22b) which use the dermal collagen fibres as a scaffolding for their growth. More solid areas may be spindle celled and mimic Kaposi's sarcoma or form undifferentiated cell masses simulating metastatic carcinoma or melanoma. Reticulin stains may be helpful in drawing attention to the vascular pattern in the more solid areas while at the periphery of lesions, well beyond their macroscopic extent, dilated channels may contain buds of endothelial cells. It is uncertain whether the vascular channels in angiosarcoma are of lymphatic or blood vessel origin. The lesion described is grossly and microscopically identical to the so-called lymphangiosarcoma arising in lymphoedematous limbs, usually in the arm many years after mastectomy (Fig. 17.22a).

The diagnosis of cutaneous angiosarcoma should be made with caution in younger patients and in sites other than the head and neck. Occasionally the actively growing immature capillary haemangioma of infants (benign haemangioendothelioma) may be mistaken for a malignant tumour. Another source of confusion is so-called *intravascular papillary endothelial hyperplasia* (vegetant intravascular haemangioendothelioma).[19]

This condition simply represents one form of organisation of thrombus where, following partial retraction from the vessel wall, cellular invasion breaks up the thrombus into small ovoid fragments or papillary tufts covered by plump but not pleomorphic endothelial cells (Fig. 17.23). The process may be seen within leg veins or involving all or part of vascular tumours or malformations in the skin or deeper tissues. This reactive process is always intravascular, and usually remaining thrombus is still identifiable.

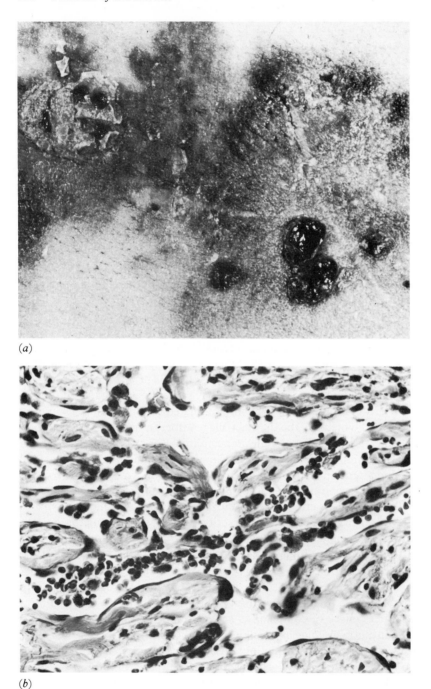

(a)

(b)

Fig. 17.22 (*a*) Lymphangiosarcoma in a lymphoedematous limb. The tumour presents as a dark purple bruise-like discoloration of the skin with 'blood blisters' and more solid raised nodules. The gross appearances are similar in haemangiosarcoma. (*b*) Angiosarcoma of scalp in a 74-year-old man. The tumour presented as a group of haemorrhagic skin nodules. Atypical, pleomorphic endothelial cells cover strands of dermal collagen. (Section by courtesy of Dr F.M. McGregor.)

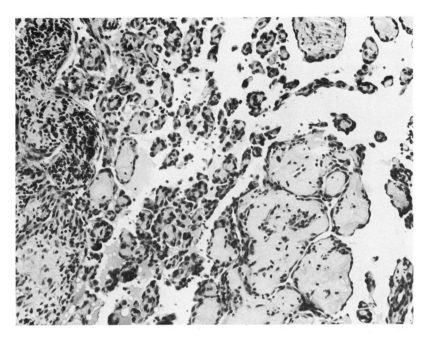

Fig. 17.23 Intravascular papillary endothelial hyperplasia. Thrombus within the lumen of a cavernous haemangioma is undergoing organisation. Papillary tufts are covered by plump endothelial cells. Clumps of pale, inspissated fibrin are still recognisable (especially lower right). (See p. 337)

Lymphangioma[20]

Lymphangioma may involve any part of the skin but the most common sites are the neck, axillae, chest, buttocks and thighs.

Two main types are described. The *superficial lymphangioma circumscriptum* may be congenital or acquired; more than half appear in the first 5 years of life. The lesion presents as a scattering or group of small vesicles, graphically described as like frog-spawn and involving one or several areas of skin. Microscopy reveals within the papillary layer of the dermis cystic spaces which bulge above the skin surface and may be mistaken for intradermal vesicles (Fig. 17.24). They are lined by flattened endothelial cells and contain coagulated lymph often with some red blood cells. Sometimes the overlying epidermis is papillomatous and hyperkeratotic. Histologically indistinguishable lesions resulting from ectasia of pre-existing lymphatics may follow lymphatic obstruction after surgery or radiotherapy. A number of the superficial lymphangiomata recur and this may be associated with communicating muscular-walled lymphatic cisterns deep in the subcutaneous tissue.[21]

Cavernous lymphangioma is a more deeply seated sponge-like lesion consisting of dilated lymphatic vessels which ramify in the deeper dermis and subcutaneous fat, sometimes destroying underlying muscle. The walls may be surrounded by delicate myxoid stroma, by denser collagen or by smooth muscle bundles. Lymphoid aggregates are sometimes conspicuous in the stroma. Histologically these lesions are similar to the clinically identified cystic hygromata of infants occurring as large fluid-filled cystic masses in the neck, axillae or groins. Recurrence occurs in about a quarter of lymphangiomata, more often in the deep than in the superficial lesions and perhaps associated with the opening up and extension of pre-existing

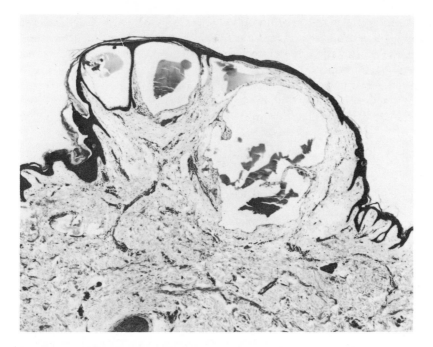

Fig. 17.24   Superficial lymphangioma. Thin-walled cystic lymphatic spaces within the papillary dermis contain a little lymph. One space appears to be completely surrounded by epidermis.

lymphatic channels. Although cystic hygromata may extend widely, malignant change has not been reported in surgically treated lymphangiomata.

Kaposi's idiopathic haemorrhagic sarcoma[22]

In parts of Africa Kaposi's sarcoma accounts for almost 10 per cent of malignant tumours. The onset is often in childhood or young adult life and the patient frequently presents with a single or a crop of purplish macules, plaques or nodules on the legs. These may coalesce and ulcerate. The development of more proximal lesions in skin or deeper tissues may be accompanied by partial regression of older lesions. The disease tends to run an aggressive course, sometimes with later visceral involvement. About 10 per cent of African patients suffer from a rapidly fatal lymphadenopathic form where extensive lymph node or visceral involvement may occur in the absence of, or precede the development of, a few scattered skin lesions.

Until recently Kaposi's sarcoma was rare in Europe and North America where it mostly affected elderly Jewish or Italian men and was mainly confined to the skin and subcutaneous tissue. In contrast to the African form, the disease in this group of patients runs a protracted course, occasionally with spontaneous remission and is rarely fatal though there is a 20-fold increased risk of developing a second primary lymphoreticular malignancy.

Immunosuppression predisposes to Kaposi's sarcoma and a few patients have developed the tumour following renal transplantation. However, recently in several of the big cities in the USA an alarming number of cases of the more aggressive, frequently fatal forms of Kaposi's sarcoma have been reported chiefly in young homosexual males with depression of their cell-mediated immunity. The acquired immunodeficiency syndrome (AIDS) has also affected other groups such as drug abusers and a few haemophiliacs. Most reported cases could be explained by the transmission of an infective agent (as yet unidentified), by sexual contact, or by blood or blood products.[23]

Biopsy of an early cutaneous lesion of Kaposi's sarcoma may show only vascular granulation tissue in the dermis, the diagnosis being made in retrospect (Fig. 17.25). As the lesion progresses the capillary endothelium becomes prominent and projects into the lumen of the

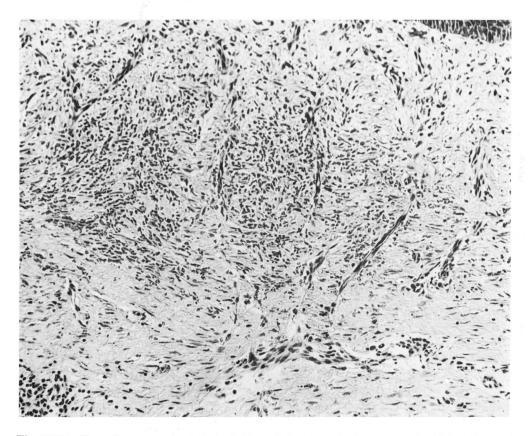

Fig. 17.25 Kaposi's sarcoma (early lesion). Granulation tissue in the upper and mid-dermis contains many new capillary vessels lined by prominent endothelial cells with hyperchromatic nuclei. The biopsy was from a solitary 'blood blister' on the dorsum of the foot of a middle-aged woman. There was no history of trauma. Nine months later multiple lesions developed on the feet and legs.

vessel. The surrounding fibroblasts enlarge, with some nuclear hyperchromatism and an occasional mitotic figure. Small areas of haemorrhage, perivascular infiltrates of plasma cells, lymphocytes and histiocytes, some containing haemosiderin, appear. There may be increased collagenisation of the dermis. While these changes are still within the bounds of a reactive process the exuberance of the capillary endothelium and pericapillary fibroblasts and the prominence of haemorrhage and haemosiderin should arouse suspicion. The appearance of ulcerated nodules may mimic pyogenic granuloma. The presence in Kaposi's sarcoma of a neoplastic fibroblastic element in the deeper tissue, of surrounding haemosiderin and of

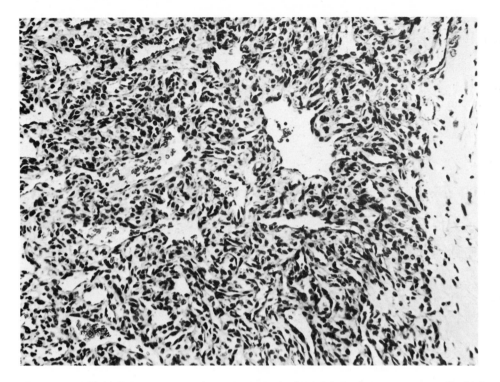

Fig. 17.26 Kaposi's sarcoma (angiosarcoma type). A number of spaces, some of which contain erythrocytes, are lined by prominent endothelium with hyperchromatic nuclei. Between these vascular channels there are solid areas of aberrant endothelial cells showing considerable variation in nuclear size and chromatin content. (Section, from the skin of an African child, by courtesy of Dr A.D. Bremner, Glasgow).

clusters of intracellular eosinophilic hyalin bodies well seen in phloxine-tartrazine stained sections help in the differential diagnosis.

In fully developed lesions, neoplastic vascular (Fig. 17.26) or fibroblastic elements (Fig. 17.27) may predominate in different parts of the same tumour. The differentiation from fibrosarcoma is best made where the spindle cells are seen in cross-section, when delicate vascular channels containing red blood cells may be made out lying between the cells and giving the tissue a sieve-like appearance. The vascular component varies from numerous endothelium-lined spaces to frank angiosarcoma with solid areas of aberrant endothelium. Visceral lesions have a similar spectrum of histological changes.

Tumours of adipose tissue

Lipoma

Lipomata are found more often in the subcutaneous than in the deeper tissues, and in this site they are well circumscribed and often encapsulated. They consist of mature adipose tissue broken up by fibrous trabeculae which are usually delicate but occasionally consist of broad bundles of dense collagen (so-called fibrolipoma). Foci of myxoid change, of necrosis, calcification or infarction may be seen.

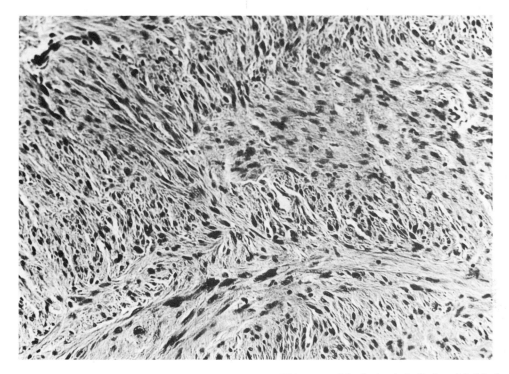

Fig. 17.27   Kaposi's sarcoma (fibrosarcoma type). This part of the lesion is indistinguishable from a fibrosarcoma. Bundles of aberrant fibroblasts, with nuclei of varying size and hyperchromasia, run in different directions. The section is from the periphery of a lesion of arm of an elderly central European. The central part of the lesion was angiosarcomatous and similar to Fig. 17.26. (See p. 342)

Angiolipoma

Angiolipoma usually presents in adolescents and young adults as single or multiple well-circumscribed, painful, small subcutaneous nodules especially in the arms and trunk. They consist of lipomata with a marked capillary component often most striking in, or sometimes confined to, the margin of the nodule. Hyaline microthrombi may be seen in some vessels. Recurrence is rare.

Spindle cell lipoma[24] and pleomorphic lipoma[25]

These are two well-circumscribed benign tumours which may readily be mistaken histologically for liposarcomata. They each occur most often in middle-aged and elderly men in the posterior part of the neck, the shoulder and the back. Occasionally a small area of spindle cell lipoma may be included within a pleomorphic lipoma. Both tumours contain mature lipocytes with a rather mucinous background, a scattering of mast cells and few if any mitotic figures. In the spindle cell lipoma randomly arranged bundles of collagen are associated with uniform fibroblast-like spindle cells (Fig. 17.28). The amount of spindle cells and collagen may be small or so great that the lipomatous component is overlooked. Usually the tumours are not very vascular but a few contain dilated branching sinusoids resembling a lymphangioma.

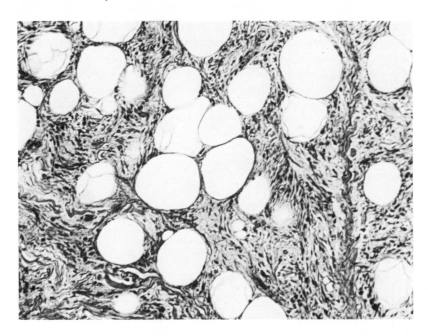

Fig. 17.28   Spindle cell lipoma. The fat cells are separated by randomly arranged corrugated strands of hyaline collagen and by rather uniform spindle cells. Blood vessels are scanty and mitotic figures are absent.

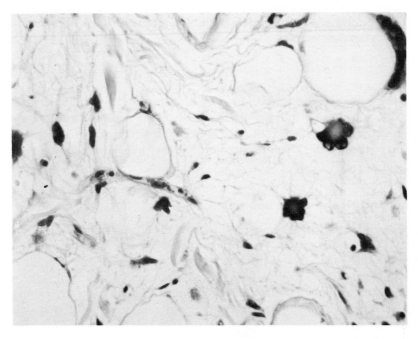

Fig. 17.29   Pleomorphic lipoma. Between the variably sized fat cells there are strands of collagen, spindle cells and multinucleated giant cells. In most of the giant cells the nuclei ring the margin of the cell.

The striking feature of the pleomorphic lipoma is the bizarre multinucleated giant cells often associated with strands of collagen. The nuclei are at the periphery of the giant cell and may overlap each other like flower petals (floret pattern) (Fig. 17.29). Lipocytes vary in size with some nuclear atypia, while an occasional vacuolated lipoblast-like cell may be seen.

In spite of the rather alarming features in both types of tumour, recurrence is unusual.

Tumours and tumour-like lesions of uncertain histogenesis

Granular cell tumour (granular cell myoblastoma)

Granular cell tumour is an uncommon but important benign lesion which occurs in many sites, including the skin and mucous membranes. There is still debate as to whether it originates from muscle, as its original name of myoblastoma suggests, or, more probably, from Schwann cells of the nerve sheath. Histologically the lesion is characterised by packets of large, polyhedral cells with acidophilic granular cytoplasm and small, round, darkly staining nuclei (Fig. 17.30). These collections occupy the dermis and extend to the under-surface of the epidermis. The intracellular granules may be overlooked in haematoxylin and eosin preparations but are made obvious by the use of one of the modifications of Mallory's trichrome stain. Electron microscopy shows that they consist of lysosomes.

A constant feature of these lesions is the pseudoepitheliomatous hyperplasia of the overlying epidermis (Fig. 17.31), which may be so striking as to be interpreted as infiltrating

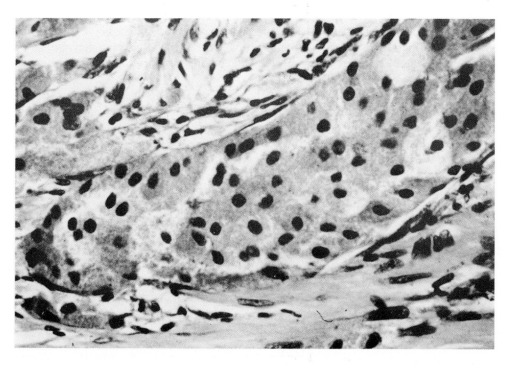

Fig. 17.30 Granular cell tumour (granular cell myoblastoma). In this strand of polyhedral cells the granular nature of the cytoplasm and the small darkly staining nuclei can be seen. (Masson's trichrome).

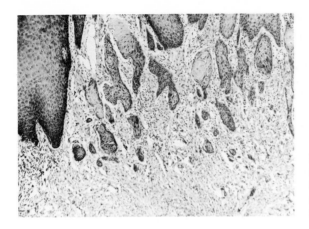

Fig. 17.31   Granular cell tumour (granular cell myoblastoma). There is marked pseudo-epitheliomatous hyperplasia of the epi-dermis overlying the clumps of granular cells in the dermis.

squamous carcinoma. In the oral cavity especially, from where biopsies are often small and badly orientated, it is only too easy to make this mistake. It is thus of paramount importance to recognise the granular cell tumour underneath the hyperplastic epithelium.

Epithelioid sarcoma[26, 27]

Attention is drawn to this relatively uncommon sarcoma, for it has often been misdiagnosed both clinically and microscopically as a necrotising granuloma or as primary or metastatic carcinoma. Although the tumour may be deep seated and ill-defined it more often presents as slowly growing, woody-hard subcutaneous lumps, as ulcerated skin nodules or occasion-ally as an annular plaque. The lesion is usually painful and tender. If a nerve is involved there may be numbness, sensory changes and muscle wasting. The sarcoma may appear at any age though predominantly in young adults, and the finger, palm, forearm and shin are the most common sites.

Microscopically the tumour is commonly nodular or lobulated, sometimes forming ribbon-like festoons of cells. Central degeneration within the tumour masses is characteristic (Fig. 17.32*a*) but may be absent at the first excision. Where there is a marked desmoplastic reaction the tumour cells may lie in cords between dense collagen strands mimicking epithelial infiltration (Fig. 17.32*b*). The tumour cells are rounded, polygonal or spindle shaped with eosinophilic cytoplasm, little nuclear pleomorphism and sometimes few mitoses. Lymphocytes may be prominent at the margin of the tumour. Local excision is usually followed by recurrence, often more proximally along tendons or fascial planes, and although the course may be protracted more than half the patients die with metastases to lymph nodes, lungs and skin. Tumour infiltration of blood vessel walls is usually followed by metastases.[27]

Clear cell sarcoma[28]

Although this rare sarcoma arises primarily in tendons or aponeuroses of the limbs, it may involve the dermis and present difficulty in differential diagnosis from metastatic malignant melanoma (Fig. 17.33*b*) especially in a minority where intracellular melanin is present.[29]

Microscopically, clear cell sarcoma consists of compact nests of fusiform cells with pale or finely granular eosinophilic cytoplasm and small round nuclei, each with a very prominent basophilic nucleolus (Fig. 17.33*a*). Reticulin stains are helpful in drawing attention to the

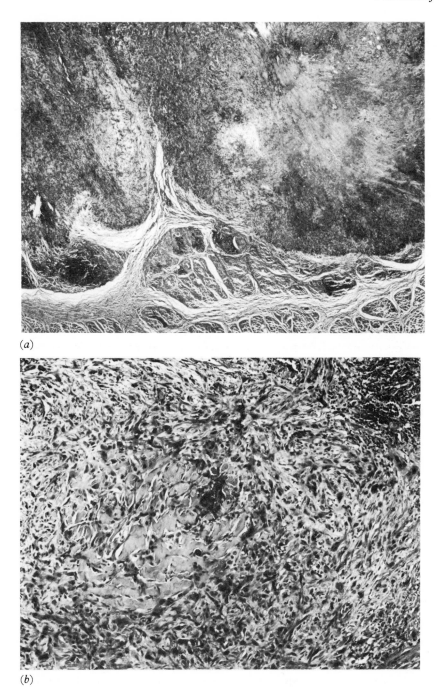

(a)

(b)

Fig. 17.32 Epithelioid sarcoma. (*a*) This cellular tumour shows a multinodular pattern with extensive central necrosis. (*b*) A hyaline collagenised area of necrosis is seen on the left, and surrounding this cords of tumour cells extend into the fibrous tissue giving the false impression of an infiltrating carcinoma. On the right, part of the inflammatory cell infiltrate at the margin of the nodule is recognisable.

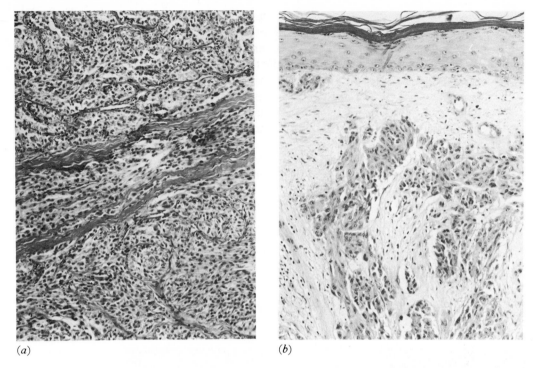

(a) (b)

Fig. 17.33 Clear cell sarcoma. (*a*) Packets of pale fusiform cells are splitting up the dense collagen strands of fascia. (*b*) The packeted cells have a less clear cytoplasm than in (*a*) and the nucleoli are prominent. The resemblance to malignant melanoma is striking.

packeted pattern. Benign-looking giant cells with a peripheral wreath of nuclei are sometimes seen and mitoses are usually scanty. Intra- and extra-cellular iron pigment is frequently present, and some tumours contain intracellular glycogen. Most tumours recur, usually as a nodule at the original site, but later there may be more diffuse extension along tendons or fascia and eventually more than half metastasise to lymph nodes and lung. The recurrences often have a less characteristic microscopic pattern with loss of cellular cohesion and increased pleomorphism.

Localised nodular synovitis (giant cell tumour, fibrous histiocytoma or xanthofibroma of tendon sheath, benign synovioma)

Many pathologists regard this lesion as reactive rather than neoplastic, though the stimulus to its formation remains obscure. More than 90 per cent of lesions occur in the fingers, chiefly in middle-aged women. Localised nodular synovitis presents as a slowly growing painless subcutaneous lump; occasionally more than one nodule develops in the same or in different fingers. On naked eye examination the creamy white nodules characteristically contain yellow or tan foci; they are multilobed, sometimes with small extensions alongside the main mass. Adjacent bone may be eroded. Nodules on the flexor surface of the finger are often associated with local villous involvement of the flexor sheath while those on the extensor surface may arise from the adjacent interphalangeal joint. The multilobed pattern and the sometimes unsuspected origin from joint or tendon sheath explains the 10–20 per cent recurrence following surgical excision. Metastases are not seen.

Microscopically the lesions consist of osteoclast-like multinucleated giant cells, histiocytes which are sometimes pale and foamy due to intracellular lipid (xanthoma cells), intra- and extracellular haemosiderin, and strands of collagen (Fig. 17.34). The proportion of these components varies from one lesion to another and within different lobules of the same lesion. Dense, branching strands of hyalinised collagen are often a striking feature. When the nodules have a sponge-like pattern a mistaken diagnosis of synovial sarcoma may be entertained. However, the clefts are lined by histiocytes and not by pseudoepithelial cells.

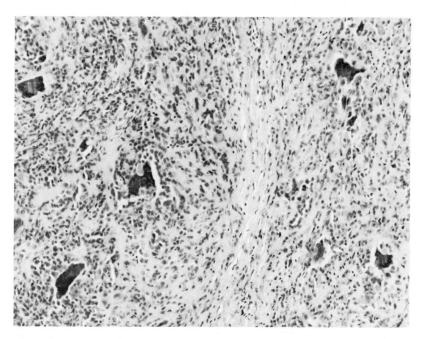

Fig. 17.34 Localised nodular synovitis. This multilobular nodule from the finger consists of histiocytes and osteoclast-like multinucleate giant cells separated by strands of hyaline collagen. Low power.

References

1. Enzinger FM, Weiss SW. *Soft Tissue Tumors*. St Louis: C.V. Mosby, 1983.
2. Pickren JW, Smith AG, Stevenson JW Jr, Stout AP. Fibromatosis of the plantar fascia. *Cancer* 1951; **4**: 846–56.
3. Allen PW. The fibromatoses: a clinicopathologic classification based on 140 cases. *Am J Surg Pathol* 1977; **1**: (a) Part I. 255–70. (b) Part II. 305–21.
4. Allen PW, Enzinger FM. Juvenile aponeurotic fibroma. *Cancer* 1970; **26**: 857–67.
5. Price EB, Silliphant WM, Shuman R. Nodular fasciitis: a clinicopathologic analysis of 65 cases. *Am J Clin Pathol* 1961; **35**: 122–36.
6. Bernstein KE, Lattes R. Nodular (pseudosarcomatous) fasciitis, a non-recurrent lesion. Clinico-pathologic study of 134 cases. *Cancer* 1982; **49**: 1668–78.
7. Johnson WC, Helwig EB. Cutaneous focal mucinosis. *Arch Dermatol* 1966; **93**: 13–20.
8. Taylor HB, Helwig EB. Dermatofibrosarcoma protuberans. A study of 115 cases. *Cancer* 1962, **15**: 717–25
9. Fretzin DF, Helwig EB. Atypical fibroxanthoma of the skin. A clinicopathologic study of 140 cases. *Cancer* 1973; **31**: 1541–52.
10. Harkin JC, Reed RJ. *Tumors of the Peripheral Nervous System*. 2nd series. Washington DC: Armed Forces Institute of Pathology, 1969.
11. Voutsinas S, Wynne-Davies R. The infrequency of malignant disease in diaphyseal aclasis and neurofibromatosis. *J med Genet* 1983; **20**: 345–49.
12. Fields JP, Helwig EB. Leiomyosarcoma of the skin and subcutaneous tissue. *Cancer* 1981; **47**: 156–69.
13. Stout AP, Hill WT. Leiomyosarcoma of the superficial soft tissues. *Cancer* 1958; **11**: 844–54.
14. Mills SE, Cooper PH, Fechner RE. Lobular capillary hemangioma: the underlying lesion of pyogenic granuloma. *Am J Surg Pathol* 1980; **4**: 471–9.
15. Enzinger FM, Smith BH. Hemangiopericytoma. An analysis of 106 cases. *Hum Pathol* 1976; **7**: 61–82.
16. Rosai J, Sumner HW, Kostianovsky M, Perez-Mesa C. Angiosarcoma of skin. A clinicopathologic and fine structural study. *Hum Pathol* 1976; **7**: 83–109.
17. Wilson Jones E. Malignant vascular tumours. *Clin Exp Dermatol* 1976; **1**: 287–312.
18. Maddox JC, Evans HL. Angiosarcoma of skin and soft tissue. A study of forty four cases. *Cancer* 1981; **48**: 1907–21.
19. Clearkin KP, Enzinger FM. Intravascular papillary endothelial hyperplasia. *Arch Pathol* 1976; **100**: 441–4.
20. Flanagan BP, Helwig EB. Cutaneous lymphangioma. *Arch Dermatol* 1977; **113**: 24–30.
21. Whimster IW. The pathology of lymphangioma circumscriptum. *Br J Dermatol* 1976; **94**: 473–86.
22. O'Connell KM. Kaposi's sarcoma: histopathological study of 159 cases from Malawi. *J Clin Pathol* 1977; **30**: 687–95.
23. Curran JW. AIDS—two years later. (Editorial) *N Engl J Med* 1983; **309**: 609–11.
24. Enzinger FM, Harvey DA. Spindle cell lipoma. *Cancer* 1975; **36**: 1852–9.
25. Shmookler BM, Enzinger FM. Pleomorphic lipoma: a benign tumor simulating liposarcoma. *Cancer* 1981; **47**: 126–33.
26. Enzinger FM. Epithelioid sarcoma. A sarcoma simulating a granuloma or a carcinoma. *Cancer* 1970; **26**: 1029–41.
27. Prat J, Woodruff JM, Marcove RC. Epithelioid sarcoma. An analysis of 22 cases indicating the prognostic significance of vascular invasion and regional lymph node metastasis. *Cancer* 1978; **41**: 1472–87.
28. Enzinger FM. Clear cell sarcoma of tendons and aponeuroses. *Cancer* 1965; **18**: 1163–74.
29. Chung EB, Enzinger FM. Malignant melanoma of soft parts. A reassessment of clear cell sarcoma. *Am. J. Surg. Pathol.* 1983; **7**: 405–13.

Index